Practice Safe Neonatology: A Clinical Survival Guide

Dr.Ahmed Badawy

Copyright © 2026 Dr. Ahmed Badawy. All rights reserved.

No part of this publication may be reproduced, distributed, or transmitted in any form or by any means, including photocopying, recording, or other electronic or mechanical methods, without the prior written permission of the author, except in the case of brief quotations embodied in critical reviews and certain other noncommercial uses permitted by copyright law.

For permission requests, contact: a.m.b.hassane@gmail.com

Published by Talented LLC, Wyoming, USA.

First Edition: 2026

ISBN: 979-8-9963420-0-6 (paperback)

Library of Congress Control Number (LCCN): 2026913882

Disclaimer: This publication is provided for educational purposes. See the Disclaimer section for complete terms, conditions, and limitations of liability.

Contents

Chapter One

PRACTICE SAFE NEONATOLOGY

A Clinical Survival Guide

First Edition, 2026

Dr. Ahmed Badawy

MRCPCH.UK | EBP | EPIC Diploma

"Safe neonatology begins with knowledge, continues with judgment, and succeeds through collaboration."

Talented LLC | Wyoming, USA

© 2026 Dr. Ahmed Badawy. All rights reserved.

No part of this publication may be reproduced, distributed, or transmitted in any form or by any means, including photocopying, recording, or other electronic or mechanical methods, without the prior written permission of the author, except in the case of brief quotations embodied in critical reviews and certain other noncommercial uses permitted by copyright law.

For permission requests, contact:a.m.b.hassane@gmail.com

Author Information:Dr. Ahmed Badawy

- M.B.,CH.B - Tanta Faculty of Medicine, Egypt
- MRCPCH.UK - Membership of the Royal College of Paediatrics and Child Health, United Kingdom
- EBP - European Board of Paediatrics
- EPIC Diploma - European Board of Paediatrics and Neonatal Intensive Care Diploma

First Edition: 2026

Published by Talented LLC, Wyoming, USA

Library of Congress Control Number (LCCN): 2026913882

ISBN: 979-8-9963420-0-6 (Paperback)

Disclaimer: This publication is provided for educational purposes. See the Disclaimer section for complete terms, conditions, and limitations of liability.

Chapter Two

ACKNOWLEDGMENTS

This clinical guide would not have been possible without the love,patience,support and kindness conveyed from my family , notably my decent wife , my lovely daughters and sons , Mena,Abdulla, Noura,Marim,Nadein,Mohamed,and Yahia . As well as the invaluable input and mentorship of the exceptional neonatal consultants with whom I have had the privilege to work. Arranged by age/seniority, I gratefully acknowledge: Dr. Ali Aqeel, Dr. Mustafa Rehawi, Dr. M. Abdelazem, Dr. Siraj El Sabea, Dr. Amal Ababdullah, Dr. Ali Al Mudeer, Dr. M. Aziabi, Dr. Majed Al Ibrahim, Dr. Fahd Somili, and Dr. Muneera Najmi. Moreover , I would like to thank all of my neonatal specialists, specially Dr.Yasser Fathy, Dr.Salah Metwaly , nurses , respiratory therapists , and the different pediatric subspecialities I worked with . Each of these colleagues has demonstrated exceptional clinical knowledge, unwavering commitment to patient safety, and generous willingness to share their expertise. Their collective wisdom, clinical judgment, and dedication to neonatal care have profoundly shaped my approach to this specialty . I am deeply grateful for their support, mentorship, and friendship.

Chapter Three

ABOUT THE AUTHOR

Dr. Ahmed Badawy is a pediatrician with extensive clinical experience in neonatal intensive care. He holds the Membership of the Royal College of Paediatrics and Child Health, United Kingdom (), European Board of Paediatrics (EBP), and the European Diploma of Paediatrics and Neonatal Intensive Care (EPIC Dip.)—qualifica tions reflecting his commitment to evidence-based pediatric practice and continuous professional development in neonatal medicine.

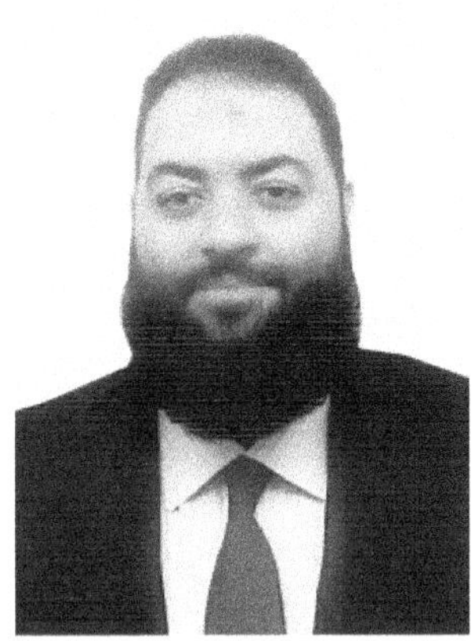

With over a decade of dedicated practice in neonatal intensive care, Dr. Badawy has developed expertise across the full spectrum of neonatal emergencies: respiratory distress, sepsis, metabolic disorders, congenital anomalies, neurological emergencies, and complex surgical conditions. His clinical experience spans tertiary care settings where advanced diagnostic capabilities, multidisciplinary consultations, and comprehensive therapeutic options are available—environments that demand both systematic clinical reasoning and the ability to synthesize complex decisions rapidly.

Dr. Badawy's approach to neonatal care is grounded in the principle that clinical safety emerges from the integration of evidence-based knowledge, meticulous attention to physiological detail, effective multidisciplinary collaboration, as well as clear communication with families. He has witnessed first-hand how the most sophisticated facilities can fail to prevent errors when clinical judgment is compromised, and conversely, how systematic thinking and teamwork could prevent catastrophic events even in challenging circumstances..

His work in a tertiary care NICU in Saudi Arabia has exposed him to the diversity of neonatal pathology, the complexity of managing critically ill newborns with multiple comorbidities, in addition to the critical importance of having structured protocols and decision-making frameworks. These experiences have shaped his conviction that neonatal care must be systematic, evidence-based, and grounded in a deep understanding of neonatal physiology.

Dr. Badawy is committed to clinical education and believes that sharing practical experience through case-based teaching improves outcomes for future patients and strengthens the practice of neonatal medicine"The real time to learn medicine is at the patient's bed-side". This manual represents his effort to distill years of clinical practice into a structured resource that will help pediatricians, neonatologists, and multidisciplinary team members to recognize, diagnose, as well as safely manage the most challenging neonatal morbidities and notably emergencies.

He continues to practice neonatal medicine, teach medical students and residents, collaborate with multidisciplinary teams, and advocate for systematic approaches to clinical safety in neonatal intensive care.

Professional qualifications

- MRCPCH (UK), Membership of the Royal College of Paediatrics and Child Health — 2015

-European Board of Paediatrics, 2021

-European Paediatric and Neonatal Intensive Care Diploma – 2022

Researcher identifiers

Google Scholar: WrUDwzUAAAAJ

ORCID: 0009-0007-7662-840X (https://orcid.org/0009-0007-7662-840X)

Scopus Author ID: 57205355058

WOS (WEB OF SCIENCE) : NGR-3092-2025

Selected publications (Vancouver style)

-Badawy A, Elfadul M, Aziabi M, Ageel HI, Aqeel A. The challenges of microvillus inclusion disease in the neonatal intensive care unit. NeoReviews. 2020;21(9):e600–e604.

- Case 1: Methylergometrin Maleate Toxicity in Neonates — Badawy A, Darwich M, Aqeel A. NeoReviews. 2018;19(12):e762–e764.

-Dhayhi NS, Aqeel A, Ghazwani S, Gosadi IM, AlQassimi HM, Thubab A,... Badawy A et al. Five Years' Experience on RSV Among Hospitalized Patients: A Retrospective Study from Jazan, Saudi Arabia. Infection and Drug Resistance. 2024;5179–5187.

Institution: King Fahd Central Hospital, Jazan, Saudi Arabia .Contact: a.m.b.hassane@gmail.com

Chapter Four

How to Use This Manual for clinical safety

The Reality of Neonatal Emergencies

Neonatal intensive care is a specialty where decisions made in seconds determine outcomes that last a lifetime. A neonate cannot tell you what is wrong. Their physiology is profoundly different from older children and adults,thus having a unique path. Their margin for error affection is microscopically small. And the pressure to act quickly, combined with the emotional weight of caring for the most vulnerable patients, creates an environment where errors are not just possible—they are inevitable unless we have systematic frameworks to prevent them . In other words , you need to learn deeply before touching these delicate creatures.

This manual exists because I have witnessed too many medical errors that were not due to lack of intelligence or dedication, but due to lack of systematic thinking, incomplete knowledge of neonatal physiology, or absence of clear protocols. For instance , I have seen clinicians make decisions that seemed reasonable in the moment but were catastrophically wrong because they misunderstood the underlying pathophysiology. Moreover,I have seen families suffer unnecessary anguish because communication was unclear or incomplete. Hence I have learned that the best defense against error is not individual brilliance—it is systematic thinking, clear protocols, multidisciplinary collaboration, and the humility to recognize the limits of our knowledge.

What This Manual Is—And Is Not

This is not a comprehensive textbook attempting to cover every rare disease or exotic complication. Excellent textbooks exist for that purpose.

This is a practical, case-based clinical survival guide that teaches you how to:

- Recognize the sick neonate and understand what is happening physiologically
- Stabilize the critically ill newborn using evidence-based protocols and systematic approaches
- Diagnose common and critical neonatal emergencies through structured clinical reasoning

- Manage the conditions you will encounter most frequently in a tertiary NICU
- Communicate with families in ways that build trust, reduce anxiety, and support informed decision-making
- Work effectively with multidisciplinary teams to optimize outcomes
- Prevent medical errors through systematic thinking and adherence to evidence-based protocols

The Philosophy Behind This Manual

This manual is built on five core principles:

1. Clinical Safety Through Systematic Thinking

Medical errors in neonatal care service often result not from lack of knowledge, but from failure to think systematically. This manual teaches you how to approach any clinical problem methodically: What is pathophysiology? What are the differential diagnoses? What investigations narrow the differential? What is my management plan, and what are the potential complications? Systematic thinking prevents cognitive errors and improves diagnostic accuracy.

2. Physiology First, Pathology Second

If you internalise neonatal physiology , you could predict what would go wrong, anticipate complications, and adapt to new situations. This manual emphasizes the "why" behind recommendations. When you understand the mechanism of disease, you know not just what to do, but why you are doing it.

3. Evidence-Based Practice

The recommendations in this manual are grounded in current evidence and guidelines, up to our knowledge at the moment. However, evidence must be interpreted in the clinical context. This manual teaches you how to evaluate evidence critically, understand its limitations, and apply it appropriately to your patients.

4. Multidisciplinary Collaboration Is Essential

Neonatal care cannot be delivered by physicians alone. Nurses, respiratory therapists, pharmacists, radiologists, surgeons, and other specialities each bring essential expertise at hand. The best outcomes occur when these professionals work as a true team with effective communication, mutual respect, and shared decision-making.

5. Families Are Partners in Care

Parents are not passive observers. They are essential partners who provide vital clinical information, help in making critical decisions about their infant's care, and provide comfort that no medication can replicate. Clear, honest, compassionate communication with families is as important as any other clinical intervention.

How to Use This Manual

Structure of Each Chapter

Most chapters follow a consistent structure, however some has a different path just to not let you “bored” , hence mostly you will see this structure:

1. Clinical Case Opening – A representative case that illustrates the condition or emergency being discussed

2. Pathophysiology – What is happening at the cellular and

organ system level

3. Clinical Recognition – What signs and symptoms should warn you

4. Differential Diagnosis – What else could this be

5. Management Framework – Systematic step-by-step guidance

6. Complications & Red Flags – What can go wrong

7. Family Communication – How to explain this condition to parents effectively

8. Key Takeaways "Summary"– The essential points you must remember

How to Read This Manual

Option 1: Sequential Reading "cover-to-cover" – Read from beginning to end. This approach gives you the complete foundation and helps you understand how different topics connect.

Option 2: Problem-Based Reading – If your neonate is critically ill right now, go directly to the relevant chapter. Each chapter is designed to stand alone.

Option 3: Reference Use – Use the index and quick reference sections to find specific information rapidly. This manual is written to be useful at 3 AM when you need an answer immediately."Save Our Self" approach

Important Notes

On Evidence & Updates: This manual reflects evidence and guidelines current as of 2026. Medical knowledge evolves continuously. Before implementing any recommendation from this manual, verify that it aligns with your current institutional protocols, local guidelines, and your professional judgment.

On Institutional Variation: Your NICU may have different protocols, different available medications, or different equipment. Adapt everything in this manual to your institutional context. What matters is the principle, not the specific protocol."Approaches are different but the goal is same"

On Your Clinical Judgment: This manual provides guidance, not dogma. Your clinical judgment, informed by this knowledge, or combined with knowledge of your individual patient, is what matters. Trust on your judgment. Question recommendations that don't make sense. Ask colleagues. Admit uncertainty.

Chapter Five

ABBREVIATIONS & SYMBOLS – QUICK REFERENCE DECODER

Respiratory & Oxygenation

- RDS = Respiratory Distress Syndrome
- TTN = Transient Tachypnea of the Newborn
- MAS = Meconium Aspiration Syndrome
- PPHN = Persistent Pulmonary Hypertension of the Newborn

- PDA = Patent Ductus Arteriosus
- BPD = Bronchopulmonary Dysplasia
- CLD = Chronic Lung Disease
- CPAP = Continuous Positive Airway Pressure
- BiPAP = Bilevel Positive Airway Pressure
- HFOV = High-Frequency Oscillatory Ventilation
- HFJV = High-Frequency Jet Ventilation
- SIMV = Synchronized Intermittent Mandatory Ventilation
- PIP = Peak Inspiratory Pressure
- PEEP = Positive End-Expiratory Pressure
- FiO_2 = Fraction of Inspired Oxygen
- SpO_2 = Peripheral Oxygen Saturation
- PaO_2 = Partial Pressure of Oxygen (arterial)
- $PaCO_2$ = Partial Pressure of Carbon Dioxide (arterial)
- pH = Hydrogen Ion Concentration
- BE = Base Excess
- A-a Gradient = Alveolar-Arterial Oxygen Gradient
- OI = Oxygenation Index
- iNO = Inhaled Nitric Oxide

Cardiovascular

- BP = Blood Pressure
- HR = Heart Rate
- MAP = Mean Arterial Pressure
- SVR = Systemic Vascular Resistance
- PVR = Pulmonary Vascular Resistance
- CO = Cardiac Output
- CHD = Congenital Heart Disease
- ASD = Atrial Septal Defect
- VSD = Ventricular Septal Defect
- PFO = Patent Foramen Ovale
- TGA = Transposition of the Great Arteries
- TOF = Tetralogy of Fallot
- HLHS = Hypoplastic Left Heart Syndrome
- TAPVR = Total Anomalous Pulmonary Venous Return
- CoA = Coarctation of the Aorta
- IAA = Interrupted Aortic Arch

Neurological

- HIE = Hypoxic-Ischemic Encephalopathy
- IVH = Intraventricular Hemorrhage
- PVL = Periventricular Leukomalacia
- NEC = Necrotizing Enterocolitis
- EEG = Electroencephalogram
- aEEG = Amplitude-Integrated Electroencephalogram
- MRI = Magnetic Resonance Imaging
- CT = Computed Tomography
- US = Ultrasound
- TH = Therapeutic Hypothermia

Metabolic & Endocrine

- Glu = Glucose
- Na = Sodium
- K = Potassium
- Ca = Calcium
- Mg = Magnesium
- Cl = Chloride

- HCO_3 = Bicarbonate
- Hgb = Hemoglobin
- Hct = Hematocrit
- TSH = Thyroid-Stimulating Hormone
- T4 = Thyroxine
- ACTH = Adrenocorticotropic Hormone

Infectious Disease

- EOS = Early-Onset Sepsis
- LOS = Late-Onset Sepsis
- GBS = Group B Streptococcus
- TORCH = Toxoplasmosis, Other, Rubella, Cytomegalovirus, Herpes Simplex
- CMV = Cytomegalovirus
- HSV = Herpes Simplex Virus
- RSV = Respiratory Syncytial Virus
- ROP = Retinopathy of Prematurity
- CRP = C-Reactive Protein
- PCT = Procalcitonin

- CBC = Complete Blood Count
- CSF = Cerebrospinal Fluid
- UTI = Urinary Tract Infection

Gastrointestinal

- NEC = Necrotizing Enterocolitis
- SIP = Spontaneous Intestinal Perforation
- GI = Gastrointestinal
- GER = Gastroesophageal Reflux
- GERD = Gastroesophageal Reflux Disease
- TPN = Total Parenteral Nutrition
- EN = Enteral Nutrition
- NG = Nasogastric
- OG = Orogastric

Hematology & Hemostasis

- Hgb = Hemoglobin
- Hct = Hematocrit
- WBC = White Blood Cell

- Plt = Platelet
- PT = Prothrombin Time
- aPTT = Activated Partial Thromboplastin Time
- INR = International Normalized Ratio
- DIC = Disseminated Intravascular Coagulation
- IUGR = Intrauterine Growth Restriction
- HDN = Hemolytic Disease of the Newborn
- ABO = ABO Blood Group
- Rh = Rhesus Factor
- DAT = Direct Antiglobulin Test (Coombs)

Obstetric & Maternal

- ROM = Rupture of Membranes
- PROM = Premature Rupture of Membranes
- PPROM = Preterm Premature Rupture of Membranes
- GA = Gestational Age
- EGA = Estimated Gestational Age
- PTL = Preterm Labor
- PIH = Pregnancy-Induced Hypertension

- PE = Preeclampsia
- GDM = Gestational Diabetes Mellitus
- SGA = Small for Gestational Age
- LGA = Large for Gestational Age
- AGA = Appropriate for Gestational Age
- IDM = Infant of Diabetic Mother

Neonatal Classification

- VLBW = Very Low Birth Weight (<1500 g)
- ELBW = Extremely Low Birth Weight (<1000 g)
- LBW = Low Birth Weight (<2500 g)
- NICU = Neonatal Intensive Care Unit
- PICU = Pediatric Intensive Care Unit

Monitoring & Procedures

- ECG = Electrocardiogram
- RR = Respiratory Rate
- Temp = Temperature
- CVP = Central Venous Pressure

- PICC = Peripherally Inserted Central Catheter
- UAC = Umbilical Arterial Catheter
- UVC = Umbilical Venous Catheter
- ETT = Endotracheal Tube
- IO = Intraosseous
- IV = Intravenous
- IM = Intramuscular
- SC = Subcutaneous
- LP = Lumbar Puncture

General Terms

Pt = Patient

Hx = History

Sx = Symptoms

Dx = Diagnosis

Tx = Treatment

Rx = Prescription

Prx = Prognosis

Px = Physical Examination

Labs = Laboratory Tests

Imaging = Radiological Imaging

QD = Once Daily

BID = Twice Daily

TID = Three Times Daily

QID = Four Times Daily

Q4H = Every 4 Hours

PRN = As Needed

NPO = Nothing by Mouth

PO = By Mouth

kg = Kilogram

g = Gram

mg = Milligram

mcg = Microgram

mL = Milliliter

L = Liter

↑ = Increased

↓ = Decreased

→ = Leads to / Causes

± = Plus or Minus

≈ = Approximately

< = Less Than

= Greater Than

Chapter Six

OVERVIEW OF FETOMATERNAL MEDICINE

Clinical Case Opening

A 34-year-old primigravida presents to labor and delivery at 38 weeks gestation with a blood pressure of 165/110 mmHg, proteinuria of 3+, and complaints of right upper quadrant pain and visual disturbances. She is in active labor. Within 2 hours of delivery via emergency cesarean section, a 3.2 kg male infant is born with an APGAR score of 6 at 1 minute and 8 at 5 minutes. The infant is brought to the NICU for observation. Within the first 6 hours of life, the baby develops severe metabolic acidosis, hypoglycemia, and signs of poor perfusion.

This case illustrates a fundamental principle: the newborn baby does not exist in isolation. The maternal condition, the intrauterine environment, the circumstances at delivery, and the transition from fetal to neonatal life all profoundly form what happens in the first hours and days after birth. Understanding fetomaternal medicine is not optional for neonatal practitioners—it is essential."Scrutiny the factory production line to know exactly how the product would be "

Why Fetomaternal Medicine Matters in Neonatal Care

Many neonatal emergencies have their origins in the intrauterine environment or in maternal pathology. A newborn baby presenting with respiratory distress may not have primary lung disorder—the problem may be maternal diabetes, maternal infection, or intrauterine growth restriction. A neonate with poor perfusion and metabolic acidosis may not have sepsis—the problem may be intrauterine hypoxia from placental insufficiency. A neonate with seizures may not have primary neurological disease—the problem may be hypoxic-ischemic encephalopathy resulting from maternal preeclampsia and fetal distress.

When you understand the maternal and fetal context, you:

- Anticipate what complications the neonate is likely to develop
- Recognize patterns that help you diagnose neonatal problems more accurately
- Prevent medical errors by understanding the underlying pathophysiology
- Communicate more effectively with obstetric colleagues and

with families

- Optimize your management plan by understanding what exactly the baby has

Section 1: The Fetal-to-Neonatal Transition

Understanding Fetal Physiology

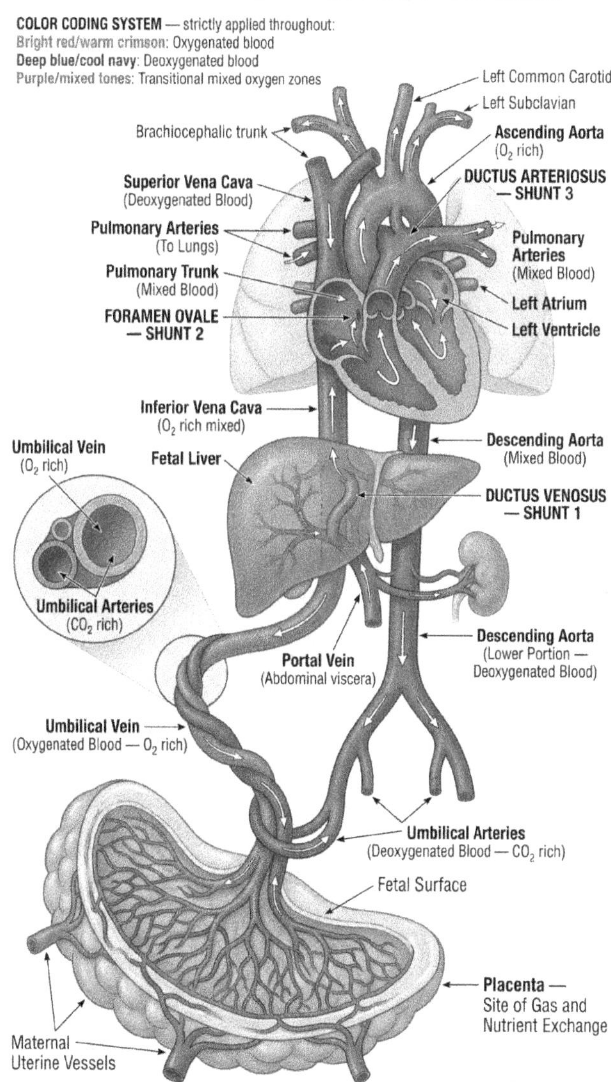
FETAL CIRCULATION SYSTEM
Anatomical Pathway and Three Major Fetal Shunts
COLOR CODING SYSTEM — strictly applied throughout:
Bright red/warm crimson: Oxygenated blood
Deep blue/cool navy: Deoxygenated blood
Purple/mixed tones: Transitional mixed oxygen zones
Left Common Carotid
Left Subclavian
Brachiocephalic trunk
Ascending Aorta
(O_2 rich)
Superior Vena Cava
(Deoxygenated Blood)
DUCTUS ARTERIOSUS — SHUNT 3
Pulmonary Arteries
(To Lungs)
Pulmonary Arteries
(Mixed Blood)
Pulmonary Trunk
(Mixed Blood)
Left Atrium
FORAMEN OVALE — SHUNT 2
Left Ventricle
Inferior Vena Cava
(O_2 rich mixed)
Umbilical Vein
(O_2 rich)
Fetal Liver
Descending Aorta
(Mixed Blood)
DUCTUS VENOSUS — SHUNT 1
Umbilical Arteries
(CO_2 rich)
Portal Vein
(Abdominal viscera)
Descending Aorta
(Lower Portion — Deoxygenated Blood)
Umbilical Vein
(Oxygenated Blood — O_2 rich)
Umbilical Arteries
(Deoxygenated Blood — CO_2 rich)
Fetal Surface
Placenta —
Site of Gas and
Nutrient Exchange
Maternal
Uterine Vessels

The fetus exists in a profoundly different physiological state than the newborn. Understanding these differences is essential:

Oxygenation in the Fetus:

- Fetal PaO_2 is approximately 30-35 mmHg (compared to postnatal PaO_2 of 80-100 mmHg)
- The fetus is NOT hypoxic despite these low oxygen tensions because:
    - Fetal hemoglobin has higher oxygen affinity than adult hemoglobin
    - Fetal cardiac output is higher relative to body weight
    - The placenta proposes efficient oxygen exchange

Circulation in the Fetus:

- The fetus has three shunts that bypass the non-functioning lungs and liver:
    a. Foramen ovale – shunts blood from right atrium to left atrium
    b. Ductus venosus – shunts umbilical venous blood past the liver
    c. Ductus arteriosus – shunts blood from pulmonary artery to aorta
- Right-to-left shunting in the fetus means the lungs receive only 5-10% of cardiac output
- The placenta, not the lungs, is the organ of gas exchange

Metabolism in the Fetus:

- The fetus is primarily dependent on glucose from the mother
- Fetal glucose production is minimal
- The fetus stores glycogen in liver and muscle during the third trimester
- Intrauterine growth-restricted fetuses have depleted glycogen stores

Hemoglobin and Oxygen Carrying:

- Fetal hemoglobin (HbF) comprises 70-80% of total hemoglobin at birth
- HbF has higher oxygen affinity than adult hemoglobin (HbA)
- This higher affinity facilitates oxygen transfer from maternal to fetal blood across the placenta

The Transition at Birth

When the umbilical cord is clamped and the neonate takes the first breath, multiple physiological changes occur simultaneously:

Respiratory Changes:

- Fluid in the fetal lungs is absorbed or expelled
- The lungs expand with air
- Pulmonary vascular resistance drops dramatically
- Pulmonary blood flow increases dramatically
- Gas exchange shifts from placenta to lungs

Cardiovascular Changes:

- Loss of placental circulation eliminates the low-resistance placental bed
- Systemic vascular resistance increases
- Foramen ovale functionally closes as left atrial pressure exceeds right atrial pressure
- Ductus arteriosus begins to close (functional closure within hours to days)

Metabolic Changes:

- Exogenous feeding begins
- Hepatic glucose production increases
- Glycogen stores are mobilized
- The neonate transitions from maternal glucose dependence to self-sufficiency

When This Transition Goes Wrong

Many neonatal emergencies represent failure or delay in this normal transition:

- Persistent pulmonary hypertension = failure of pulmonary vascular resistance to drop
- Respiratory distress = inability of lungs to expand adequately
- Hypoglycemia = inadequate hepatic glucose production or excessive glucose utilization

- Poor perfusion = inadequate systemic blood pressure or cardiac output
- Persistent right-to-left shunting = failure of fetal shunts to close

Section 2: Maternal Conditions That Impact the Neonate

Maternal Hypertension and Preeclampsia

Pathophysiology:

- Preeclampsia is characterized by maternal endothelial dysfunction
- Placental insufficiency results from abnormal trophoblastic invasion
- Fetal perfusion is compromised
- Intrauterine hypoxia develops

Neonatal Consequences:

- Intrauterine growth restriction (IUGR)
- Prematurity (if delivery is indicated)
- Intrauterine hypoxia leading to metabolic acidosis, poor perfusion, hypoglycemia, and potential HIE
- Thrombocytopenia and/or leucopenia

- Respiratory distress

Neonatal Recognition:

- Small for gestational age (SGA) infant
- Signs of intrauterine distress: meconium-stained amniotic fluid, low APGAR score
- Metabolic acidosis on cord blood gas
- Poor perfusion, weak cry, decreased tone
- Hypoglycemia in first hours of life

Neonatal Management Implications:

- Anticipate hypoglycemia—check glucose early and frequently
- Anticipate metabolic acidosis—obtain cord blood gas
- Anticipate poor perfusion—have resuscitation team ready
- Anticipate need for therapeutic hypothermia if HIE develops

Maternal Diabetes

Pathophysiology:

- Maternal hyperglycemia leads to fetal hyperglycemia
- Fetal pancreas responds with hyperinsulinemia
- Excessive fetal insulin promotes increased glucose utiliza-

tion, fat deposition, and organomegaly

Neonatal Consequences:

- Large for gestational age (LGA) infant
- Macrosomia with associated birth trauma risk
- Hypoglycemia (most common metabolic complication)
- Respiratory distress
- Cardiomyopathy
- Polycythemia
- Hyperbilirubinemia
- Congenital anomalies

Neonatal Management Implications:

- Aggressive hypoglycemia screening: check glucose at 30 minutes, 1 hour, 2 hours, then every 2-4 hours and continue monitoring for the first 24 hours of age
- Start early feeding as soon as possible
- Have IV dextrose available for rapid treatment
- Monitor for birth trauma complications
- Screen for congenital anomalies

Maternal Infection (Chorioamnionitis)

Neonatal Consequences:

- Early-onset sepsis (especially Group B Streptococcus, Gram-negative organisms)
- Prematurity
- Respiratory distress
- Metabolic acidosis
- Poor perfusion and shock
- Potential meningitis

Neonatal Management Implications:

- Empiric antibiotics should be started immediately (Ampicillin + Gentamicin)
- Obtain blood culture before antibiotics
- Lumbar puncture should be considered
- Monitor vital signs closely

Section 3: Obstetric Complications That Impact the Neonate

Meconium-Stained Amniotic Fluid

Pathophysiology:

- Meconium passage in utero indicates fetal stress

- Meconium aspiration causes airway obstruction, chemical pneumonitis, surfactant inactivation, and severe hypoxemia

Neonatal Consequences:

- Meconium aspiration syndrome (MAS)
- Severe respiratory distress " secondary to possible surfactant deficiency due to meconium"
- Persistent pulmonary hypertension (PPHN)
- Pneumothorax
- Metabolic acidosis

Prolonged Rupture of Membranes (PROM)

Neonatal Consequences:

- Early-onset sepsis (significant if >18 hours rupture)
- Chorioamnionitis-related complications
- Prematurity
- Respiratory distress

Cord Prolapse and Fetal Distress

Neonatal Consequences:

- Low APGAR score
- Severe metabolic acidosis

- Poor perfusion
- Potential HIE
- Seizures

Neonatal Management Implications:

- Aggressive resuscitation
- Consider therapeutic hypothermia if HIE criteria are met
- Monitor for seizures

Section 4: Prematurity and Its Consequences

Gestational Age Categories:

- Extremely preterm: <28 weeks
- Very preterm: 28-32 weeks
- Preterm: 32-36 weeks+6 days
- Late preterm: 34-36 weeks+6 days
- Term: ≥37 weeks

Organ System Maturation by Gestational Age:

Pulmonary System:

- 24 weeks: Type II pneumocytes begin surfactant production

- 28 weeks: Minimal but present surfactant
- 32 weeks: Improved surfactant production
- 34-35 weeks: Adequate surfactant for most infants

Hepatic System:

- Preterm infants at high risk for hypoglycemia, hyperbilirubinemia, and impaired drug metabolism

Renal System:

- Preterm infants at high risk for electrolyte abnormalities, fluid overload, and impaired drug clearance

Gastrointestinal System:

- Preterm infants at high risk for feeding intolerance, necrotizing enterocolitis, and poor nutritional intake

Neurological System:

- Preterm infants at high risk for intraventricular hemorrhage

Section 5: The Umbilical Cord and Placental Pathology

Cord Blood Gas Interpretation

Normal Values"Accepted values":

- pH: 7.25-7.35 (arterial), 7.30-7.40 (venous)
- $PaCO_2$: 45-55 mmHg (arterial), 35-45 mmHg (venous)

- PaO_2: 15-25 mmHg (arterial), 25-35 mmHg (venous)
- Base excess: -5 to +5 mEq/L

Interpretation:

- Metabolic acidosis (low pH, negative base excess, normal/high $PaCO_2$) = indicates intrauterine hypoxia
- Respiratory acidosis (low pH, high $PaCO_2$, normal base excess) = indicates acute hypoxia near delivery
- Mixed acidosis (low pH, high $PaCO_2$, negative base excess) = indicates prolonged hypoxia

Section 6: Key Principles for Neonatal Management Based on Fetomaternal History

1. Obtain Detailed Maternal and Obstetric History
2. Anticipate Problems Based on Maternal/Obstetric Context
3. Interpret Clinical Findings in Context
4. Communicate with Obstetric Colleagues
5. Communicate with Families

Key Takeaways

✓ The newborn baby does not exist in isolation—maternal and obstetric factors profoundly reflected on neonatal pathology

✓ Understanding fetal physiology and the transition to neonatal life helps you recognize when things go wrong

✓ Maternal conditions (diabetes, hypertension, infection) foresee neonatal complications

✓ Cord blood gas, APGAR score, and maternal/obstetric history together depict a picture of what the neonate has endured

✓ Anticipation based on maternal/obstetric context allows you to prevent complications and optimize care

Chapter Seven

FOUNDATIONS OF NEONATAL PHYSIOLOGY AND STABILIZATION

Clinical Case Opening

A 34-week gestational age male infant is delivered via emergency cesarean section for fetal bradycardia. Birth weight is 2100 grams. In the delivery room, the infant is limp, not breathing, with a heart rate of 60 bpm. Immediate positive pressure ventilation is initiated. Within 60 seconds, the heart rate rises up to 120 bpm ,hence spontaneous respiratory effort begins. The infant is transferred to the NICU on nasal cannula oxygen supplementation.

In the NICU, you notice the infant's respiratory rate is 80 breaths per minute, with moderate retractions and grunting. Oxygen saturation is 88% on 40% FiO_2 . Peripheral perfusion is delayed (capillary refill 3 seconds). Blood pressure is 45/28 mmHg. The temperature is 36.2°C.

You recognize that this infant is not simply "recovering" from delivery—this infant is unstable yet and requires immediate stabilization. But what exactly is happening ? Why is the heart rate elevated? Why is the infant struggling to breathe? Why is perfusion poor? Understanding the answers to these questions will guide every intervention you make.

Understanding Neonatal Physiology: The Foundation for Safe Practice

Neonatal medicine differs fundamentally from pediatric or adult medicine because neonatal physiology is profoundly different. The transition from intrauterine to extrauterine life represents the most dramatic physiological changes . Understanding this transition—and what can go wrong during this sensitive time—is essential for safe neonatal practice.

The Intrauterine Environment

In utero, the fetus exists in a fluid-filled environment with unique circulatory and respiratory characteristics:

- Gas exchange occurs across the placenta, not through the lungs. Maternal blood in the placenta exchanges oxygen and carbon dioxide with fetal blood.

- Fetal lungs are fluid-filled and collapsed.Hence they do not participate in gas exchange.
- Fetal hemoglobin (HbF) has higher oxygen affinity than adult hemoglobin(It loves hugging more oxygen coming from the mother-side and hates releasing it back to mother). This facilitates oxygen transfer from maternal to fetal blood across the placenta.
- The fetal circulation is organized to bypass the lungs and liver:
    - The foramen ovale permits right-to-left shunting of blood from the right atrium to the left atrium, bypassing the lungs.
    - The ductus venosus allows umbilical venous blood to bypass the liver.
    - The ductus arteriosus facilitates pulmonary arterial blood to bypass the lungs and flow directly into the descending aorta.
- Pulmonary vascular resistance is very high because the lungs are fluid-filled and collapsed,while Systemic one is relatively low because of the minimal resistance offered by placenta.
- Oxygen content of fetal blood is lower than postnatal blood (fetal PaO_2 is approximately 30-35 mmHg, in comparison to postnatal PaO_2 which is approximately 80-100 mmHg), however fetal tissues extract oxygen efficiently and fetal hemoglobin's high affinity augments oxygen delivery.

The Transition at Birth: The First Minutes

At birth, the most dramatic physiological transitions occur:

1. Onset of Breathing(First cry)

With the first breath, the lungs expand and fluid is commencing washing out. This expansion:

- Drastically diminishes pulmonary vascular resistance
- Increases pulmonary blood flow
- Pushing up left atrial return
- Augments left ventricular preload and cardiac output

2. Clamping of the Umbilical Cord:

- Eliminates the low-resistance placental circulation from the equation
- Rockets systemic vascular resistance
- Declines right-to-left shunting through the foramen ovale
- Increases pulmonary blood flow

3. Changes in Intracardiac Shunting

As pulmonary vascular resistance drops and systemic vascular resistance rises:

- The pressure gradient across the foramen ovale reverses
- Left atrial pressure exceeds right atrial pressure
- The foramen ovale functionally closes (Even though anatomically it remains probe-patent in most newborns)

- Right-to-left shunting ceases

4. Closure of Fetal Shunts

Over hours to days:

- The ductus venosus closes as umbilical venous flow stops
- The ductus arteriosus closes as pulmonary vascular resistance inclines and systemic vascular resistance rises, eliminating the pressure gradient that drove right-to-left shunting
- The foramen ovale remains functionally closed but could reopen transiently with increased right atrial pressure (For instance , during crying)

5. Changes in Oxygen Content and Hemoglobin

- Postnatal PaO_2 rises from 30-35 mmHg up to 80-100 mmHg
- This increased PaO_2 triggers for closing the fetal shunts
- Fetal hemoglobin (HbF) gradually decreases and is replaced by adult hemoglobin (HbA)
- This transition takes weeks to months

Why Neonates Are Physiologically Vulnerable

Understanding why neonates are vulnerable aids you to anticipate problems and recognize early deterioration.(Newborn babies are stigmatized as vulnerable group, they are so delicate that needs wise approach for handling)

1. Immature Respiratory System

- Surfactant deficiency: Surfactant, the substance that reduces surface tension in alveoli, is not produced in adequate quantities until approximately 34:35 weeks gestation. Without surfactant, alveoli collapse at the end of expiration, requiring enormous effort to re-expand them with each breath. This is the pathophysiology of Respiratory Distress Syndrome (RDS).

- Fewer alveoli: Neonates have approximately 50 million alveoli at birth, compared to 300 million in adults. Alveolar development continues until approximately 8 years of age.

- Compliant chest wall: The neonatal chest wall is highly compliant (easily deformable) because the ribs are cartilaginous and the intercostal muscles are weak. This means that when the infant generates negative intrathoracic pressure to breathe, the chest wall collapses inward rather than expanding outward. This is why you see retractions (intercostal, subcostal, suprasternal) in distressed neonates.

- Obligate nasal breathing: Neonates are obligate nasal breathers. Nasal obstruction (from secretions, edema, or anatomic abnormality) can cause severe respiratory distress. (Remember here , the baby who has bilateral choanal atresia , only breaths while crying intermittently, otherwise becomes apneic and needs immediate respiratory support)

- Immature higher respiratory control: The respiratory centers in the brainstem are immature. Hence prematures might have irregular breathing patterns and are prone to apnea (cessation of breathing for >20 seconds , or less with association with bradycardia).

2. Immature Cardiovascular System

- Limited cardiac reserve: The neonatal heart operates near the top of the Frank-Starling curve. This means that small increases in preload increase cardiac output significantly, but small decreases in preload cause dramatic decreases in cardiac output. In other words, newborn babies are preload-depen dent.(Remember here the judicious use of volume expansion fluids to fix early signs of hypotension)

- Immature myocardium: The neonatal myocardium has fewer contractile fibers and less developed sarcoplasmic reticulum. This limits the ability to increase contractility in response to stress.

- Immature autonomic nervous system: The neonatal sympathetic nervous system is kept immature,that newborns cannot mount an effective sympathetic response to shock. This is why neonates in shock often appear deceptively well—they do not develop tachycardia and peripheral vasoconstriction as effectively as older children.

- Patent fetal shunts: The foramen ovale, ductus venosus, and ductus arteriosus are patent at birth. If pulmonary vascular resistance rises (due to hypoxia, acidosis, or lung pathology), right-to-left shunting can resume,hence worsening hypoxemia.

- Immature baroreceptor reflex: The baroreceptor reflex (which maintains blood pressure) is immature. Therefore neonates cannot compensate for blood pressure changes as effectively as older children.

3. Immature Thermoregulation

- Large surface area to body weight ratio: Newborns lose heat rapidly to the environment.
- Limited ability to generate heat: Neonates cannot shiver. Heat generation occurs primarily through non-shivering thermogenesis (brown fat metabolism), which is triggered by norepinephrine release in response to cold.
- Immature vasoconstriction: babies cannot vasoconstrict effectively in response to cold.
- Hypothermia consequences: Even mild hypothermia (35-36°C) increases metabolic rate, increases oxygen consumption, causes metabolic acidosis, and impairs immune function.

4. Immature Metabolic System

- Rapid glucose consumption: Newborns have high metabolic rates and rapidly deplete glycogen stores. Hypoglycemia can develop easily within minutes to hours of birth.
- Limited gluconeogenesis: The enzymatic pathways for glu-

coneogenesis are immature, limiting the ability to generate glucose when glycogen is depleted.

- Immature thermoregulation increases metabolic demand: Cold stress increases metabolic rate and oxygen consumption, worsening hypoglycemia and acidosis.
- Immature kidney function: Neonatal kidneys cannot concentrate or dilute urine effectively, limiting the ability to regulate fluid and electrolyte balance.

5. Immature Immune System

- Immune system vulnerabilities: Neonatal neutrophils have reduced chemotaxis, phagocytosis, and killing capacity.
- Immature adaptive immunity: Neonates have minimal IgM and IgA. IgG is passively transferred from the mother, but this protection is limited to organisms against which the mother has immunity.
- Immature complement system: Complement levels are reduced, limiting opsonization and killing of bacteria.
- Immature barrier function: The babies' skin is thin and permeable, allowing bacterial colonization and transepidermal water loss.

The Concept of Physiological Stabilization

When you encounter a sick newborn, your first priority is not diagnosis—it is stabilization. Stabilization means creating an internal physiological environment that is compatible with life and allows time for diagnosis and definitive treatment.(Stabilize you patient first then take your time to navigate through diagnosis and tailoring your management plan)

The acronym ABCDE guides stabilization:

A – Airway

- Is the airway patent?
- Is the infant breathing?
- Is ventilation adequate (chest rise, bilateral breath sounds)?
- Does the infant need intubation?

B – Breathing

- What is the respiratory rate?
- What does the work of breathing look like (retractions, grunting, flaring)?
- What is oxygen saturation?
- What supplemental oxygen is needed?
- Does the infant need mechanical ventilation?

C – Circulation

- What is the heart rate?
- What is the blood pressure?
- What is the capillary refill time?

- Is perfusion adequate (warm extremities, brisk capillary refill, good urine output)?
- Does the infant need fluid resuscitation or inotropic support?

D – Disability (Neurological)

- What is the level of consciousness?
- Are there seizures?
- What is the glucose level?
- What is the temperature?

E – Exposure

- Examine the entire infant
- Prevent heat loss
- Look for signs of trauma, infection, or congenital anomalies

Oxygen Delivery: The Central Concept

Understanding oxygen delivery is essential because most neonatal emergencies involve inadequate oxygen delivery to tissues.

Oxygen Delivery (DO_2) = Cardiac Output (CO) × Arterial Oxygen Content (CaO_2)

Where:

- Cardiac Output = Heart Rate × Stroke Volume
- Arterial Oxygen Content = (Hemoglobin × 1.34 × SaO_2) + (PaO_2 × 0.003)

This equation tells you that oxygen delivery depends on:

1. Cardiac output (determined by heart rate and stroke volume)

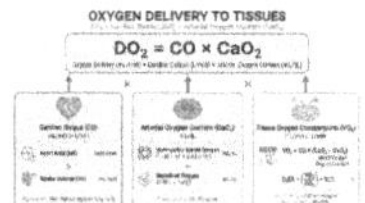

2. Hemoglobin concentration (oxygen-carrying capacity)

3. Oxygen saturation (percentage of hemoglobin carrying oxygen)

4. Partial pressure of oxygen (minimal contribution to total oxygen content)

Clinical Implications:

- Tachycardia is a compensatory mechanism: When oxygen delivery is threatened (due to low hemoglobin, low saturation, or low cardiac output), the heart rate increases to maintain cardiac output. Tachycardia in a sick neonate is NOT normal—it is a sign of physiological stress.

- Anemia reduces oxygen delivery: Even if saturation is 100%, if hemoglobin is low, oxygen delivery is reduced. This is why transfusion is sometimes necessary in critically ill neonates.

- Hypoxemia reduces oxygen delivery: Even if cardiac output is normal, if saturation is low, oxygen delivery is reduced. This is why supplemental oxygen is essential.

- Low cardiac output reduces oxygen delivery: Even if saturation and hemoglobin are normal, if cardiac output is low (due to hypovolemia, poor contractility, or arrhythmia), oxygen delivery is reduced.

Acid-Base Balance in Neonates

Acidosis is a common problem in sick neonates and reflects inadequate tissue oxygenation and perfusion.

Types of Acidosis

1. Metabolic Acidosis
    - Caused by accumulation of organic acids (lactate, ketones) due to anaerobic metabolism
    - Reflects tissue hypoxia and inadequate perfusion
    - Biochemically pH < 7.35, HCO_3 < 22 mEq/L , however a slightly lower range could be accepted notably if pH is a bit higher than 7.25.
    - Base excess (BE) < -2

2. Respiratory Acidosis
    - Caused by inadequate ventilation and CO_2 retention
    - Reflects inadequate minute ventilation
    - pH < 7.35, $PaCO_2$ > 45 mmHg , however a slightly lower range could be accepted notably if pH is a bit higher than 7.25.

3. Mixed Acidosis
    - Combination of metabolic and respiratory acidosis
    - Most common in critically ill neonates

- Reflects both inadequate perfusion and inadequate ventilation

Clinical Significance

- Mild acidosis (pH 7.25-7.35) is common in sick neonates and usually reflects the transition from intrauterine to extrauterine life
- Moderate acidosis (pH 7.15-7.25) indicates significant physiological stress and requires intervention
- Severe acidosis (pH < 7.15) indicates severe shock and requires aggressive resuscitation

Management of Acidosis(Treat the cause)

- Metabolic acidosis: Improve tissue perfusion and oxygenation. Sodium bicarbonate is rarely used in acute resuscitation because it generates CO_2, which can worsen acidosis if ventilation is inadequate, unless the primary cause is one of inborn error of metabolism that necessitates replacement , or the pH is lower than 7.00 , to guard against severe myocardial depression and impending cardio-pulmonary arrest.
- Respiratory acidosis: Improve ventilation. Increase minute ventilation by increasing respiratory rate or tidal volume.
- Mixed acidosis: Simultaneously improve perfusion (fluids, inotropes) and ventilation (mechanical support).

Principles of Neonatal Stabilization

1. Maintain Body Temperature
   - Place the infant under a radiant warmer immediately
   - Dry the infant thoroughly, unless less than 32 weeks (put in plastic bag)
   - Avoid unnecessary exposure
   - Target core temperature 36.5-37.5°C
   - Hypothermia increases metabolic rate, oxygen consumption, and acidosis
   - Hyperthermia increases metabolic rate and can worsen neurological injury

2. Establish Vascular Access
   - Establish IV access early (peripheral IV, PICC line, or umbilical catheter)
   - Do not delay resuscitation , commence as per Neonatal resuscitation program
   - Emergency low-line UVC or intraosseous line placement is adequate for initial resuscitation (CPR)

3. Correct Hypoglycemia
   - Check blood glucose immediately in any sick neonate
   - Hypoglycemia (< 40 mg/dL in first 4 hours, < 50 mg/dL after 4 hours) requires immediate correction

- Give 10% dextrose IV bouls(0.3-0.6 g/kg = 3-6 mL/kg of 10% dextrose)(try to avoid many boluses and start your maintenance glucose infusion as needed)

- Recheck glucose in 15-30 minutes

- Start continuous dextrose infusion (maintenance fluids with 10-12.5% dextrose)

4. Correct Anemia
   - Check hemoglobin in any infant with respiratory distress or poor perfusion

   - Severe anemia (Hgb < 10 g/dL in a critically ill infant) reduces oxygen delivery

   - Transfuse if hemoglobin is low and the infant is in shock or has severe respiratory distress

5. Optimize Ventilation
   - Ensure adequate oxygenation (target SpO_2 > 94% in term infants, 90:94% in preterm infants)

   - Ensure adequate ventilation (target $PaCO_2$ 45-55 mmHg in most conditions)

   - Avoid hyperoxia notably in preterm babies(SpO_2 > 95%) which increases risk of retinopathy of prematurity

   - Avoid hypoxia (SpO_2 < 85%) which causes tissue hypoxia

6. Optimize Perfusion
   - Establish IV access

- Give fluid boluses (10 mL/kg of normal saline or Ringer's lactate) if signs of hypovolemic shock appreciated

- Start inotropic support (eg:dobutamine) if signs of cardiogenic shock or if blood pressure is low despite fluid resuscitation

- Target mean arterial pressure ≥ gestational age in weeks (e.g., 28 mmHg for 28-week infant, 35 mmHg for 35-week infant)(this numerical guidance is not optimal all the time , thus monitor the clinical context in terms of perfusion , urine output and the status of the metabolic element of blood gases is paramount)

7. Obtain Initial Investigations
   - Blood gas (arterial, capillary, or venous)
   - Complete blood count
   - Blood glucose
   - Blood culture (if sepsis suspected)
   - Chest X-ray (if respiratory distress)
   - Other imaging as clinically indicated

8. Start Monitoring
   - Continuous cardiorespiratory monitoring (heart rate, respiratory rate, SpO_2)
   - Continuous temperature monitoring
   - Frequent blood pressure monitoring

- Frequent clinical assessment

The Sick Neonate: Recognition of Physiological Compromise

Signs of Respiratory Compromise

- Respiratory rate > 60 breaths/min (tachypnea)
- Retractions (intercostal, subcostal, suprasternal)
- Grunting (expiratory grunt indicates attempt to maintain positive end-expiratory pressure)
- Nasal flaring
- Cyanosis
- Decreased breath sounds
- Asymmetric breath sounds (suggests pneumothorax or other air leak)
- Gasping or irregular breathing pattern

Signs of Circulatory Compromise

- Heart rate < 100 or > 160 bpm (abnormal)
- Blood pressure low for gestational age

- Capillary refill > 2 seconds
- Cool extremities
- Pallor or mottling
- Poor urine output (< 1 mL/kg/hr)
- Metabolic acidosis
- Altered mental status

Signs of Metabolic Compromise

- Hypoglycemia (< 40 mg/dL)
- Hypothermia (< 36.5°C)
- Severe acidosis (pH < 7.15)
- Hyperkalemia or hypokalemia
- Hyponatremia or hypernatremia

Signs of Neurological Compromise

- Seizures
- Altered consciousness
- Hypotonia or hypertonia
- Poor feeding

- Vomiting
- Bulging fontanelle

Key Takeaways

✓ Neonatal physiology is profoundly different from older children. Understanding the transition from intrauterine to extrauterine life is essential for safe practice.

✓ Newborn babies are physiologically vulnerable due to immature respiratory, cardiovascular, metabolic, and immune systems.

✓ Stabilization before diagnosis: Your first priority is to create a physiological environment compatible with life, not establishing a diagnosis.

✓ Use the ABCDE framework for systematic stabilization.

✓ Oxygen delivery is the central concept: Adequate oxygen delivery depends on cardiac output, hemoglobin, and oxygen saturation.

✓ Tachycardia is a sign of stress, not normality: Compensatory tachycardia indicates that oxygen delivery is threatened.

✓ Acidosis reflects tissue hypoxia: Metabolic acidosis indicates inadequate perfusion and oxygenation.

✓ Temperature, glucose, and perfusion are non-negotiable: Every sick neonate needs correction of hypothermia, hypoglycemia, and hypoperfusion.

✓ Multidisciplinary collaboration is essential: Nurses, respiratory therapists, and physicians must work together to optimize outcomes.

✓ Continuous reassessment is critical: Neonates change rapidly. Frequent clinical assessment and adjustment of interventions are essential.

Chapter Eight

ETHICAL APPROACH IN NICU

Introduction: Why Ethics Matters in Neonatal Care

Ethics in the NICU is not abstract philosophy. It is the practical framework that guides us when we face difficult decisions: Should we resuscitate this extremely premature infant? How do we honor parental wishes when they conflict with our medical judgment? When do we transition from curative to palliative care? How do we allocate our resources fairly? What do we do when we make a medical error?

These are not theoretical questions. It is happening every day in our neonatal intensive care, often in circumstances where there is no "right" answer, only competing values and uncertain outcomes. The ethical approach provides a systematic way to think through these dilemmas, to involve the right people in decision-making, and to act in ways that respect the dignity and autonomy of patients and families.

Without an ethical framework, decisions become reactive, inconsistent, and sometimes harmful. With a clear ethical approach, we can navigate complexity with integrity.

The Four Pillars of Neonatal Ethics

1. Autonomy: Respecting Parental Decision-Making

What It Means

Autonomy is the right of parents to make decisions about their infant's care based on their own values, beliefs, and preferences. It is grounded in the principle that parents are the legitimate decision-makers for their child, not the medical team.

In Practice

Respecting autonomy means:

- Providing complete information – Parents cannot make autonomous decisions without understanding their child's condition, the treatment options available, the risks and benefits of each option, and the likely outcomes. This information must be presented in language they understand, not medical jargon.(clear simple language)

- Ensuring voluntary choice – Decisions must be free from intended manipulation, or pressure. Parents should never feel that they are being forced into a particular decision by the medical team.

- Honoring parental values – Even when parental choices conflict with what the medical team believes is best, we must respect those choices if they are informed and voluntary, provided they do not constitute abuse or neglect.
- Involving parents in decision-making – Major decisions about resuscitation, life support, transition to palliative care, and other critical issues should be made collaboratively with parents, not imposed by physicians.

Common Challenges

Challenge 1: Information Overload

Parents are often overwhelmed by medical information delivered in crisis situations. They may not retain what they hear, may misunderstand, or may feel pressured to make decisions before they are ready.(Do not confuse them)

Solution: Provide information in stages. Start with the most critical information. Check understanding. Repeat information as needed. Provide written materials. Allow time for questions. Involve a social worker, or patient advocate if available.

Challenge 2: Conflicting Parental Wishes

When parents disagree with each other about their infant's care, the medical team is caught in the middle.

Solution: Facilitate communication between parents. Help them understand each other's values and concerns. Involve ethics consultation if needed. Document the discussion. If parents cannot reach agreement, continue life-sustaining care while efforts to reach consensus continue.

Challenge 3: Cultural and Religious Considerations

Parental decisions are often grounded in cultural or religious beliefs that may differ from the medical team's values. For example, some families may refuse blood products, others may request aggressive resuscitation despite a terminal prognosis, and others may have specific rituals around death and dying.

Solution: Ask about cultural and religious values early. Respect these values unless they constitute clear abuse. Involve religious or cultural advisors if appropriate. Document conversations about values and preferences.

2. Beneficence: Acting in the Infant's Best Interest

What It Means

Beneficence is the obligation to act in the best interest of the patient—to do good, to heal, to relieve suffering, to promote well-being. It is the fundamental principle underlying medical practice.

In Practice

Beneficence in neonatal care means:

- Accurate diagnosis – We cannot act in the infant's best interest if we do not understand what is wrong. Systematic clinical reasoning, appropriate investigations, and specialist consultation when needed are essential.

- Evidence-based treatment – We should offer treatments that have evidence of benefit and avoid treatments that are futile or harmful.

- Anticipating complications – Understanding neonatal physiology allows us to anticipate what might go wrong and take preventive measures.

- Relieving suffering – Pain management, comfort care, and palliative measures are part of beneficence, not contrary to it.

- Honest clarification about the real prognosis – Families cannot make good decisions without understanding the likely outcomes. We have an obligation to provide honest, realistic prognostication based on the best available evidence.

Common Challenges

Challenge 1: Determining "Best Interest" When Prognosis Is Uncertain

Often we do not know whether an infant will survive or what quality of life they will have. In these circumstances, how do we determine "best interest"?

Solution: Acknowledge uncertainty explicitly. Present the range of possible outcomes. Discuss what quality of life means to the family. Make decisions based on the infant's current condition and trajectory, not on speculation about the future. Revisit decisions as new information becomes available.

Challenge 2: Balancing Aggressive Treatment With Comfort Care

Sometimes aggressive treatment and comfort are in tension. For example, aggressive resuscitation may prolong dying rather than restore health. Aggressive pain management may suppress respiratory drive. How do we balance these competing goods?

Solution: Clarify the goal of care. If the goal is cure, pursue aggressive treatment. If the goal is comfort, prioritize comfort even if it means accepting earlier death. These goals can coexist at different times in the course of illness.

Challenge 3: Resource Allocation

In a tertiary NICU with limited beds, staff, and equipment, how do we allocate resources fairly when demand exceeds supply?

Solution: Have institutional policies about resource allocation. Base allocation on medical need, likelihood of benefit, and fair distribution principles, not on ability to pay or social status. When resources are truly scarce, involve the ethics committee.

3. Non-Maleficence: "First, Do No Harm"

What It Means

Non-maleficence is the obligation to avoid causing harm. It is the foundation of the Hippocratic Oath and remains central to medical ethics. However, in neonatal medicine, "harm" is complex. Sometimes we must cause short-term harm (pain from procedures, side effects of medications) to prevent greater harm (death, severe disability).

In Practice

Non-maleficence in neonatal care means:

- Minimizing iatrogenic harm – Every intervention carries risk. We should use the minimum necessary intervention to achieve the therapeutic goal. For example, we use the smallest endotracheal tube that allows adequate ventilation, the lowest FiO_2 that maintains adequate oxygenation, and the shortest duration of mechanical ventilation possible.

- Avoiding futile treatment – Continuing treatment that offers no realistic hope of benefit is a form of harm. It prolongs suffering without purpose.

- Pain management – Procedures cause pain. We have an obligation to minimize pain through appropriate anesthesia, analgesia, and comfort measures.

- Preventing medical errors – Systematic approaches to safety, double-checking, clear communication, and adherence to protocols prevent errors that harm patients.

- Recognizing complications early – Many complications can be prevented or minimized if recognized early. Vigilant monitoring and willingness to act on subtle signs of deterioration are essential.

Common Challenges

Challenge 1: Balancing Aggressive Treatment With Harm Prevention

Sometimes the treatment necessary to prevent death or severe disability carries significant risk of harm. For example, mechanical ventilation can cause barotrauma and volutrauma. How aggressive should we be?

Solution: Use lung-protective ventilation strategies. Use the minimum pressure and volume necessary. Monitor for complications. Transition to less invasive support as soon as possible. Involve parents in discussions about acceptable risk.

Challenge 2: Recognizing When Treatment Is Futile

When is continued treatment futile? When should we transition to comfort care? These decisions are often unclear.

Solution: Define futility clearly. Futility means the treatment will not achieve its physiological goal, not that the outcome will be bad. For example, antibiotics are futile in a dying infant with overwhelming sepsis and multiorgan failure, but they are not futile in a stable infant with possible early sepsis. Involve the ethics committee when there is disagreement about futility.

Challenge 3: Medication Errors and Adverse Events

Errors happen. A dose is calculated incorrectly. A medication is given to the wrong patient. A procedure is performed on the wrong side. How do we respond ethically?

Solution: Disclose errors to families honestly and promptly. Explain what happened, why it happened, and what is being done to prevent recurrence. Apologize. Provide appropriate care to mitigate harm. Report the error through institutional channels. Learn from the error to prevent future occurrences.

4. Justice: Fair and Equitable Care

What It Means

Justice in healthcare means treating people fairly, allocating resources equitably, and ensuring that benefits and burdens are distributed according to principles of fairness. In neonatal care, justice means that every infant receives excellent care regardless of their social status, ability to pay, ethnicity, or other non-medical factors.

In Practice

Justice in neonatal care means:

- Equal access – Every infant born at your hospital should have access to the same level of NICU care. Social status, insurance status, or other non-medical factors should not determine who receives care.

- Fair allocation of resources – When resources are limited, they should be allocated based on medical need and likelihood of benefit, not on ability to pay.

- Culturally sensitive care – Different families have different values, beliefs, and communication styles. We should adapt our approach to respect cultural differences while maintaining standards of care.

- Advocacy for vulnerable populations – Some infants are

particularly vulnerable: extremely premature infants, infants with severe congenital anomalies, infants born to families with limited resources or social support. We have an obligation to advocate for their interests.

- Transparency in decision-making – Families should understand how decisions are made and should have access to the same information regardless of their background or ability to advocate.

Common Challenges

Challenge 1: Resource Allocation in a Tertiary NICU

Your NICU has limited beds. Two infants need NICU admission, but only one bed is available. How do you decide?

Solution: Have explicit institutional criteria for admission. Base decisions on medical need and likelihood of benefit. Do not base decisions on social factors. Involve the ethics committee if needed. Document the decision and the reasoning.

Challenge 2: Cultural Conflicts

A family's cultural or religious beliefs about medical care differ significantly from the medical team's recommendations. For example, a family may refuse a necessary blood transfusion, or may request resuscitation that the team believes is futile.

Solution: Approach with respect and curiosity. Understand the family's values and beliefs. Explain the medical perspective clearly. Look for common ground. Involve religious or cultural advisors if appropriate. If the family's choice would constitute abuse or neglect, involve institutional ethics and legal resources.

Challenge 3: Advocacy for Infants Without Family Support

Some infants are born to families with limited resources, limited understanding of medical care, or limited ability to advocate for their infant. How do we ensure these infants receive fair treatment?

Solution: Assign a primary care team that develops continuity with the family. Involve social work, chaplaincy, and patient advocacy. Ensure communication is clear and accessible. Do not assume families understand the medical system or their rights. Advocate actively for the infant's interests.

Ethical Frameworks for Decision-Making

The Four-Box Method

When facing an ethical dilemma, use this systematic approach:

Box 1: Medical Indications

- What is the patient's diagnosis?
- What is the prognosis with and without treatment?
- What are the treatment options?
- What are the risks and benefits of each option?
- Is the proposed treatment medically indicated?

Box 2: Patient/Family Preferences

- What does the family want?
- Do they understand the medical situation?
- Are their preferences informed and voluntary?

- Are there cultural or religious factors influencing their preferences?
- What are their values regarding quality of life, acceptable risk, and acceptable outcomes?

Box 3: Quality of Life

- What is the likely quality of life if treatment is pursued?
- What is the likely quality of life if treatment is withheld?
- What does quality of life mean to this family?
- Are there interventions that could improve quality of life?
- Is the infant experiencing pain or suffering?

Box 4: Contextual Factors

- Are there resource constraints?
- Are there legal or regulatory considerations?
- What is the impact on other patients or the institution?
- Are there conflicts of interest?
- What is the family's social support?

Using the Framework

Work through each box systematically. Often, the boxes align and the ethical path is clear. When boxes conflict—for example, when medical indications suggest aggressive treatment but family preferences and quality of life considerations suggest comfort care—the conflict must be addressed through dialogue, ethics consultation, or other institutional mechanisms.

Specific Ethical Issues in Neonatal Care

Resuscitation Decisions

When Should We Resuscitate?

Not every newborn should be resuscitated. Resuscitation is appropriate when there is a reasonable chance of survival with acceptable quality of life. Resuscitation is not appropriate when the infant will not survive or will survive with severe disability incompatible with the family's values.

Periviable Birth (22-24 weeks gestation)

Infants born at 22-24 weeks gestation have uncertain prognosis. Survival is possible but not guaranteed, and survivors often have significant morbidity. Resuscitation decisions should be individualized based on:

- Exact gestational age (22 weeks vs. 24 weeks makes a significant difference)
- Birth weight (larger infants have better outcomes)
- Singleton vs. multiple gestation
- Maternal factors (antenatal steroids, maternal infection)
- Parental preferences and values

Counseling Approach: Provide honest, evidence-based prognostication. Discuss the range of possible outcomes. Discuss what quality of life means to the family. Make a plan together about resuscitation, and document it clearly. Recognize that parents may change their minds as the situation evolves.

- Extreme Prematurity (22-23 weeks): At 22-23 weeks, survival is rare and morbidity is severe. Many institutions offer "comfort care" as the primary option, with resuscitation available if parents strongly desire it after full counseling about likely outcomes.

- Moderate Prematurity (24-28 weeks): At 24-28 weeks, survival is likely but morbidity is common. Resuscitation is usually offered, with discussion about the likely need for prolonged NICU stay and possible long-term complications.

- Late Prematurity (28-37 weeks) and Term Infants: Resuscitation is standard unless there is a known lethal condition or the infant is stillborn.

Withholding and Withdrawing Life Support

Ethical Equivalence

Withholding life support (not starting it) and withdrawing life support (stopping it) are ethically equivalent. Both are appropriate when treatment is futile, when the burden of treatment outweighs benefit, or when it no longer aligns with the infant's or family's goals.

Common Situations

Situation 1: The Infant With No Chance of Survival

Some infants have conditions incompatible with life: anencephaly, severe hydrops fetalis with severe cardiac anomalies, extreme prematurity with massive intraventricular hemorrhage and multiorgan failure.

Approach: Offer comfort care. Provide pain management, warmth, feeding if possible, and family time. Do not pursue aggressive interventions that prolong dying without hope of recovery.

Situation 2: The Infant With Severe Disability

Some infants survive but with severe disability: profound developmental delay, inability to breathe without mechanical ventilation, inability to feed, severe pain.

Approach: Discuss with parents what quality of life is acceptable to them. Some families choose aggressive treatment despite severe disability. Others choose comfort care. Both choices are ethically valid if informed and voluntary.

Situation 3: The Chronically Ill Infant

Some infants spend months in the NICU with ongoing medical complexity, recurrent infections, and slow progress toward discharge.

Approach: Regularly reassess goals of care. Discuss with parents whether current treatment aligns with their values and the infant's best interest. Consider palliative care approaches even while pursuing curative treatment.

Palliative and Comfort Care

What Is Palliative Care?

Palliative care is an approach to care focused on relieving suffering and supporting quality of life, rather than on curing disease. It can be provided alongside curative treatment or as the primary approach when cure is not possible.

Principles of Palliative Care in Neonates

- Pain and symptom management – Aggressive management of pain, respiratory distress, and other symptoms

- Family support – Emotional, spiritual, and practical support for parents and siblings
- Honest communication – Clear, compassionate discussion about prognosis and goals
- Respect for dignity – Treating the infant and family with respect and compassion
- Bereavement support – Support for families after the infant's death

Transitioning to Palliative Care

Transitioning to palliative care does not mean "giving up." It means changing the focus from cure to comfort. This transition should be discussed with families before crisis situations force the decision.

Conversation Starter: "We want to make sure we are doing what is best for your baby. Let's talk about what 'best' means to you. If your baby's condition does not improve, what would be most important to you—trying every possible treatment, or focusing on comfort and time together as a family?"

Disclosure of Medical Errors

When an Error Occurs

Medical errors happen. A medication dose is calculated incorrectly. A procedure is performed on the wrong patient. An important finding is missed. What is the ethical response?

The Ethical Obligation

You have an ethical obligation to:

1. Disclose the error to the family – Families have a right to

know what happened. Disclosure should be prompt, honest, and compassionate.

2. Explain what happened – Describe the error clearly, without jargon. Explain how it occurred.

3. Explain the impact – Discuss what harm, if any, resulted from the error. If the infant was harmed, explain what is being done to mitigate that harm.

4. Apologize – Say "I'm sorry" or "We're sorry." Apologizing for the error is not an admission of guilt; it is an expression of compassion.

5. Explain prevention – Discuss what is being done to prevent similar errors in the future.

6. Provide support – Offer resources: social work, chaplaincy, ethics consultation, legal advice.

Documentation

Document the error in the medical record. Describe what happened, when it was discovered, what harm resulted, and what was done. Also document the disclosure conversation with the family.

Institutional Response

Report the error through your institution's incident reporting system. Participate in root cause analysis. Implement system changes to prevent recurrence.

Building an Ethical NICU Culture

Ethics Rounds and Case Discussions

Regularly discuss ethical issues in your NICU. Use case conferences to work through difficult situations. Discuss not just the medical facts, but the ethical dimensions: What are the family's values? What does the family want? What does the medical team believe is best? How do we navigate conflict?

Ethics Consultation

Most institutions have an ethics committee or ethics consultant available. Use this resource when:

- There is conflict between the family and the medical team
- There is conflict among team members
- A decision is particularly complex or high-stakes
- You are unsure about the ethical path forward

Communication Training

Good communication prevents many ethical conflicts. Invest in training on:

- Delivering bad news
- Shared decision-making
- Cultural competency
- Conflict resolution

- Family-centered care

Moral Distress

Moral distress occurs when you believe you know the right thing to do, but institutional constraints, resource limitations, or other factors prevent you from doing it. Moral distress is common in neonatal care and can lead to burnout and decreased job satisfaction.

Addressing Moral Distress

- Acknowledge it – Recognize that moral distress is real and valid
- Discuss it – Talk with colleagues, mentors, or ethics consultants
- Act on it – Advocate for changes that reduce moral distress
- Support colleagues – Create a culture where moral distress can be discussed openly

Key Takeaways

✓ Ethics is not abstract – It is the practical framework that guides decision-making in complex situations

✓ The four pillars – Autonomy, beneficence, non-maleficence, and justice provide a foundation for ethical practice

✓ Families are partners – Respect parental autonomy while providing honest medical guidance

✓ Acknowledge uncertainty – Be honest about what you don't know and what you can't predict

✓ Systematic decision-making – Use frameworks like the four-box method to work through ethical dilemmas

✓ Palliative care is not failure – It is an appropriate and compassionate approach when cure is not possible

✓ Disclose errors honestly – Transparency builds trust and prevents harm

✓ Build an ethical culture – Regular ethics discussions, ethics consultation, and communication training strengthen ethical practice

✓ Recognize moral distress – Create space for team members to discuss ethical concerns and advocate for change

✓ Humility matters – Recognize the limits of your knowledge and the complexity of ethical decision-making

Chapter Nine

DELIVERY ROOM MANAGEMENT AND INITIAL RESUSCITATION

Introduction: The Golden Minutes "For successful Neonatal Golden Hour"

The delivery room is where neonatal life begins. The first minutes after birth are critical.Hence decisions made in these moments, actions taken or not taken, set the trajectory for the entire NICU course. A neonate who is effectively resuscitated and stabilized in the delivery room has a fundamentally different outcome than one who arrives in the NICU hypoxic, hypothermic, and acidotic.

Yet the delivery room is chaotic. Multiple health care providers are present. Communication is often unclear. Equipment may not be readily available. The pressure to act quickly is intense. Emotions run high. In this environment, systematic preparation and clear protocols are essential." Follow a systematic algorithm as the Neonatal Resuscitation Program "

This chapter teaches you how to prepare for delivery, how to rapidly assess the newborn, and how to initiate resuscitation using evidence-based algorithms. The goal is not to memorize a protocol, but to understand the physiological principles underlying resuscitation so you can adapt to any situation.

Preparation: Before the Delivery

Know the Maternal and Obstetric History

Before the infant arrives, you should know:

Maternal Factors

- Maternal age and medical history
- Infections (GBS, chorioamnionitis, maternal fever)
- Medications (magnesium sulfate, opioids, antibiotics)
- Substance use (drugs, alcohol)
- Diabetes or other metabolic disorders

Obstetric Factors

- Gestational age (critical for resuscitation decisions)

- Single vs. multiple gestation
- Rupture of membranes and duration
- Labor progression
- Umbilical cord management plan
- Fetal monitoring (reassuring vs. concerning)
- Vaginal delivery vs. cesarean section
- Indication for delivery (elective vs. emergency)

Placental and Cord Factors

- Placental abnormalities (previa, abruption, insufficiency)
- Cord abnormalities (nuchal cord, true knot, oligohydramnios)
- Meconium-stained amniotic fluid

Expected Neonatal Factors

- Expected gestational age and estimated weight
- Known or suspected congenital anomalies
- Expected complications (IUGR, hydrops, etc.)

Why This Matters

This information allows you to anticipate problems. If you know the infant is extremely premature, you prepare for respiratory distress and temperature management. If you know there is meconium, you prepare for meconium aspiration. If you know there is a suspected congenital anomaly, you prepare for potential airway or cardiac issues.

Prepare the Delivery Room

Equipment Check

Before every delivery, verify that the delivery room has:

Thermal Management

- Radiant warmer on and functioning
- Warm blankets
- Plastic wrap or bag for extremely premature infants
- Hats and gloves

Airway Equipment

- Suction apparatus (wall and portable)
- Suction catheters (10F, 12F, 14F)
- Laryngoscopes (straight blade, appropriate sizes)
- Endotracheal tubes (sizes 2.5, 3.0, 3.5)
- Laryngeal mask airway (LMA)
- Bag and mask (term size and preterm size)
- Oxygen source and tubing
- Pulse oximetry probe
- Cardiac monitor and leads

Medication and IV Access

- Epinephrine (1:10,000)

- Normal saline
- Sodium bicarbonate
- Dextrose
- IV catheters (umbilical venous catheter, peripheral IV)
- Syringes and needles
- Medication labels

Other Equipment

- Cord clamp and scissors
- Bulb syringe
- Towels and drapes
- Gloves and personal protective equipment
- Clock (for timing)
- Delivery record and resuscitation documentation

Checklist Approach

Use a formal checklist before every delivery. Assign one person to verify equipment. Do not assume equipment is present or functioning. Check it yourself.

Assemble the Team

Team Composition

For a high-risk delivery, have:

- Neonatology team leader – Responsible for overall management and decision-making
- Airway specialist – Prepared to intubate if needed
- Chest compressions provider – Prepared to initiate CPR
- IV access provider – Prepared to place UVC or IO line
- Medication provider – Prepares and administers medications
- Scribe – Documents resuscitation events and times
- Obstetric team – Remains available for complications

For Lower-Risk Deliveries

One experienced person may be sufficient, but know who will be called if resuscitation is needed.

Team Communication

- Designate a team leader before delivery begins
- Brief the team on the anticipated situation
- Use clear, direct communication during resuscitation
- Call out roles and responsibilities
- Communicate findings ("No spontaneous respirations", "Heart rate 80 and dropping")
- Use closed-loop communication ("I'm going to intubate" → "Ready to intubate")

Initial Assessment: The First 30 Seconds

The Three Critical Questions

When the infant is born, immediately ask three questions:

Question 1: Is the infant term?Termness determines management. A term infant with no spontaneous respirations requires immediate resuscitation. A 22-week infant with no spontaneous respirations may not, depending on parental preferences and institutional policy.

Question 2: Is the amniotic fluid clear?If meconium is present, prepare for meconium aspiration. If amniotic fluid is clear, proceed with standard resuscitation.

Question 3: Is the infant breathing or crying?If the infant is breathing vigorously and crying, place skin-to-skin with mother and observe. If the infant is not breathing or breathing is weak, begin resuscitation.

The Apgar Score: Useful But Not for Resuscitation Decisions

The Apgar score (Appearance, Pulse, Grimace, Activity, Respiration) is assigned at 1 minute and 5 minutes. It is useful for describing the infant's condition and predicting outcome, but it should not be used to guide resuscitation decisions.

Why Not?Resuscitation decisions must be made in real-time, often before the 1-minute Apgar is assigned. The Apgar score is retrospective and does not guide management.

What To Do InsteadUse the assessment algorithm below, which is based on the infant's response to interventions in real-time.

Resuscitation Algorithm: The Systematic Approach

Step 1: Initial Stabilization (First 30 Seconds)

For All Infants

1. Dry the infant – Remove wet blankets. Dry skin prevents heat loss.

2. Assess tone – If the infant has poor tone, place on radiant warmer. If tone is good, skin-to-skin with mother is appropriate.

3. Position the airway – Place the infant supine with head in neutral position (not hyperextended). A small roll under the shoulders may help.

4. Suction if needed – Suction the mouth first, then nose. Do not deep suction unless meconium is present. Aggressive suctioning can cause vagal stimulation and bradycardia.

5. Stimulate – Dry the infant, rub the back, or slap the soles of the feet. Most infants respond to this stimulation.

6. Assess response – Does the infant have spontaneous breathing? Is the heart rate >100? Is there a good tone?

Decision Point After 30 Seconds

After initial stabilization and stimulation, assess:

- Spontaneous breathing present? YES
  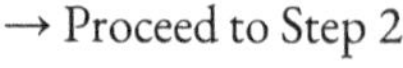
  → Proceed to Step 2

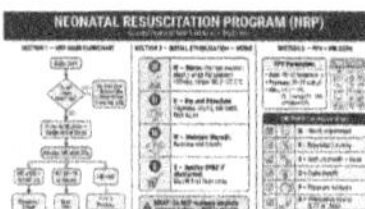

- Spontaneous breathing present? NO

→ Proceed to PPV

- Heart rate >100? YES → Observe and reassess
- Heart rate >100? NO → Proceed to PPV
- Good tone and color? YES → Observe and reassess
- Poor tone or cyanosis? → Proceed to PPV

Step 2: Positive Pressure Ventilation (PPV)

When to Start PPV

Start PPV if:

- Spontaneous breathing is absent or gasping
- Heart rate is <100 bpm
- Persistent cyanosis despite adequate oxygenation

Initial Settings

- Rate: 40-60 breaths per minute (for term infant)
- Pressure: Start with 20 cm H_2O, titrate to achieve chest rise
- FiO_2: Start with 21% (room air) for term infants. For preterm infants <30 weeks, consider starting with 30% FiO_2. Titrate based on pulse oximetry.

Technique

1. Seal the mask – Use appropriately sized mask (should cover nose and mouth but not eyes or chin)

2. Position the head – Neutral position, not hyperextended

3. Apply gentle pressure – Watch for chest rise

4. Deliver breaths – Synchronize with any spontaneous breathing if possible

5. Assess response – After 15 seconds of PPV, reassess heart rate and breathing

Response to PPV

Good Response (Heart Rate >100, Spontaneous Breathing)

- Continue PPV at lower rate (20-30 bpm) while spontaneous breathing increases
- Wean to room air or lower FiO_2 as SpO_2 improves
- Transition to observation

Inadequate Response (Heart Rate <100 or No Improvement in Breathing)

- Check seal of mask
- Reposition head
- Clear airway of secretions
- Open mouth
- Increase pressure slightly
- Consider intubation
- Proceed to chest compressions if heart rate remains <60

Step 3: Chest Compressions

When to Start

Start chest compressions if heart rate remains <60 bpm after 15 seconds of effective PPV (with good chest rise).

Technique: Two-Thumb Method (Preferred)

- Hand position – Place both thumbs on the lower third of the sternum, just below the nipple line

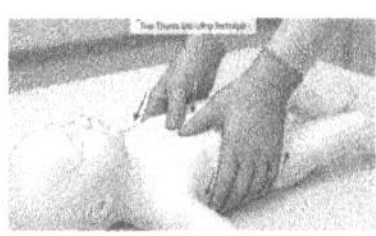

- Finger position – Wrap fingers around the chest, supporting the back
- Compression depth – Compress to 1/3 the depth of the chest (approximately 1.5 inches for a term infant)
- Rate – 90 compressions per minute
- Coordination – Coordinate with ventilations at a 3:1 ratio (3 compressions to 1 ventilation)

Alternative: Two-Finger Method

If only one provider is present:

- Place two fingers on the lower sternum
- Compress to 1/3 chest depth
- Maintain 3:1 compression-to-ventilation ratio

Reassessment

After 10 cycles of CPR (approximately 10 seconds), reassess heart rate:

- Heart rate >60? → Continue PPV alone, discontinue compressions
- Heart rate <60? → Continue CPR, proceed to medications

Step 4: Medications

When to Administer

Administer medications if:

- Heart rate remains <60 after 10 cycles of CPR with effective PPV
- Asystole or severe bradycardia despite resuscitation
- Need for specific reversal agents (naloxone for opioids)

Epinephrine (First-Line Medication)

- Dose: 0.01-0.03 mg/kg IV (0.1-0.3 mL/kg of 1:10,000 concentration)
- Route: Intravenous (preferred) or intraosseous
- Timing: Every 3-5 minutes if needed
- Effect: Increases heart rate and blood pressure through alpha and beta-adrenergic stimulation

Administration via Umbilical Venous Catheter (UVC)

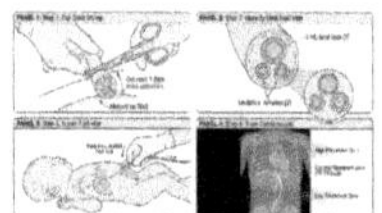

If IV access cannot be obtained quickly:

1. Place UVC in the lower third of umbilical vein

2. Flush with normal saline

3. Administer medication

4. Flush with saline to push medication into circulation

Other Medications

Sodium Bicarbonate

- Dose: 1 mEq/kg IV

- Indication: Metabolic acidosis (use only if resuscitation is prolonged and pH is severely low)

- Note: Not recommended in first 10 minutes of resuscitation

Glucose (Dextrose)

- Dose: 0.25-0.5 g/kg IV (2.5-5 mL/kg of 10% dextrose)

- Indication: Hypoglycemia (check glucose if available, but do not delay resuscitation)

- Note: Check glucose after resuscitation is successful

Naloxone (Narcan)"Not strongly recommended , otherwise with expert clinician"

- Dose: 0.1 mg/kg IV or IM

- Indication: Respiratory depression from maternal opioid use

- Note: Do not give if mother has opioid dependency (risk of acute withdrawal)

Atropine

- Dose: 0.02 mg/kg IV
- Indication: Bradycardia from vagal stimulation (rare in neonatal resuscitation)
- Note: Not recommended for routine use

Special Situations in Delivery Room Resuscitation

Meconium Aspiration

ScenarioAmniotic fluid is stained with meconium. Either The infant is vigorous Or NOT , .Both will require same approach as per NRP approach

Management

- Fulfill initial steps with emphasis on suctioning mouth and nose
- Do NOT intubate for suctioning
- Monitor for respiratory distress
- If baby is in apnea or have bradycardia and not improved with bag-mask ventilation , then Intubate for delivering effective ventilation
- If meconium is thick and you face difficulty to ventilate the lung well then you could try doing meconium suctioning via meconium aspirator device attached to the ETT , then reintubate and continue CPR measures .

Extremely Premature Infants (22-24 Weeks)

Decision-Making

Before delivery, discuss with parents and obstetric team:

- Will resuscitation be offered?
- What is the goal of resuscitation (full support vs. comfort care)?
- What should happen if the infant is born without a heartbeat?

Management if Resuscitation Is Chosen

- Provide full resuscitation as outlined above
- Gentle handling to prevent intraventricular hemorrhage
- Minimize heat loss (plastic wrap, hat)
- Defer cord clamping if stable (30-60 seconds)"Needs judicious order by the most expert clinician in the team "
- Transfer to NICU urgently

Management if Comfort Care Is Chosen

- Provide warmth and comfort
- Dry and wrap the infant
- Allow parents to hold and spend time
- Provide pain management if needed

- Provide support to parents

Multiple Gestation

Preparation

- Have a resuscitation team for each infant
- Identify each infant clearly
- Communicate with obstetric team about delivery order and any complications

Management

- Proceed with standard resuscitation for each infant
- Prioritize based on need (more compromised infant may need more intensive intervention)
- Communicate clearly about which infant is being managed

Congenital Anomalies

Known Anomalies (Prenatal Diagnosis)

If a congenital anomaly is known prenatally:

1. Discuss with parents and obstetric team
2. Plan delivery and resuscitation accordingly
3. Assemble appropriate specialists (surgery, cardiology, etc.)

4. Prepare equipment specific to the anomaly

Examples:

Congenital Diaphragmatic Hernia

- Do NOT use bag and mask (inflates stomach, compromises lungs)
- Intubate immediately
- Place NG tube to decompress stomach

Gastroschisis

- Do NOT place infant skin-to-skin
- Wrap exposed bowel in warm, sterile plastic wrap
- Establish IV access
- Prepare for urgent surgical consultation

Anencephaly or Other Lethal Anomalies

- Discuss with parents about goals of care
- Provide comfort care
- Allow family time

Cord Complications

Nuchal Cord (Cord Around Neck)

- If loose, slip over the infant's head
- If tight, clamp and cut before delivery of the body

- Proceed with standard resuscitation if needed

True Knot or Cord Prolapse

- Obstetric team manages delivery
- Be prepared for possible fetal distress
- Have resuscitation team ready

Maternal Substance Use

Opioids

- Infant may have respiratory depression
- Provide PPV as needed
- Have naloxone available
- Use naloxone only if respiratory depression is severe and mother does not have opioid dependency

Benzodiazepines or Barbiturates

- Infant may have decreased tone and respiratory depression
- Provide PPV as needed
- No specific antidote available
- Supportive care

Cocaine or Amphetamines

- Infant may be jittery or irritable
- May have tachycardia or hypertension

- Provide supportive care
- Monitor for seizures

Transition From Delivery Room to NICU

Handoff Communication

When transferring the infant to the NICU, provide clear communication using SBAR Format:

- Situation: "This is a term infant born by vaginal delivery at 2:15 PM"
- Background: "Mother had prolonged labor, fetal heart rate showed late decelerations. Amniotic fluid was clear."
- Assessment: "Infant was apneic at birth, required PPV for 2 minutes, now breathing spontaneously with heart rate 140."
- Recommendation: "Recommend continuous monitoring, pulse oximetry, and close observation for respiratory distress."

Documentation

Document in the delivery room record:

- Time of delivery
- Apgar scores at 1, 5, and 10 minutes

- Resuscitation interventions and times
- Response to interventions
- Medications administered
- Vital signs
- Any complications or concerns
- Parental presence and response

Key Takeaways

✓ Preparation prevents problems – Know the maternal and obstetric history, check equipment, and assemble the team

✓ The first 30 seconds are critical – Dry, position, stimulate, and assess response

✓ Use the algorithm – Systematic approach to PPV, compressions, and medications improves outcomes

✓ Meconium management – Suction only if meconium is present AND infant is not vigorous

✓ Chest compressions are rare – Most infants respond to PPV; compressions are needed in <1% of deliveries

✓ Medications are last resort – Effective PPV and compressions are more important than medications

✓ Communicate clearly – Use SBAR format for handoff to NICU team

✓ Document thoroughly – Accurate documentation is essential for continuity of care and quality improvement

✓ Adapt to context – Adjust management based on gestational age, known anomalies, and parental preferences

✓ Humility and teamwork – Resuscitation is a team effort; ask for help, communicate clearly, and support colleagues

Chapter Ten

NEWBORN NUTRITION FUNDAMENTALS

Introduction

Nutrition is not a luxury in the NICU—it is a critical component of survival and neurodevelopment. Every hour of suboptimal nutrition in the first weeks of life has measurable consequences for growth, brain development, and long-term outcomes. This chapter provides a systematic approach to feeding decisions in the NICU, from the extremely premature infant to the term newborn with complications.

Nutritional Physiology of the Newborn

Energy Requirements

- Basal metabolic rate: 40-50 kcal/kg/day
- Thermoregulation: 10-15 kcal/kg/day
- Growth: 15-20 kcal/kg/day
- Activity and stress: 5-10 kcal/kg/day

Total requirement: 80-120 kcal/kg/day (varies by gestational age, illness, and growth goals)

Macronutrient Requirements

Micronutrient Considerations

Critical micronutrients in preterm infants:

- Iron (for hemoglobin synthesis and myelination)
- Calcium and phosphorus (bone mineralization)
- Vitamins A, D, E (antioxidant and immune function)
- Zinc (immune function, wound healing)

Feeding Route Decision Algorithm

Step 1: Assess Gastrointestinal Maturity and Function

Can the infant tolerate enteral feeding?

✓ YES → Proceed to enteral feeding (preferred)✗ NO → Start parenteral nutrition; reassess daily

Contraindications to enteral feeding:

- Hemodynamic instability (shock, severe hypotension)
- Severe respiratory distress (FiO_2 >0.60, alongside severe acidosis)
- Active necrotizing enterocolitis (NEC) or suspected NEC
- Abdominal distension with bilious gastric residuals
- Acute surgical abdomen
- Severe thrombocytopenia (<20,000) with abdominal bleeding tendensy

Step 2: Determine Feeding Type

Enteral feeding options:

1. Breast milk (mother's own or donor)"Fortification could be added "
   - First choice for all infants
   - Provides immunologic protection, optimal nutrient bioavailability
   - Fortification needed for preterm <32 weeks

2. Formula (standard or specialized)
    - When breast milk unavailable
    - Preterm formula for <34 weeks
    - Term formula for ≥34 weeks
    - Specialized formulas for specific conditions (hydrolyzed protein, amino acid-based)
3. Combination (breast milk + formula)
    - Common in NICU
    - Maximize breast milk while meeting caloric needs

Step 3: Determine Feeding Route

Oral feeding:

- Term or near-term infants with intact suck-swallow-breathe coordination
- Typically ≥34 weeks gestation
- Assess readiness: alertness, rooting reflex, coordination

Orogastric/nasogastric tube feeding:

- <34 weeks gestation
- Infants with weak suck or coordination issues
- Allows continuous or intermittent feeding

- Assess tube placement: gastric aspirate pH, X-ray if uncertain

Transpyloric feeding:

- Reserved for specific indications (severe gastroesophageal reflux, gastric dysmotility)
- Higher risk of complications (perforation, malabsorption)
- Not routine

Parenteral Nutrition (PN)

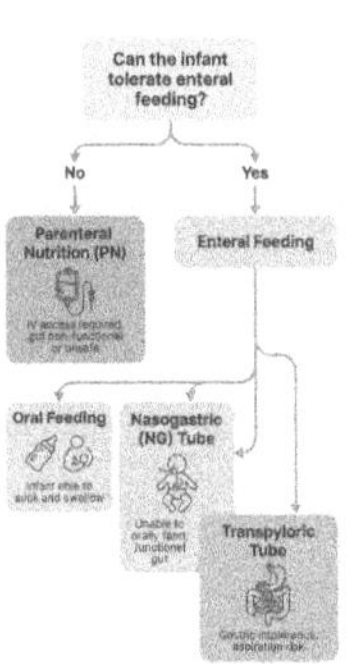

Indications for PN

- Gestational age <28 weeks (until enteral feeding established)
- Birth weight <1000g (until enteral feeding established)
- Contraindications to enteral feeding (see Section 8.2)
- Surgical conditions (NEC, intestinal obstruction, abdominal wall defects)
- Severe malabsorption (short bowel, cholestasis)

PN Composition

Macronutrients:

- Dextrose: Start 5-8 g/kg/day; advance by 2-3 g/kg/day to maximum usual goal 12-14 g/kg/day
- Amino acids: Start 1-2 g/kg/day; advance by 1 g/kg/day to goal 3-4 g/kg/day
- Lipids: Start 1-2 g/kg/day; advance by 0.5-1 g/kg/day to goal 3-4 g/kg/day (hold if triglycerides >400 mg/dL)

Micronutrients:

- Vitamins (MVI-Pediatric or equivalent)
- Trace elements (zinc, copper, selenium, chromium, manganese)
- Calcium, phosphorus, magnesium
- Adjust based on labs and renal function

PN Monitoring

Labs to obtain:

- Baseline: Glucose, electrolytes, BUN, creatinine, liver function tests, triglycerides
- During advancement: Glucose daily until stable; electrolytes every 2-3 days; liver function weekly
- Ongoing: Triglycerides weekly; phosphorus, calcium, magnesium weekly

Clinical monitoring:

- Fluid balance (input/output, weight trend)

- Glucose control (target 100-150 mg/dL)
- Signs of infection (central line care essential)
- Hepatic dysfunction (cholestasis, elevated bilirubin)

Enteral Feeding Advancement Protocol

Phase 1: Trophic Feeding (Days 1-3)

Goal: Stimulate gastrointestinal development, not nutrition

- Volume: 10-20 mL/kg/day (divided into 8-12 feeds)
- Frequency: Every 2-3 hours
- Type: Breast milk preferred; formula if unavailable
- Method: Continuous or intermittent tube feeding

Monitoring:

- Gastric residuals before each feed (discard if >50% of previous feed volume or bilious)
- Abdominal distension, tenderness
- Stool output
- Feeding tolerance

Phase 2: Progressive Advancement (Days 3-7)

Criteria to advance:

- Tolerating trophic feeds (residuals <50%, no distension)
- Stable vital signs, no sepsis signs
- Normal abdominal exam

Advancement protocol:

- Increase by 20-30 mL/kg/day every 1-2 days
- Target: 120-150 mL/kg/day by day 7-10
- Transition from continuous to intermittent feeding (8-12 feeds/day)

Feeding volume by gestational age (mL/kg/day):

Phase 3: Full Enteral Feeding (Days 7-14)

Goal: Achieve full caloric intake (120-150 kcal/kg/day) enterally

Feeding schedule:

- 8-12 times daily for preterm
- Ad libitum for term infants

Fortification (for preterm <32 weeks):

- Add human milk fortifier to breast milk (increases protein, calories, minerals)
- Start at 50% fortification; advance to full fortification
- Reassess need as infant grows

Transition to bottle/breast:

- Begin at 32-34 weeks
- Start with 1-2 oral feeds daily
- Gradually replace tube feeds
- Assess for fatigue, desaturation during feeds

Feeding Intolerance: Recognition and Management

Red Flags for Feeding Intolerance

Gastric signs:

- Gastric residuals >50% of feed volume or bilious
- Persistent gastric distension
- Vomiting

Abdominal signs:

- Abdominal distension (measure abdominal girth)
- Tenderness, guarding
- Visible loops, erythema

Systemic signs:

- Apnea, bradycardia during feeding
- Temperature instability
- Lethargy or irritability

- Metabolic acidosis

Differential Diagnosis

1. Immature gut motility (most common in preterm)
    - *Management:* Slow advancement, consider prokinetics (domperidone)
2. Necrotizing enterocolitis (NEC) (medical emergency)
    - *Signs:* Pneumatosis, portal venous gas, perforation
    - *Management:* NPO, NG decompression, antibiotics, surgery if needed
3. Gastroesophageal reflux (GER)
    - *Signs:* Vomiting, aspiration risk
    - *Management:* Positional, smaller more frequent feeds, thickening agents
4. Infection (sepsis, NEC, meningitis)
    - *Management:* Hold feeds, investigate, treat underlying infection
5. Surgical abdomen (obstruction, perforation, appendicitis)
    - *Management:* NPO, imaging, surgical consultation

Special Feeding Situations

Extremely Premature Infants (<28 Weeks)

Challenges:

- Immature suck-swallow-breathe coordination
- High aspiration risk
- Increased NEC risk
- Rapid growth requirements

Strategy:

- Start PN on day 1 (amino acids + dextrose + lipids)
- Begin trophic breast milk feeds on day 3-5
- Slow advancement (20 mL/kg/day every 2-3 days)
- Continue PN until 120+ mL/kg/day enteral achieved
- Fortify breast milk when at goal volume

Growth-Restricted Infants (IUGR)

Challenges:

- Depleted glycogen stores
- Increased metabolic rate
- Hypoglycemia risk

- Feeding intolerance common

Strategy:

- Aggressive early glucose support (dextrose infusions)
- Early trophic feeds to stimulate gut
- Careful advancement (avoid overfeeding)
- Higher caloric density feeds (fortified breast milk or formula)
- Monitor for NEC (increased risk with rapid advancement)

Infants with Congenital Heart Disease

Challenges:

- Increased caloric requirements (150-200 kcal/kg/day)
- Feeding-related desaturation
- Fluid restriction (depending on lesion)
- Increased work of breathing with feeds

Strategy:

- Coordinate with cardiology
- Higher caloric density feeds (fortified breast milk, high-calorie formula)
- Smaller, more frequent feeds
- Monitor for signs of heart failure

- Consider gastric tube if oral feeding causes desaturation

Infants with Gastroesophageal Reflux

Non-pharmacologic management:

- Smaller, more frequent feeds
- Thickened feeds (rice cereal, commercial thickener)
- Upright positioning 30 minutes post-feed
- Left lateral decubitus position

Pharmacologic management:

- Omeprazole or Ranitidine"If registered in your country formulary " (reduce gastric acid)
- Domperidone or metoclopramide (enhance motility)
- Use only if conservative measures fail

Infants with Cleft Palate/Lip

Feeding challenges:

- Difficulty creating adequate suction
- Increased aspiration risk
- Milk leakage from nose

Strategies:

- Specialized bottles (Pigeon, Haberman)

- Increased milk flow
- Tube feeding if unable to meet needs orally
- Coordinate with cleft team regarding surgical timing

Breast Milk and Lactation Support

Benefits of Breast Milk

- Immunologic: IgA, lactoferrin, lysozyme, white blood cells
- Nutritional: Optimal protein-to-calorie ratio, bioavailable nutrients
- Developmental: Enhanced neurodevelopment, reduced NEC risk
- Maternal: Bonding, reduced postpartum bleeding, lower cancer risk

Lactation Management

Initiation:

- Begin pumping within 2-4 hours of delivery
- Pump 8-10 times daily (including night)
- Electric double pump recommended

Supply optimization:

- Frequent, effective milk removal
- Skin-to-skin contact
- Adequate maternal nutrition and hydration
- Lactation consultant involvement
- Medications if needed (domperidone for low supply)

Milk storage:

- Room temperature: 4 hours
- Refrigerator: 4 days at 4°C
- Freezer: 3-6 months at -20°C
- Thaw in warm water, never microwave

Fortification Strategies

Human milk fortifier (HMF):

- Start when infant tolerating 100 mL/kg/day
- Provides additional protein, calories, minerals
- Types: Cow's milk-based (standard), human milk-based (premium)

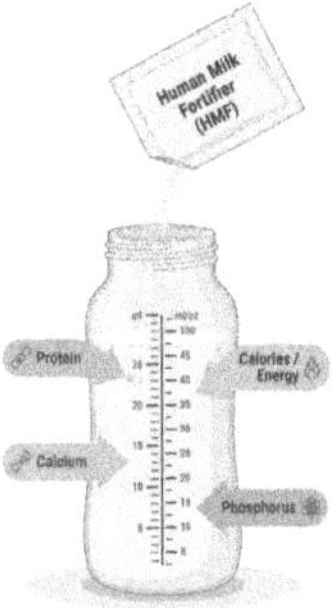

Targeted fortification:

- Measure breast milk nutrient content

- Add specific nutrients based on analysis
- More individualized but labor-intensive

Adjustments:

- Reduce fortification as infant grows
- Monitor growth velocity
- Reassess at 34 weeks, 36 weeks, discharge

Formula Feeding

Types of Formula

Standard preterm formula (22-24 kcal/oz):

- For infants <34 weeks or <1800g
- Higher protein, calcium, phosphorus than term formula

Standard term formula (20 kcal/oz):

- For infants ≥34 weeks or >2000g
- Lower mineral content than preterm

Specialized formulas:

- Hydrolyzed protein: For allergy/intolerance
- Amino acid-based: For severe allergy or malabsorption
- MCT oil-enriched: For fat malabsorption

- Lactose-free: For lactose intolerance

Formula Preparation and Safety

Sterile technique:

- Use sterile water for mixing
- Wash hands before preparation
- Use clean, sterile bottles
- Discard unused formula after 2 hours at room temperature

Osmolarity considerations:

- Standard formula: ~300 mOsm/L
- High osmolarity increases NEC risk
- Avoid adding supplements unless medically indicated

Monitoring Growth and Nutritional Adequacy

Growth Metrics

Weight:

- Expected loss: 5-10% by day 3-5
- Return to birth weight: By day 10-14
- Growth velocity: 15-20 g/kg/day in preterm

Length and head circumference:

- Length growth: 0.8-1.0 cm/week
- Head circumference: 0.5-0.75 cm/week
- Critical for neurodevelopment

Plotting growth:

- Use appropriate growth charts (Fenton for preterm, WHO for term)
- Plot weekly
- Assess trajectory, not absolute values

Laboratory Monitoring

Routine labs:

- Glucose (daily until stable, then as needed)
- Electrolytes (sodium, potassium, chloride, CO_2)
- Minerals (calcium, phosphorus, magnesium)
- Liver function (AST, ALT, bilirubin, albumin)
- Albumin (marker of protein status)

Frequency:

- Baseline (day 1)
- During PN advancement (2-3 times weekly)
- Once stable (weekly)

- Before discharge (to confirm adequate nutrition)

Metabolic Markers

Adequate protein intake:

- BUN 10-20 mg/dL
- Albumin >2.5 g/dL (indicates adequate recent protein intake)
- Prealbumin >20 mg/dL (sensitive marker of protein status)

Adequate caloric intake:

- Weight gain curve
- Albumin maintenance
- Normal glucose, electrolytes

Transition to Discharge Feeding

Readiness Criteria

✓ Infant tolerating full enteral feeds (120-150 mL/kg/day)✓ Stable growth trajectory✓ Coordinated oral feeding (if appropriate for age/condition)✓ No significant cardiorespiratory compromise with feeds✓ Adequate weight gain (15+ g/kg/day)

Discharge Feeding Plan

Document:

- Type of feeding (breast milk, formula, combination)
- Volume and frequency
- Fortification (if applicable)
- Special feeding techniques or precautions
- Growth goals
- Follow-up nutrition assessment timeline

Parent education:

- Proper formula preparation and storage
- Feeding techniques and positioning
- Recognition of adequate intake (wet diapers, stools)
- When to contact provider (vomiting, poor intake, weight loss)
- Lactation support resources (if breastfeeding)

Follow-up:

- Pediatrician visit within 3-5 days
- Weight check at 1-2 weeks
- Reassess feeding plan at 2-4 weeks
- Refer to pediatric dietitian if growth concerns

Key Takeaways

✓ Nutrition is foundational: Every day of inadequate nutrition affects growth and neurodevelopment

✓ Breast milk first: Maximize breast milk for all infants; fortify preterm breast milk

✓ Enteral over parenteral: Advance enteral feeds as soon as tolerated; PN as bridge only

✓ Systematic advancement: Trophic → progressive → full feeds; monitor tolerance at each step

✓ Individual assessment: Feeding strategy varies by gestational age, illness, growth needs

✓ Monitor closely: Weight, labs, growth trajectory guide adequacy of nutrition

✓ Recognize intolerance early: Residuals, distension, systemic signs warrant reassessment

✓ Prepare for discharge: Clear feeding plan, parent education, close follow-up essential

Chapter Eleven

COMMON NICU COMPLICATIONS AND MANAGEMENT

Respiratory Distress Syndrome (RDS)

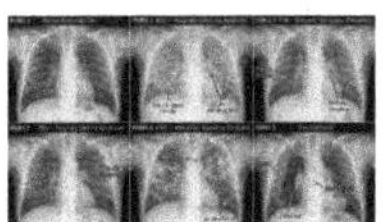

Pathophysiology

- Deficiency of pulmonary surfactant
- Increased alveolar surface tension
- Atelectasis and ventilation-perfusion mismatch

- Most common in preterm infants <34 weeks

Clinical Presentation

- Tachypnea (>60 breaths/min)
- Grunting, nasal flaring, intercostal retractions
- Cyanosis
- Decreased air entry on auscultation
- Chest X-ray: ground-glass appearance, air bronchograms

Management

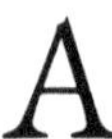ntenatal:

- Corticosteroids (betamethasone/dexamethasone) at 24-34 weeks
- Accelerates fetal lung maturity
- Reduces RDS incidence by 30-60%

Postnatal:

- Continuous positive airway pressure (CPAP): 5-8 cmH_2O
- Exogenous surfactant replacement (Calfactant , Beractant)
- Mechanical ventilation if CPAP failure
- Oxygen therapy titrated to SpO_2 targets (90-94% preterm,

95-98% term)

- Supportive care: temperature control, fluid management

Complications

- Barotrauma/volutrauma
- Oxygen toxicity
- Bronchopulmonary dysplasia (BPD)
- Pneumothorax

Bronchopulmonary Dysplasia (BPD)

Definition

- Chronic lung disease of prematurity
- Oxygen requirement at 36 weeks postmenstrual age (PMA)
- Classified as mild, moderate, or severe based on oxygen/ventilator dependence

Risk Factors

- Prematurity (<28 weeks)
- RDS requiring mechanical ventilation

- Prolonged oxygen exposure
- Barotrauma/volutrauma
- Sepsis/inflammation
- Patent ductus arteriosus (PDA)
- Pulmonary edema

Pathophysiology

- Disrupted alveolarization
- Abnormal vascularization
- Chronic inflammation
- Fibrosis and remodeling

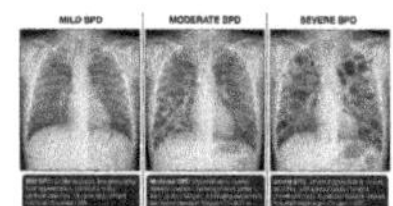

Clinical Features

- Persistent oxygen requirement
- Tachypnea
- Retractions and increased work of breathing
- Recurrent respiratory infections
- Cor pulmonale in severe cases

Management

Prevention:

- Gentle ventilation strategies (permissive hypercapnia)"Provided that pH kept 7.25 or more "
- Volume-targeted ventilation
- Early CPAP initiation
- Surfactant replacement
- Avoid excessive oxygen exposure
- Fluid restriction if applicable as per the clinical context "Judicious fluid management is paramount"

Treatment:

- Diuretics (furosemide) for pulmonary edema
- Bronchodilators (albuterol, ipratropium)
- Corticosteroids (dexamethasone, hydrocortisone) – short course"DART protocol"
- Nutritional optimization
- Pulmonary vasodilators (inhaled nitric oxide – iNO) for pulmonary hypertension
- Caffeine for apnea of prematurity"moreover , has a mild diuretic effect"

Patent Ductus Arteriosus (PDA)

Pathophysiology

- Failure of ductus arteriosus closure after birth
- Left-to-right shunt
- Increased pulmonary blood flow
- Decreased systemic perfusion

Risk Factors

- Prematurity
- RDS
- Sepsis
- Fluid overload
- Maternal indomethacin use

Clinical Presentation

Hemodynamically Significant PDA (hsPDA):

- Wide pulse pressure (bounding pulses)
- Continuous "machinery" murmur " rarely heard in neonates" " instead systolic murmur is appreciated "

- Hyperactive precordium
- Pulmonary edema
- Feeding intolerance
- Oliguria
- Metabolic acidosis
- Left ventricular hypertrophy on echo

Diagnosis

- Echocardiography (gold standard)
- Chest X-ray: cardiomegaly, pulmonary edema
- Clinical assessment

Management

Conservative:

- Judicious Fluid management
- Supportive care , ventilatory support if needed
- Medical management in hemodynamically significant PDA
- Try to avoid Diuretics (furosemide) unless truly needed

Pharmacological:

- Indomethacin: 0.1 mg/kg IV every 12-24 hours (3 doses)

- Ibuprofen: 10 mg/kg loading, then 5 mg/kg at 24 and 48 hours
- Acetaminophen: 15 mg/kg every 6 hours (5:7 days)
- *Contraindicated:* active infection, thrombocytopenia, renal dysfunction, NEC

Surgical:

- Surgical ligation if medical management fails
- Catheter-based closure in selected cases

Necrotizing Enterocolitis (NEC)

Pathophysiology

- Multifactorial: immature intestinal barrier, abnormal microbiota, ischemia
- Inflammatory cascade leading to mucosal necrosis
- Most common in preterm infants 32-34 weeks

Risk Factors

- Prematurity (<32 weeks)
- Intrauterine growth restriction (IUGR)
- Hypoxia-ischemia

- Rapid feeding advancement
- Formula feeding (vs. breast milk)
- Sepsis
- Polycythemia
- Patent ductus arteriosus

Clinical Presentation

Stage I (Suspected NEC):

- Feeding intolerance
- Abdominal distension
- Gastric residuals
- Mild diarrhea

Stage II (Definite NEC):

- Persistent abdominal distension
- Bilious vomiting
- Blood in stools
- Abdominal tenderness
- Pneumatosis intestinalis on X-ray

Stage III (Advanced NEC):

- Peritonitis

- Septic shock
- Perforation
- Portal venous gas
- Free air on X-ray

Diagnosis

- Clinical assessment
- Abdominal X-ray: pneumatosis, portal venous gas, free air
- Laboratory: elevated CRP, thrombocytopenia, metabolic acidosis
- Ultrasound: echogenic bowel, ascites"Point Of Care US "

Management

Medical:

- NPO (nothing by mouth)
- Nasogastric decompression
- Broad-spectrum antibiotics (ampicillin, gentamicin, consider metronidazole if perforated)
- IV fluids and electrolyte management
- Supportive care: oxygen, ventilation as needed

- Probiotics (controversial) "better to avoid"
- Lactoferrin supplementation

Surgical:

- Indications: perforation, peritonitis, clinical deterioration despite medical management
- Primary peritoneal drainage vs. resection
- Ostomy creation if extensive necrosis

Prevention:

- Trophic feeding (minimal enteral nutrition)
- Slow feeding advancement
- Breast milk feeding
- Avoid hyperosmolar feeds
- Optimize perfusion

Intraventricular Hemorrhage (IVH)

Classification (Papile Grade)

- Grade I: Isolated germinal matrix hemorrhage
- Grade II: IVH without ventricular dilatation
- Grade III: IVH with ventricular dilatation

- Grade IV: Periventricular leukomalacia (PVL) – now considered white matter injury

Pathophysiology

- Germinal matrix fragility
- Fluctuating cerebral blood flow
- Impaired autoregulation
- Venous obstruction

Risk Factors

- Prematurity (<32 weeks)
- Respiratory distress
- Hypoxia-ischemia
- Hypotension
- Seizures
- Rapid fluid administration
- Patent ductus arteriosus
- Sepsis
- Coagulopathy

Clinical Presentation

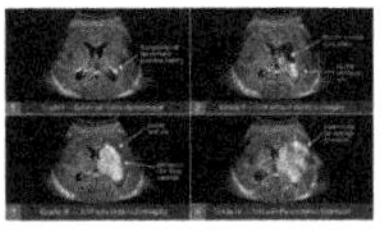

- Often asymptomatic
- Acute: seizures, bulging fontanelle, posturing
- Chronic: hydrocephalus, developmental delay

Diagnosis

- Cranial ultrasound (screening)
- MRI (better for white matter injury)
- Head CT (if hemorrhage suspected)

Management

Prevention:

- Antenatal corticosteroids
- Delayed cord clamping
- Gentle resuscitation
- Avoid rapid fluid boluses
- Maintain normothermia
- Avoid hypoxia, hypercapnia, hypoglycemia

Treatment:

- Supportive care
- Seizure management
- Hydrocephalus management: head positioning, fluid restriction, diuretics
- Neurosurgical intervention if progressive ventriculomegaly

Retinopathy of Prematurity (ROP)

Classification (International Classification)

- Zone: Location (central to peripheral)
- Stage: Severity (1-5)
- Plus disease: Vascular tortuosity and dilation

Risk Factors

- Prematurity (<30 weeks)
- Low birth weight (<1500g)
- Oxygen exposure
- Sepsis
- Transfusions

- Apnea
- Intraventricular hemorrhage

Pathophysiology

- Abnormal retinal vascularization
- Oxygen-induced vasoconstriction
- Hypoxia-induced neovascularization
- Traction and retinal detachment

Screening

- First exam: 31 weeks PMA or 4 weeks after birth (whichever is later)
- Infants <30 weeks or <1500g birth weight
- High-risk infants with unstable course

Management

Prevention:

- Oxygen saturation targets: 91-95% in preterm infants
- Avoid hyperoxia and hypoxia
- Minimize sepsis

- Nutritional optimization

Treatment:

- Anti-VEGF agents (bevacizumab, aflibercept, ranibizumab)
- Laser photocoagulation
- Vitrectomy for advanced disease
- Referral to pediatric ophthalmology

Sepsis and Infection

Early-Onset Sepsis (EOS)

- Onset: 0-72 hours after birth
- Transmission: Vertical from mother
- Common organisms: GBS, E. coli, Listeria

Late-Onset Sepsis (LOS)

- Onset: >72 hours after birth
- Transmission: Nosocomial or environmental
- Common organisms: Coagulase-negative Staphylococcus, Candida, Pseudomonas

Risk Factors

- Prematurity
- Prolonged rupture of membranes
- Maternal fever/chorioamnionitis
- Low birth weight
- Invasive procedures
- Central lines
- Prolonged hospitalization

Clinical Presentation

- Temperature instability
- Poor feeding
- Lethargy or irritability
- Apnea and bradycardia
- Hypoglycemia
- Jaundice
- Hepatosplenomegaly
- Rash
- Shock

Diagnosis

- Blood culture (gold standard)
- CBC: WBC abnormalities, left shift, thrombocytopenia
- CRP and procalcitonin
- Lactate
- Cerebrospinal fluid culture if meningitis suspected
- Urine culture

Management

Empiric Antibiotics:

- EOS: Ampicillin + Gentamicin ± "Acyclovir if there is strong possibility of herpes infection"
- LOS: Vancomycin + Gentamicin ± Fluconazole
- Duration: 7-10 days if culture-positive, 48 hours if negative

Supportive Care:

- IV fluids
- Oxygen/ventilation as needed
- Vasopressors for shock
- Glucose management

- Thermal regulation

Prevention:

- Hand hygiene
- Aseptic technique
- Minimize line duration
- Selective decontamination (controversial)
- Probiotics (limited evidence)

Hypoglycemia

Pathophysiology

- Inadequate glucose production
- Excessive glucose utilization
- Impaired counterregulatory response

Risk Factors

- Prematurity
- Small for gestational age (SGA)
- Intrauterine growth restriction

- Maternal diabetes
- Hypothermia
- Sepsis
- Delayed feeding

Clinical Presentation

- Often asymptomatic
- Jitteriness, tremors
- Poor feeding
- Lethargy
- Seizures (severe)
- Apnea and bradycardia

Diagnosis

- Point-of-care glucose testing
- Plasma glucose <40 mg/dL in preterm, <45 mg/dL in term
- Confirm with laboratory measurement

Management

Prevention:

- Early feeding (within 1-2 hours)
- Frequent feeds (every 2-3 hours)
- Breast milk or formula
- Skin-to-skin contact

Treatment:

- Asymptomatic, can feed: breast/formula feed
- Cannot feed: IV dextrose (D10W 2 mL/kg bolus)
- Continuous IV dextrose infusion
- Recheck glucose 30 minutes after intervention
- Treat underlying cause

Hyperbilirubinemia and Jaundice

Pathophysiology

- Increased bilirubin production (hemolysis, polycythemia)
- Decreased bilirubin conjugation (immature liver)
- Increased enterohepatic circulation

Risk Factors

- Prematurity
- Hemolytic disease (ABO/Rh incompatibility)
- G6PD deficiency
- Sepsis
- Delayed feeding
- Dehydration
- Acidosis

Clinical Presentation

- Jaundice (cephalocaudal progression)
- Poor feeding
- Lethargy
- Hypotonia (kernicterus)
- High-pitched cry
- Seizures (severe)

Diagnosis

- Transcutaneous bilirubinometry (screening)
- Serum total bilirubin

- Direct/indirect bilirubin
- Reticulocyte count
- Blood type and Coombs test
- G6PD screening if indicated

Management

Phototherapy:

- Indicated based on age-specific nomogram
- Intensive phototherapy for severe hyperbilirubinemia
- Blue-green spectrum light (460-490 nm)
- Monitor bilirubin levels every 4-8 hours

Exchange Transfusion:

- Indicated for severe hyperbilirubinemia or hemolytic disease
- Removes 85% of bilirubin
- Complications: infection, electrolyte abnormalities

Supportive Care:

- Frequent feeding (8-12 times/day)
- Adequate hydration
- Monitor urine output
- Treat underlying cause

Apnea of Prematurity

Pathophysiology

- Immature respiratory control centers
- Decreased chemoreceptor sensitivity
- Periodic breathing pattern

Types

- Central apnea: No respiratory effort
- Obstructive apnea: Airway obstruction despite effort
- Mixed apnea: Central + obstructive components

Clinical Presentation

- Cessation of breathing >20 seconds
- Bradycardia (<100 bpm)
- Cyanosis or desaturation
- Pallor or hypotonia
- Typically resolves by 34-36 weeks PMA

Management

Non-pharmacological:

- Thermal management
- Gentle tactile stimulation
- Continuous pulse oximetry/cardiorespiratory monitoring
- Positioning (prone or semi-prone)
- Avoid gastric distension

Pharmacological:

- Caffeine citrate: 20 mg/kg loading, 5-10 mg/kg daily maintenance
- Theophylline (less commonly used)
- Duration: until 34-36 weeks PMA

Respiratory Support:

- CPAP or high-flow nasal cannula
- Mechanical ventilation if severe

Key Takeaways

Common NICU complications require:

- Early recognition and diagnosis
- Evidence-based management protocols

- Prevention strategies when possible
- Multidisciplinary team coordination
- Close monitoring and reassessment
- Family-centered communication

Mastery of these conditions is essential for optimal neonatal intensive care delivery.

Chapter Twelve

METABOLIC DISORDERS AND ENDOCRINE ISSUES

Neonatal Hypoglycemia

Classification

Transient Neonatal Hypoglycemia:

- Self-limiting, resolves within first week
- Most common type

- Associated with poor feeding, stress

Persistent Neonatal Hypoglycemia:

- Lasts >7-10 days
- Requires investigation"Endocrinologist consultation is needed in most scenarios"
- May indicate serious metabolic disorder

Etiology

Decreased Glucose Production:

- Prematurity
- Intrauterine growth restriction (IUGR)
- Hypopituitarism
- Cortisol deficiency
- Growth hormone deficiency
- Glycogen storage diseases
- Fatty acid oxidation disorders

Increased Glucose Utilization:

- Sepsis/infection
- Polycythemia
- Hyperthermia

- Seizures
- Hyperinsulinism (persistent hyperinsulinemic hypoglycemia of infancy – PHHI)

Impaired Counterregulation:

- Prematurity
- Perinatal stress
- Maternal diabetes

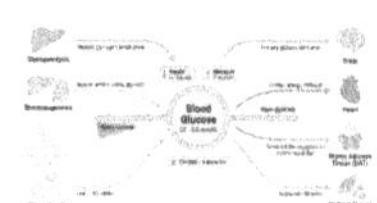

Risk Stratification

High-Risk Infants:

- Preterm <35 weeks
- SGA or IUGR
- Maternal diabetes
- Sepsis
- Polycythemia
- Hypothermia

Clinical Assessment

- Symptoms: jitteriness, tremors, poor feeding, lethargy, seizures, apnea

- Often asymptomatic
- Symptomatic hypoglycemia requires urgent intervention

Diagnostic Approach

Initial Testing:

- Point-of-care glucose (POC) testing
- Confirm with plasma glucose
- Threshold: <40 mg/dL preterm, <45 mg/dL term"after 24 hours of age keep it > 60 mg/dl"

Further Investigation (if persistent):

- Insulin level during hypoglycemia
- C-peptide level
- Free fatty acids and ketones
- Lactate and pyruvate
- Amino acids
- Acylcarnitine profile
- Cortisol and growth hormone
- Genetic testing if indicated

Management Algorithm

Prevention (First-Line):

- Early feeding within 1-2 hours

- Frequent feeds: every 2-3 hours
- Breast milk or formula
- Skin-to-skin contact to maintain temperature
- Avoid stress and hypothermia

Asymptomatic Hypoglycemia (<40 mg/dL):

- Feed immediately (breast or bottle)
- Recheck glucose in 30-60 minutes
- If unable to feed: IV dextrose

Symptomatic Hypoglycemia:

- IV dextrose: 2 mL/kg of 10% dextrose (200 mg/kg) IV push
- Followed by continuous infusion: D10W at 5-8 mg/kg/min
- Recheck glucose in 15-30 minutes
- Titrate infusion based on glucose levels

Persistent Hypoglycemia:

- Increase dextrose infusion rate
- Add glucagon: 0.03 mg/kg IM/IV if dextrose ineffective
- Hydrocortisone: 5 mg/kg every 6 hours if cortisol deficiency
- Diazoxide or somatostatin for hyperinsulinism
- Consider transfer to tertiary center

Monitoring

- Glucose checks: every 30-60 minutes until stable
- Then every 4-6 hours
- Transition to feeding when stable

Neonatal Hyperglycemia

Pathophysiology

- Relative insulin deficiency
- Increased hepatic glucose production
- Stress-induced hyperglycemia
- Impaired glucose utilization

Risk Factors

- Prematurity (<28 weeks)
- Critical illness/sepsis
- Medications (corticosteroids, theophylline)
- High dextrose infusion rates
- Parenteral nutrition

- Pancreatic immaturity

Clinical Presentation

- Often asymptomatic
- Osmotic diuresis
- Polyuria
- Dehydration
- Hyperglycemic hyperosmolar state (rare)

Diagnosis

- Plasma glucose >150 mg/dL (preterm), >180 mg/dL (term)
- Glycosuria
- Elevated serum osmolality
- Metabolic acidosis if severe

Management

Mild Hyperglycemia (150-200 mg/dL):

- Reduce dextrose infusion rate
- Increase caloric intake via enteral feeding

- Monitor glucose levels
- Usually self-limited

Moderate to Severe Hyperglycemia (>200 mg/dL):

- Reduce dextrose concentration or infusion rate
- Insulin infusion: 0.01-0.1 units/kg/hour
- Start at low dose, titrate based on glucose response
- Monitor glucose every 1-2 hours
- Electrolyte monitoring
- Treat underlying cause (sepsis, stress)

Prevention:

- Avoid excessive dextrose infusion
- Gradual advancement of feeds
- Early enteral nutrition
- Minimize stress

Hypocalcemia and Hypomagnesemia

Pathophysiology of Hypocalcemia

- Decreased parathyroid hormone (PTH) secretion
- End-organ resistance to PTH

- Vitamin D deficiency
- Phosphate retention
- Hypomagnesemia (prevents PTH secretion)

Classification

Early Hypocalcemia (24-72 hours):

- Associated with perinatal stress
- Birth asphyxia
- Maternal diabetes
- Prematurity
- Transient hypoparathyroidism

Late Hypocalcemia (>72 hours):

- High phosphate feeding
- Vitamin D deficiency
- Hypomagnesemia
- Chronic kidney disease
- Persistent hypoparathyroidism

Risk Factors

- Prematurity

- Birth asphyxia
- Maternal diabetes
- Maternal hypercalcemia (suppresses fetal PTH)
- Sepsis
- Renal failure
- Malabsorption
- Inadequate vitamin D intake

Clinical Presentation

- Often asymptomatic
- Jitteriness, tremors
- Irritability
- Poor feeding
- Apnea and bradycardia
- Seizures
- Laryngospasm
- Tetany
- Prolonged QT interval on ECG

Diagnosis

- Serum total calcium <7 mg/dL or ionized calcium <3 mg/dL
- Serum magnesium <1.5 mg/dL
- Serum phosphate
- PTH level
- Vitamin D (25-hydroxyvitamin D)
- Alkaline phosphatase
- Albumin (affects total calcium)

Management

Acute Symptomatic Hypocalcemia:

- Calcium gluconate 10%: 2-4 mL/kg (200-400 mg/kg) IV slowly over 10-20 minutes"longer infusion time is suggestive" " keep under cardio-pulmonary monitoring during infusion"
- Monitor primary heart rate for bradycardia
- Repeat every 6-12 hours as needed
- Dilute IV calcium to prevent extravasation injury

Asymptomatic or Chronic Hypocalcemia:

- Calcium supplementation: 50-100 mg/kg/day divided doses
- Oral calcium gluconate or lactate

- Vitamin D supplementation: 400-1000 IU/day
- Correct hypomagnesemia (see below)
- Ensure adequate phosphate restriction

Hypomagnesemia Management:

- Magnesium sulfate: 25-50 mg/kg IV/IM over 20-30 minutes
- Or magnesium chloride: 10-20 mg/kg/day orally
- Monitor magnesium levels
- Correct before treating hypocalcemia

Monitoring

- Serum calcium and magnesium every 4-6 hours initially
- Then daily until stable
- ECG if severe or symptomatic
- Clinical assessment for signs of hypocalcemia

Hyponatremia and Hypernatremia

Hyponatremia

Pathophysiology:

- Excessive free water intake

- Impaired water excretion
- SIADH (syndrome of inappropriate antidiuretic hormone)
- Renal immaturity

Risk Factors:

- Excessive hypotonic fluid administration
- Maternal polyhydramnios
- Renal failure
- Sepsis
- CNS abnormalities
- Medications

Clinical Presentation:

- Lethargy, poor feeding
- Seizures
- Coma
- Cerebral edema

Management:

- Fluid restriction
- Identify and treat underlying cause
- Hypertonic saline (3%) if symptomatic: 0.5-1 mL/kg slowly
- Increase sodium gradually: <10-12 mEq/L per 24 hours

- Avoid rapid correction (risk of osmotic demyelination)
- Monitor sodium levels every 4-6 hours

Hypernatremia

Pathophysiology:

- Excessive free water loss
- Inadequate water intake
- Excessive sodium intake
- Renal immaturity

Risk Factors:

- Inadequate fluid intake
- Excessive insensible losses (phototherapy, radiant warmer)
- Diarrhea
- Vomiting
- Renal failure
- High sodium formula or medications

Clinical Presentation:

- Lethargy
- Seizures
- Hyperreflexia

- Cerebral hemorrhage

Management:

- Increase free water intake
- Hypotonic fluids IV if unable to feed
- Identify and treat underlying cause
- Decrease sodium gradually: <10-12 mEq/L per 24 hours
- Avoid rapid correction (risk of cerebral edema)
- Monitor sodium every 4-6 hours
- Maintain adequate hydration

Neonatal Thyroid Disorders

Congenital Hypothyroidism

Etiology:

- Primary hypothyroidism (95%): thyroid dysgenesis, dyshormonogenesis
- Central hypothyroidism (5%): TSH deficiency, TRH deficiency
- Transient hypothyroidism: maternal iodine deficiency, maternal antithyroid drugs

Screening:

- Newborn screening program: TSH and/or T4
- Performed on dried blood spot 24-48 hours after birth

Clinical Presentation:

- Often asymptomatic in newborn period
- Delayed manifestation: poor feeding, constipation, jaundice, hypotonia, developmental delay
- Cretinism if untreated: intellectual disability, growth retardation, coarse features

Diagnosis:

- Elevated TSH (>25 mIU/L) and/or low T4 (<6.5 mcg/dL)
- Confirm with repeat TSH and free T4
- Thyroid ultrasound
- Thyroid scan if dysgenesis suspected
- Thyroid peroxidase (TPO) antibodies if autoimmune

Management:

- Levothyroxine: 10-15 mcg/kg/day starting dose
- Adjust based on TSH and free T4 levels
- Recheck TSH at 2-4 weeks, then every 1-3 months
- Target TSH: 1-5 mIU/L
- Lifelong replacement therapy
- Early treatment prevents intellectual disability

Congenital Hyperthyroidism

Etiology:

- Maternal Graves' disease (90%)
- Neonatal Graves' disease (10%)
- TSH receptor stimulating antibodies (TRAb)

Risk Factors:

- Maternal hyperthyroidism
- Maternal antithyroid antibodies

Clinical Presentation:

- Irritability, poor feeding
- Tachycardia, arrhythmias
- Tremors
- Hepatosplenomegaly
- Jaundice
- Thyroid enlargement
- Exophthalmos (rare)
- Thyroid storm (fever, severe tachycardia, shock)

Diagnosis:

- Elevated free T4 (>2 ng/dL)

- Suppressed TSH (<0.1 mIU/L)
- Elevated T3 if severe
- Thyroid antibodies (TRAb)
- ECG for cardiac effects

Management:

- Propranolol: 2-4 mg/kg/day divided every 6-8 hours (for cardiac symptoms)
- Propylthiouracil (PTU): 5-10 mg/kg/day divided every 6-8 hours
- Methimazole: 0.5-1 mg/kg/day (reserve for PTU intolerance)
- Iodine solution (Lugol's or SSKI): 1 drop every 8 hours (after PTU/methimazole started)
- Beta-blockers for tachycardia
- Monitor free T4, TSH every 1-2 weeks
- Usually self-limited (resolves as maternal antibodies wane)
- Discontinue antithyroid drugs when TSH normalizes

Adrenal Insufficiency

Congenital Adrenal Hyperplasia (CAH)

Pathophysiology:

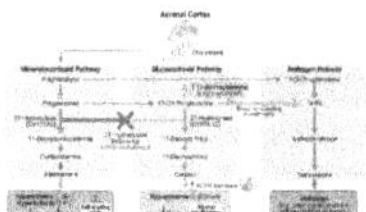

- Autosomal recessive enzyme deficiency
- Most common: 21-hydroxylase deficiency (90%)
- Impaired cortisol and aldosterone synthesis
- Accumulation of precursor steroids

Classification: Classic CAH:

- Salt-wasting form: cortisol and aldosterone deficiency
- Simple virilizing form: cortisol deficiency, excess androgens

Non-classic CAH:

- Mild enzyme deficiency
- Late-onset symptoms

Clinical Presentation (Classic):

- Salt-wasting crisis: poor feeding, vomiting, dehydration, hypotension, shock (5-14 days)
- Virilization: ambiguous genitalia in females, precocious puberty in males
- Hyponatremia, hyperkalemia, metabolic acidosis
- Hypoglycemia

Screening:

- Newborn screening: 17-hydroxyprogesterone (17-OHP)
- Elevated in classic CAH

- False positives in preterm infants

Diagnosis:

- Elevated 17-OHP (>10 ng/mL)
- Elevated ACTH
- Low cortisol
- Elevated androgens (testosterone, androstenedione)
- Genetic testing: CYP21A2 mutations
- Karyotype if ambiguous genitalia

Management: Acute Salt-Wasting Crisis:

- IV fluids: 0.9% saline bolus 20 mL/kg over 30 minutes
- Repeat as needed for hypotension
- Hydrocortisone: 50 mg/kg/day IV divided every 6 hours
- Treat electrolyte abnormalities
- Monitor closely in ICU

Chronic Management:

- Hydrocortisone: 15-20 mg/m^2/day divided 2-3 times daily
- Fludrocortisone: 0.05-0.1 mg daily (salt-wasting form)
- Sodium supplementation: 1-2 g/day (salt-wasting form)
- Increase steroid dose during stress/illness
- Genetic counseling

- Gender assignment discussion for virilized females
- Surgical consultation for genital reconstruction

Primary Adrenal Insufficiency (Other Causes)

Etiology:

- Adrenal hypoplasia congenita
- Adrenal hemorrhage
- Sepsis (Waterhouse-Friderichsen syndrome)
- Congenital infections
- Adrenoleukodystrophy

Management:

- Glucocorticoid replacement: hydrocortisone 15-20 $mg/m^2/day$
- Mineralocorticoid replacement if aldosterone deficiency: fludrocortisone 0.05-0.2 mg/day
- Sodium supplementation
- Stress-dose steroids during illness

Inborn Errors of Metabolism (IEMs)

Screening

- Tandem mass spectrometry (MS/MS)
- Newborn screening panel
- Identifies amino acid, fatty acid oxidation, and organic acid disorders
- Performed 24-48 hours after birth

Amino Acid Disorders

Phenylketonuria (PKU):

- Phenylalanine hydroxylase deficiency
- Elevated phenylalanine (>20 mg/dL)
- Screening: elevated phenylalanine on MS/MS
- Clinical: intellectual disability if untreated, light skin, musty odor, seizures
- Management: phenylalanine-restricted diet, frequent monitoring, lifelong treatment
- Early treatment prevents intellectual disability

Maple Syrup Urine Disease (MSUD):

- Branched-chain amino acid (BCAA) decarboxylase deficiency
- Accumulation of leucine, isoleucine, valine
- Screening: elevated BCAAs on MS/MS

- Clinical: poor feeding, lethargy, seizures, developmental delay, maple syrup-scented urine
- Management: BCAA-restricted diet, frequent monitoring, emergency management of acute decompensation

Homocystinuria:

- Cystathionine beta-synthase deficiency
- Elevated homocysteine
- Clinical: intellectual disability, ectopia lentis, thrombosis, marfanoid features
- Management: vitamin B6 supplementation, betaine, methionine restriction

Fatty Acid Oxidation Disorders

Medium-Chain Acyl-CoA Dehydrogenase (MCAD) Deficiency:

- Most common fatty acid oxidation disorder
- Impaired energy production during fasting
- Screening: elevated C6-C10 acylcarnitines on MS/MS
- Clinical: hypoglycemia, hypoketotic encephalopathy, sudden death
- Management: frequent feeds, avoid fasting, emergency glucose during illness
- Prognosis: excellent with appropriate management

Organic Acid Disorders

Propionic Acidemia:

- Propionyl-CoA carboxylase deficiency
- Accumulation of propionic acid
- Screening: elevated C3 acylcarnitine on MS/MS
- Clinical: poor feeding, vomiting, metabolic acidosis, developmental delay
- Management: protein-restricted diet, carnitine supplementation, frequent monitoring

Methylmalonic Acidemia:

- Methylmalonyl-CoA mutase deficiency or cobalamin metabolism defect
- Screening: elevated C3 acylcarnitine on MS/MS
- Clinical: similar to propionic acidemia
- Management: cobalamin supplementation, protein restriction, frequent monitoring

Management of IEM Acute Decompensation

- NPO (nothing by mouth)
- IV dextrose: 5-10 mg/kg/min
- Electrolyte management

- Ammonium reduction strategies
- Amino acid supplementation (if applicable)
- Consultation with metabolic specialist
- Genetic testing and counseling

Polycythemia and Hyperviscosity

Pathophysiology

- Elevated hemoglobin (>20 g/dL) or hematocrit (>65%)
- Increased blood viscosity
- Impaired microcirculation
- Tissue hypoxia paradoxically

Risk Factors

- Intrauterine growth restriction
- Maternal diabetes
- Maternal smoking
- Chronic hypoxia
- Delayed cord clamping

- Twin-twin transfusion syndrome
- Placental insufficiency

Clinical Presentation

- Often asymptomatic
- Plethora (ruddy appearance)
- Poor feeding
- Jitteriness, irritability
- Hypoglycemia
- Hypocalcemia
- Seizures
- Thrombosis
- Pulmonary hemorrhage
- Renal vein thrombosis

Diagnosis

- Venous hematocrit >65% or hemoglobin >20 g/dL
- Capillary hematocrit may be falsely elevated
- Blood viscosity measurement (if available)

- Assess for complications

Management

Asymptomatic Polycythemia:

- Monitor
- Encourage feeding
- Maintain hydration
- Recheck hematocrit in 4-6 hours

Symptomatic or Severe Polycythemia:

- Partial exchange transfusion with normal saline
- Goal: reduce hematocrit to 55%
- Calculate volume: (observed Hct – desired Hct) × blood volume × 0.9
- Perform slowly to avoid sudden hemodynamic changes
- Recheck hematocrit after exchange
- Treat complications (hypoglycemia, hypocalcemia)
- Frequent feeds
- Maintain hydration

Neonatal Hyperlipidemia

Pathophysiology

- Immature lipid metabolism
- Increased lipid infusion
- Sepsis
- Parenteral nutrition

Risk Factors

- Prematurity
- Prolonged TPN
- Sepsis
- Liver dysfunction
- Genetic lipid disorders (rare in neonates)

Clinical Presentation

- Often asymptomatic
- Lipemia (milky appearance of blood/plasma)
- Hepatomegaly
- Pancreatitis (rare)

- Thrombocytopenia
- Sepsis-like picture

Diagnosis

- Triglycerides >200 mg/dL (fasting)
- Lipemic plasma
- Elevated cholesterol (variable)
- Assess for underlying causes

Management

- Reduce or discontinue lipid infusion
- Increase dextrose calories
- Transition to enteral feeds
- Treat underlying sepsis
- Monitor triglyceride levels
- Restart lipids slowly once triglycerides normalize
- Limit lipid infusion to <3 g/kg/day

Bone Metabolism and Metabolic Bone Disease

Pathophysiology

- Inadequate mineral accretion
- Vitamin D deficiency
- Phosphate depletion
- Alkaline phosphatase elevation
- Impaired osteoblast function

Risk Factors

- Prematurity (<32 weeks)"Osteopenia of prematurity"
- Prolonged TPN
- Cholestasis
- Inadequate phosphate/calcium intake
- Vitamin D deficiency
- Chronic lung disease
- Diuretic use

Clinical Presentation

- Often asymptomatic

- Radiographic findings: osteopenia, fractures, metaphyseal lucencies
- Rickets: bowing of long bones, subperiosteal new bone formation
- Delayed fontanelle closure
- Hypocalcemia, hypophosphatemia
- Elevated alkaline phosphatase

Diagnosis

- Serum calcium, phosphate, alkaline phosphatase
- Vitamin D (25-hydroxyvitamin D): <20 ng/mL indicates deficiency
- Parathyroid hormone (PTH)
- Bone-specific alkaline phosphatase
- Radiographs: osteopenia, rickets
- DEXA scan for bone density (research)

Management

Prevention:

- Early enteral feeding
- Adequate calcium (120-150 mg/kg/day) and phosphate (60-90 mg/kg/day)
- Vitamin D supplementation: 400-1000 IU/day
- Minimize diuretic use
- Adequate protein and energy intake

Treatment:

- Calcium supplementation: 100-200 mg/kg/day
- Phosphate supplementation: 50-100 mg/kg/day
- Vitamin D: 1000-2000 IU/day
- Vitamin A supplementation
- Monitor mineral levels monthly
- Reduce diuretic use if possible
- Optimize nutrition

Key Takeaways

Metabolic and endocrine disorders in neonates require:

- High index of suspicion
- Appropriate screening and diagnostic testing
- Early recognition and intervention

- Knowledge of management protocols
- Close monitoring and reassessment
- Multidisciplinary team approach
- Family education and support
- Long-term follow-up and management

Early diagnosis and treatment of these conditions prevent serious complications and optimize neurodevelopmental outcomes.

Chapter Thirteen

NEONATAL NEUROLOGICAL DISORDERS AND SEIZURES

Neonatal Seizures: Overview

Pathophysiology

- Excessive synchronized neuronal discharge
- Immature brain with reduced inhibitory mechanisms
- Increased excitatory neurotransmission

- Altered ion channel function
- Metabolic derangements

Incidence

- 1-5 per 1,000 live births
- Higher in preterm and critically ill infants
- Most common neurological emergency in NICU

Clinical Significance

- Marker of underlying CNS or systemic disease
- Associated with adverse neurodevelopmental outcomes
- Requires urgent evaluation and treatment

Classification of Neonatal Seizures

Clinical Seizure Types

Clonic Seizures:

- Rhythmic jerking movements
- May be focal or generalized

- 50% of neonatal seizures
- Focal clonic: localized to one limb or area
- Multifocal clonic: multiple areas sequentially

Tonic Seizures:

- Sustained muscle contraction
- Extension or flexion posturing
- 5-10% of neonatal seizures
- Often associated with severe encephalopathy

Myoclonic Seizures:

- Brief jerking movements
- Single or repetitive
- 10-15% of neonatal seizures
- May be benign sleep myoclonus

Subtle Seizures:

- Most common type (50-60%)
- Oculomotor signs: eye deviation, nystagmus, eye opening
- Oral-buccal movements: lip smacking, tongue protrusion
- Limb movements: pedaling, stepping
- Autonomic signs: apnea, bradycardia, blood pressure changes

- May be accompanied by EEG seizure activity

Spasms:

- Infantile spasms (West syndrome): typically >3 months
- Rare in neonatal period"however could be seen , personally I have seen 1 case "
- Flexor or extensor spasms

Electrographic vs. Clinical Seizures

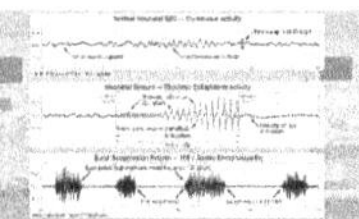

- Electrographic seizures: abnormal EEG discharge without clinical signs
- Common in preterm infants
- May indicate more severe brain injury
- Associated with worse outcomes
- Often require treatment despite lack of clinical manifestations

Etiology of Neonatal Seizures

Hypoxic-Ischemic Encephalopathy (HIE)

- Most common cause (40-50%)
- Occurs within first 72 hours

- Associated with perinatal asphyxia
- Severity correlates with seizure burden

Infection

- Sepsis/meningitis (20-30%)
- Bacterial meningitis: GBS, E. coli, Listeria
- Viral: HSV, CMV, enterovirus, coronavirus
- Congenital infections: TORCH agents
- Fungal: Candida (in immunocompromised)

Metabolic Disorders

- Hypoglycemia
- Hypocalcemia
- Hypomagnesemia
- Hyponatremia
- Hypernatremia
- Inborn errors of metabolism
- Vitamin B6 deficiency

Intracranial Hemorrhage

- Intraventricular hemorrhage (IVH)
- Subdural hemorrhage
- Subarachnoid hemorrhage
- Intracerebral hemorrhage
- Germinal matrix hemorrhage

Stroke

- Arterial ischemic stroke (AIS)"mostly detected in aEEG as asymmetrical trace between right and left hemispheres "
- Cerebral sinovenous thrombosis (CSVT)
- Associated with thrombophilia, infection, dehydration

Structural Abnormalities

- Malformations: holoprosencephaly, lissencephaly, polymicrogyria
- Hydrocephalus
- Porencephaly
- Agenesis of corpus callosum

Drug Withdrawal

- Maternal opioid use
- Maternal benzodiazepine use
- Withdrawal symptoms: irritability, tremors, seizures
- Onset: 24 hours to several days

Genetic/Inherited Disorders

- Benign familial neonatal seizures (KCNQ2/KCNQ3 mutations)
- Pyridoxine-dependent seizures
- Early infantile epileptic encephalopathy (EIEE)
- Progressive myoclonic encephalopathies

Other Causes

- Kernicterus (severe hyperbilirubinemia)
- Polycythemia
- Anemia
- Hypothermia

- Hyperthermia
- Sleep-related myoclonus (benign)

Diagnostic Approach to Neonatal Seizures

History

- Maternal history: infections, medications, substance use, diabetes
- Perinatal history: delivery complications, asphyxia, resuscitation
- Timing of seizure onset
- Description of seizure activity
- Associated symptoms
- Family history of seizures or neurological disease

Physical Examination

- General: vital signs, growth parameters, skin findings
- Neurological: alertness, tone, reflexes, cranial nerves
- Dysmorphic features
- Signs of infection: fever, rash, hepatosplenomegaly

- Metabolic signs: jaundice, hypoglycemia signs

Laboratory Investigations

Immediate:

- Blood glucose (point-of-care and serum)
- Serum electrolytes: sodium, potassium, chloride
- Serum calcium, magnesium, phosphate
- Blood gas analysis
- Complete blood count
- Blood culture
- Liver function tests

Metabolic Screening:

- Amino acids (serum and urine)
- Organic acids (urine)
- Lactate and pyruvate
- Ammonia level
- Acylcarnitine profile
- Glucose-6-phosphatase deficiency screening

Infectious Workup:

- Cerebrospinal fluid (CSF): cell count, glucose, protein, culture, viral PCR

- Blood culture
- Viral serologies: HSV, CMV, enterovirus
- Congenital infection screening: TORCH serology, PCR
- Maternal serology if indicated

Neuroimaging

- Cranial ultrasound: initial screening, can be done at bedside
- MRI brain: superior for white matter injury, stroke, malformations
- CT brain: if acute hemorrhage suspected, structural abnormality
- Timing: urgent if hemodynamically stable, after stabilization if critical

Electroencephalography (EEG)

- Gold standard for seizure diagnosis
- Continuous EEG monitoring recommended"amplitude integrated EEG "(aEEG)
- Identifies electrographic seizures

- Assesses background activity and maturation
- Prognostic value: burst-suppression indicates severe encephalopathy
- Video-EEG: correlates clinical and electrical seizures

Genetic Testing

- Indicated if: family history, dysmorphic features, suspected genetic syndrome
- Gene panels for neonatal seizures
- Whole exome sequencing (WES) for refractory seizures
- Chromosomal microarray for structural abnormalities

Management of Acute Seizures

Initial Stabilization

- Assess airway, breathing, circulation (ABCs)
- Place on continuous cardiorespiratory monitoring
- Establish IV access
- Supplemental oxygen as needed
- Maintain temperature regulation

- Position to prevent aspiration
- NPO until swallowing assessed

Acute Seizure Termination

First-Line Antiepileptic Drug (AED):

Phenobarbital: 20 mg/kg IV loading dose over 10-20 minutes

- Onset: 15-30 minutes
- Effective in 60-80% of neonatal seizures
- Long half-life (96-120 hours)
- Side effects: sedation, respiratory depression, hypotension
- Maintenance: 3-5 mg/kg/day divided every 12 hours

Second-Line AED (if seizure persists after phenobarbital):"debatable as recently most clinicians prefer Levetiracetam as second line , even advocated as first line "

Phenytoin: 15-20 mg/kg IV loading dose over 20-30 minutes

- Onset: 30-60 minutes
- Effective in additional 20-30% of cases
- Requires cardiac monitoring (risk of arrhythmias)
- Maintenance: 4-8 mg/kg/day divided every 8-12 hours

Levetiracetam: 10-50 mg/kg IV loading dose

- Emerging first-line agent

- Fewer drug interactions
- Well-tolerated
- Maintenance: 10-20 mg/kg/day divided every 12 hours

Third-Line AED (refractory seizures):
Lorazepam: 0.05-0.1 mg/kg IV over 2-5 minutes

- Rapid onset (1-5 minutes)
- Short duration (4-8 hours)
- Risk of respiratory depression
- Use with caution in preterm infants

Pyridoxine: 50-100 mg IV

- If pyridoxine-dependent seizures suspected
- Seizure cessation within minutes if responsive
- Diagnostic and therapeutic

Status Epilepticus Management

- Seizure lasting >5 minutes or recurrent seizures without recovery
- Medical emergency
- Escalate AED therapy
- Consider midazolam infusion: 0.5-1 mcg/kg/min initial, titrate to seizure cessation

- Pentobarbital coma if refractory
- Transfer to tertiary care NICU if not already
- Continuous EEG monitoring essential

Correction of Underlying Causes

- Hypoglycemia: IV dextrose
- Hypocalcemia: calcium gluconate IV
- Hypomagnesemia: magnesium sulfate IV
- Hyponatremia: fluid restriction, hypertonic saline if symptomatic
- Infection: antibiotics/antivirals
- Hypoxia: oxygen, ventilation support

Specific Seizure Etiologies and Management

Hypoxic-Ischemic Encephalopathy (HIE)

Pathophysiology:

- Perinatal asphyxia leading to brain injury
- Energy failure, excitotoxicity, oxidative stress
- Seizures indicate moderate to severe injury

Clinical Stages:

- Stage 1 (Mild): hyperalertness, normal tone, normal reflexes
- Stage 2 (Moderate): lethargy, hypotonia, decreased reflexes
- Stage 3 (Severe): coma, flaccidity, absent reflexes

Seizure Management:

- Aggressive AED therapy
- Treat underlying hypoxia, hypoglycemia, electrolyte abnormalities
- Therapeutic hypothermia: 33.5°C for 72 hours
- Reduces seizure burden and improves outcomes
- Improves neurodevelopmental prognosis

Prognosis:

- Seizures within first 72 hours indicate moderate-severe injury
- Seizure burden correlates with outcome
- Early EEG abnormalities (burst-suppression) indicate poor prognosis

Neonatal Meningitis

Common Organisms:

- Bacterial: GBS, E. coli , Listeria monocytogenes
- Viral: HSV, enterovirus, CMV

- Fungal: Candida species

Seizure Characteristics:

- Often subtle or electrographic only
- May be first sign of meningitis
- Associated with ventriculitis

Management:

- Empiric antibiotics: ampicillin + gentamicin + cefotaxime
- Add acyclovir if HSV suspected
- CSF sterilization monitoring
- Repeat LP to document CSF sterilization
- Adjunctive dexamethasone controversial in neonates
- Seizure management with AEDs
- Long-term follow-up for hearing loss, neurodevelopmental disability

Intraventricular Hemorrhage (IVH)

Seizure Characteristics:

- Usually occur 24-48 hours after hemorrhage
- May indicate extension or progression
- Associated with increased ICP

Management:

- IVH-specific treatment: maintain normothermia, avoid hypoxia
- Seizure management with AEDs
- Monitor for hydrocephalus
- Neurosurgical consultation if ventriculomegaly
- Head positioning, fluid management

Pyridoxine-Dependent Seizures

Pathophysiology:

- Rare genetic disorder
- Defect in pyridoxamine-5'-phosphate oxidase or antiquitin
- Seizures refractory to standard AEDs
- Responsive to vitamin B6 (pyridoxine)

Clinical Presentation:

- Onset: first hours to weeks of life
- Refractory seizures
- May have intrauterine seizure activity
- Family history may be present

Diagnosis:

- Clinical response to pyridoxine trial

- Elevated urine alpha-aminoadipic semialdehyde
- Genetic testing

Management:

- Pyridoxine: 50-100 mg IV or oral
- Dramatic response within minutes if positive
- Maintenance: 10-50 mg/kg/day divided doses
- Lifelong supplementation required

Benign Familial Neonatal Seizures (BFNS)

Pathophysiology:

- Autosomal dominant inheritance
- KCNQ2/KCNQ3 potassium channel mutations
- Self-limited seizures
- Excellent prognosis

Clinical Features:

- Onset: 1-3 days after birth
- Clonic or tonic seizures
- Typically brief duration
- Responsive to AEDs
- Seizures stop by 1-6 months

- Normal neurodevelopment

Diagnosis:

- Clinical presentation
- Family history
- Genetic testing
- EEG: normal background

Management:

- AED therapy during seizure period
- Phenobarbital or phenytoin
- Discontinue AEDs after seizure-free period
- Genetic counseling
- Reassurance regarding prognosis

Neonatal Stroke

Arterial Ischemic Stroke (AIS)

Pathophysiology:

- Arterial occlusion leading to cerebral infarction
- Most common type of neonatal stroke
- Often presents with seizures

Risk Factors:

- Cardiac disease (congenital heart disease, cardiomyopathy)
- Thrombophilia (factor V Leiden, prothrombin mutation)
- Infection/sepsis
- Dehydration
- Maternal diabetes
- Placental abnormalities
- IUGR

Clinical Presentation:

- Seizures (60-80%)
- Focal neurological deficits: hemiparesis, facial droop
- Irritability, poor feeding
- Hypotonia
- Asymmetric tone/reflexes
- Seizures often focal

Diagnosis:

- MRI brain: acute infarction on DWI/PWI sequences
- CT: less sensitive, used if hemorrhage excluded
- Echocardiography: cardiac source evaluation
- Thrombophilia workup

- Coagulation studies

Management:

- Seizure management with AEDs
- Supportive care
- Anticoagulation controversial (consider if cardioembolic source)
- Thrombolysis not routinely used in neonates
- Rehabilitation and follow-up

Prognosis:

- Variable, depends on stroke location and size
- Many infants have good functional outcomes
- Some develop hemiparesis, cognitive impairment
- Early intervention services important

Cerebral Sinovenous Thrombosis (CSVT)

Pathophysiology:

- Thrombosis of dural venous sinuses
- Impaired venous drainage
- Secondary hemorrhage common

Risk Factors:

- Dehydration

- Sepsis/meningitis
- Thrombophilia
- Maternal antiphospholipid syndrome
- Birth trauma

Clinical Presentation:

- Seizures (common)
- Irritability
- Bulging fontanelle
- Altered consciousness
- Focal neurological signs

Diagnosis:

- MRI/MRV: gold standard
- CT/CTV: if MRI unavailable
- Thrombophilia workup

Management:

- Seizure management
- Supportive care
- Anticoagulation: unfractionated heparin or LMWH (controversial)
- Treat underlying cause

- Monitor for complications

Hypoxic-Ischemic Encephalopathy (HIE)

Definition

- Brain injury from perinatal asphyxia
- Inadequate oxygen and perfusion
- Most common cause of neonatal seizures

Pathophysiology

Primary Phase (0-6 hours):

- Energy depletion
- Anaerobic metabolism
- Lactate accumulation
- Cell death begins

Latent Phase (6-48 hours):

- Apparent recovery
- Continued cellular injury
- Mitochondrial dysfunction
- Therapeutic window for intervention

Reperfusion Phase (>48 hours):

- Oxidative stress
- Free radical formation
- Inflammatory cascade
- Delayed cell death
- Apoptosis

Clinical Staging (Sarnat Scale)"the most usable staging"

Stage 1 (Mild):

- Hyperalertness, irritability
- Normal muscle tone
- Exaggerated reflexes
- No seizures
- Duration: <24 hours
- Prognosis: good

Stage 2 (Moderate):

- Lethargy
- Hypotonia initially, then hypertonia
- Weak suck, poor feeding
- Seizures common (>50%)

- Duration: days to weeks
- Prognosis: variable

Stage 3 (Severe):

- Coma
- Flaccidity
- Absent suck and gag reflexes
- Seizures frequent and severe
- Autonomic instability
- Duration: days to weeks
- Prognosis: poor

Diagnosis

- Clinical presentation and history of asphyxia
- Apgar scores <5 at 5 and 10 minutes
- Cord blood pH <7.0 or base deficit >12
- MRI brain: injury pattern correlates with stage
- EEG: background activity correlates with prognosis
- Biomarkers: elevated lactate, troponin, NSE (research)

Management

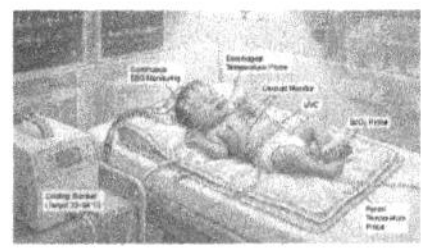

Therapeutic Hypothermia:

- Cooling to 33.5°C for 72 hours
- Initiated within 6 hours of birth (preferably <3 hours)
- Reduces death and disability by 15-20%
- Reduces seizure burden
- Slows metabolic rate, reduces secondary injury
- Rewarming gradually over 8-12 hours
- Complications: bradycardia, hypotension, coagulopathy

Seizure Management:

- Phenobarbital: first-line
- Phenytoin: if phenobarbital ineffective
- Levetiracetam: emerging option
- Aggressive treatment of electrolyte abnormalities
- Maintain normoglycemia

Supportive Care:

- Mechanical ventilation if needed
- Maintain normothermia (after cooling period)

- Fluid management
- Cardiovascular support
- Infection prevention
- Nutritional support when feasible
- Pain management

Monitoring:

- Continuous EEG
- Serial neuroimaging
- Neurodevelopmental assessment
- Long-term follow-up

Prognosis

- Mild HIE: 95% normal outcome
- Moderate HIE: 50-60% normal outcome (improved with hypothermia)
- Severe HIE: 10-15% normal outcome
- Therapeutic hypothermia most effective for moderate HIE
- Long-term sequelae: cerebral palsy, cognitive impairment, epilepsy

Neonatal Encephalopathy

Definition

- Altered level of consciousness, seizures, or abnormal tone
- Multiple etiologies beyond HIE
- Requires systematic evaluation

Differential Diagnosis

- Hypoxic-ischemic encephalopathy
- Infection (sepsis, meningitis, congenital infection)
- Metabolic disorders
- Intracranial hemorrhage
- Stroke
- Structural abnormalities
- Drug withdrawal
- Kernicterus
- Genetic/inherited disorders

Diagnostic Approach

1. Stabilize infant
2. Detailed history and examination
3. Laboratory investigations
4. Neuroimaging
5. EEG
6. Genetic testing if indicated
7. Specialist consultation

Management

- Treat identified cause
- Supportive care
- Seizure management
- Long-term follow-up and intervention

Long-Term Neurological Sequelae

Cerebral Palsy

- Motor disorder resulting from CNS injury
- Types: spastic (70%), dyskinetic (15%), ataxic (10%), mixed

(5%)

- Risk factors: severe HIE, IVH, infection, stroke
- Early identification and intervention important

Neurodevelopmental Impairment

- Cognitive delay
- Speech and language delay
- Learning disabilities
- Attention deficit disorders
- Autism spectrum disorders

Epilepsy

- Increased risk after neonatal seizures
- Depends on etiology and severity of initial injury
- Early seizure management may reduce risk

Hearing Loss

- Associated with meningitis, severe HIE, hyperbilirubinemia
- Screening essential

- Early intervention if identified

Visual Impairment

- Retinopathy of prematurity
- Cortical visual impairment from CNS injury
- Screening and management important

Intervention and Follow-Up

- Early developmental assessment
- Physical, occupational, speech therapy
- Educational support
- Family counseling and support
- Long-term neurodevelopmental follow-up

Key Takeaways

Neonatal seizures and neurological disorders require:

- High index of suspicion
- Systematic diagnostic approach
- Identification of underlying cause

- Prompt and appropriate treatment
- Continuous EEG monitoring
- Neuroimaging when indicated
- Long-term neurodevelopmental follow-up
- Family education and support
- Early intervention services

Optimal management of neonatal neurological emergencies significantly improves long-term neurodevelopmental outcomes.

Chapter Fourteen

NEONATAL JAUNDICE AND HEMOLYTIC DISEASE

Neonatal Jaundice: Overview

Pathophysiology

- Unconjugated (indirect) hyperbilirubinemia most common
- Bilirubin production exceeds excretion capacity
- Immature hepatic conjugation and excretion

- Increased enterohepatic circulation
- Shortened neonatal RBC lifespan (70-90 days vs. 120 days in adults)

Incidence

- Clinical jaundice: 50-60% of term, 80% of preterm infants
- Severe hyperbilirubinemia (>25 mg/dL): 1-2 per 1,000 live births
- Kernicterus (bilirubin encephalopathy): rare but preventable

Clinical Significance

- Most common cause of hospital readmission
- Risk of bilirubin neurotoxicity (kernicterus)
- Requires systematic screening and management
- Prevention of severe hyperbilirubinemia is key

Bilirubin Metabolism

Bilirubin Production

Sources:

- Hemoglobin degradation (80%): 1 g hemoglobin → 34 mg bilirubin
- Myoglobin and catalase (20%)
- Increased in hemolysis, polycythemia, bruising

Process:

- Heme oxygenase: heme → biliverdin + CO (carbon monoxide)
- Biliverdin reductase: biliverdin → unconjugated bilirubin
- Unconjugated bilirubin binds to albumin for transport

Hepatic Uptake and Conjugation

- Ligandin (Y protein) binds unconjugated bilirubin
- UDP-glucuronosyltransferase (UGT1A1) conjugates bilirubin
- Immature in neonates: activity increases 100-fold by 2 weeks
- Genetic variants (Gilbert syndrome, Crigler-Najjar) affect conjugation

Excretion and Enterohepatic Circulation

- Conjugated bilirubin excreted into bile

- Transported to intestine via common bile duct
- Intestinal beta-glucuronidase deconjugates bilirubin
- Reabsorbed in terminal ileum
- Recycled to liver (enterohepatic circulation)
- Fecal excretion eliminates bilirubin

Factors Increasing Enterohepatic Circulation

- Delayed passage of meconium
- Decreased intestinal motility
- Increased intestinal beta-glucuronidase activity
- Poor feeding (inadequate milk intake)
- Exclusive formula feeding (higher reabsorption than breast milk)

Classification of Hyperbilirubinemia

Unconjugated (Indirect) Hyperbilirubinemia

Physiologic Jaundice:

- Normal developmental process
- Peak: 3-5 days in term, 5-7 days in preterm

- Serum bilirubin <95th percentile for age
- Resolves by 2 weeks

Exaggerated Physiologic Jaundice:

- Bilirubin levels exceed 95th percentile
- Risk factors: prematurity, poor feeding, hemolysis
- Requires phototherapy

Pathologic Jaundice:

- Appears within first 24 hours
- Rises >0.2 mg/dL/hour
- Suggests underlying disease
- Requires investigation

Conjugated (Direct) Hyperbilirubinemia

- Direct bilirubin >1.5 mg/dL or >20% of total bilirubin
- Indicates hepatic or biliary dysfunction
- Requires investigation for cholestasis

Risk Factors for Severe Hyperbilirubinemia

Hemolytic Causes

- ABO incompatibility
- Rh incompatibility
- Other blood group incompatibilities
- G6PD deficiency
- Hereditary spherocytosis
- Alpha thalassemia
- Infection (sepsis, TORCH)
- Polycythemia
- Cephalohematoma, extensive bruising

Non-Hemolytic Causes

- Prematurity (<35 weeks)
- Delayed feeding
- Poor breastfeeding technique
- Exclusive formula feeding (early)
- Dehydration
- Acidosis
- Hypothermia
- Sepsis

- Asphyxia
- Maternal diabetes
- Genetic factors (UGT1A1 polymorphisms)

Isoimmune Hemolytic Disease Risk Factors

- Maternal blood type O, A, or B with anti-A or anti-B
- Maternal Rh negative with Rh-positive infant
- Previous affected infant
- Positive direct antiglobulin test (DAT/Coombs)

Hemolytic Disease of the Newborn (HDN)

ABO Incompatibility

Pathophysiology:

- Mother blood type O (naturally occurring anti-A and anti-B)
- Infant blood type A or B
- IgG antibodies cross placenta
- Bind to RBC antigens → RBC hemolysis → unconjugated hyperbilirubinemia

Incidence:

- 1-2% of ABO-incompatible pregnancies
- Clinical disease in 20-25% of cases
- Milder than Rh disease

Clinical Features:

- Jaundice within 24-72 hours
- Mild to moderate anemia
- Hepatosplenomegaly (variable)
- Rarely hydrops fetalis

Diagnosis:

- Positive direct antiglobulin test (DAT/Coombs)
- Elevated indirect bilirubin
- Elevated reticulocyte count
- Spherocytes on blood smear

Management:

- Phototherapy based on nomogram
- Exchange transfusion if severe
- Supportive care
- Monitor hemoglobin and bilirubin
- Usually self-limited

Rh Incompatibility (Rh Disease)

Pathophysiology:

- Rh-negative mother (lacks D antigen)
- Rh-positive infant (D antigen present)
- Maternal sensitization from previous pregnancy or transfusion
- IgG anti-D antibodies cross placenta
- RBC hemolysis in utero and postnatal
- Severe hemolytic anemia
- Unconjugated hyperbilirubinemia

Incidence:

- Rare in developed countries due to RhIG prophylaxis
- Still common in resource-limited settings
- Hydrops fetalis possible if severe

Clinical Features:

- Severe jaundice within 24 hours
- Severe anemia (hemoglobin <10 g/dL)
- Hepatosplenomegaly
- Edema, ascites (hydrops)

- Pallor, poor perfusion
- Respiratory distress

Diagnosis:

- Positive DAT (Coombs test)
- Elevated indirect bilirubin
- Severe anemia
- Elevated reticulocyte count
- Nucleated RBCs
- Maternal serology: Rh negative, anti-D positive

Management:

- Exchange transfusion (often needed)
- Phototherapy
- Supportive care: oxygen, ventilation, inotropes
- Transfusion for severe anemia if needed
- Close monitoring

Prevention:

- Rh immunoglobulin (RhIG) at 28 weeks gestation
- RhIG within 72 hours of delivery/miscarriage/invasive procedure
- Dose: 300 mcg (1500 IU) IM for US, 500 IU/mL fetal RBCs

Other Blood Group Incompatibilities

- Kell incompatibility: anti-Kell antibodies, severe hemolytic disease
- Duffy incompatibility: anti-Fya, anti-Fyb antibodies
- Kidd incompatibility: anti-Jka, anti-Jkb antibodies
- MNS incompatibility: anti-M, anti-N, anti-S antibodies

Screening and Assessment for Hyperbilirubinemia

Universal Screening Approach"it is advocated to prevent long-term handicapped yield"

Timing:

- All infants screened before discharge or by 5 days of age
- Risk stratification at birth
- Follow-up testing based on risk category

Methods:

- Transcutaneous bilirubinometry (TcB): non-invasive, rapid
- Serum total bilirubin (STB): confirmatory, more accurate"requires budget"
- Both methods acceptable for screening

Risk Stratification

Low Risk (<38 weeks gestation):

- Birthweight ≥2500g
- Well infant
- No isoimmune hemolytic disease
- Follow-up at 24 hours if discharged <24 hours

Medium Risk (<38 weeks gestation):

- Birthweight 2000-2499g
- Or well infant 38-42 weeks with risk factors
- Follow-up at 24-48 hours

High Risk (<38 weeks gestation):

- Birthweight <2000g
- Or ill infant
- Or isoimmune hemolytic disease
- Close follow-up within 24 hours

Nomogram-Based Management

AAP Phototherapy Nomogram:

- Age-specific thresholds (in hours after birth)

- Based on risk category (low, medium, high)
- Bilirubin level plotted against age
- Determines need for phototherapy
- Different thresholds for exchange transfusion

Risk Stratification by Postnatal Age:

- <24 hours: lower thresholds (higher risk)
- 24-48 hours: intermediate thresholds
- 48-96 hours: higher thresholds (lower risk)
- 96 hours: highest thresholds

Phototherapy

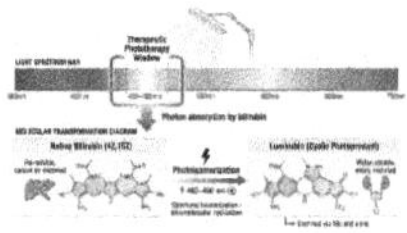

Mechanism of Action

- Photoisomerization: converts unconjugated bilirubin to lumirubin (water-soluble, excreted in urine and bile)
- Structural isomerization: converts bilirubin to less toxic forms
- Oxidative degradation: breaks down bilirubin molecule

- Reduces unconjugated bilirubin levels by 5-20%

Phototherapy Devices

Conventional Phototherapy:

- Fluorescent or halogen lamps
- Overhead or fiberoptic delivery
- Spectral output: 420-500 nm (blue-green)
- Distance: 15-30 cm from infant
- Surface area exposure important

Intensive Phototherapy:"capsule phototherapy"

- High-intensity light sources
- Multiple light sources (overhead + fiberoptic)
- Spectral irradiance >30 mcW/cm^2/nm
- Reduces bilirubin faster
- Reserved for higher bilirubin levels

Fiberoptic Phototherapy:

- Portable, can be used during feeding
- Less effective than overhead lights
- Useful for supplemental therapy
- Allows infant-parent contact

Phototherapy Indications

- Based on age-specific nomogram
- Bilirubin level ≥ phototherapy threshold
- Hemolytic disease: lower threshold
- Risk factors: consider lower threshold

Phototherapy Duration and Monitoring

- Continuous exposure until bilirubin decreases
- Recheck bilirubin every 4-6 hours initially
- Then every 6-12 hours
- Continue until bilirubin below phototherapy threshold
- Resume if rebound occurs

Complications and Concerns

- Dehydration: monitor fluid intake and output
- Hyperthermia: monitor temperature
- "Bronze baby" syndrome: rare, with cholestasis
- Retinal damage: minimal risk with current devices

- Circadian rhythm disruption: minor concern
- Loose stools: common, not harmful
- Skin rash: transient

Phototherapy Discontinuation

- When bilirubin decreases to safe level
- Risk of rebound: monitor for 24 hours
- Ensure adequate feeding
- Outpatient follow-up within 24-48 hours

Exchange Transfusion

Indications

- Bilirubin level ≥ exchange transfusion threshold (age-specific)
- Hemolytic disease with severe anemia
- Rapidly rising bilirubin (>0.2 mg/dL/hour despite phototherapy)
- Signs of bilirubin encephalopathy
- Failed phototherapy

Thresholds for Exchange Transfusion

- Age-specific nomogram used
- Lower thresholds for hemolytic disease
- Varies by risk category
- Typically 25-30 mg/dL in term infants

Procedure

Preparation:

- Obtain informed consent
- Type and crossmatch infant blood
- Prepare blood: O-negative or type-specific, crossmatched
- Warm blood to body temperature
- Gather equipment: umbilical catheter, syringes, blood warmer
- NPO 2-4 hours before procedure

Technique (Double Volume Exchange):

- Insert umbilical venous catheter
- Withdraw 5-10 mL infant blood
- Infuse equal volume donor blood

- Repeat 80-100 times (total 2× blood volume)
- Final volume: 160-180 mL/kg exchanged
- Removes 85% of bilirubin and RBCs (in HDN)
- Procedure duration: 1-2 hours

Monitoring During Procedure:

- Continuous cardiorespiratory monitoring
- Vital signs every 15-30 minutes
- Temperature maintenance
- Glucose monitoring
- Electrolyte monitoring

Complications

- Umbilical catheter: perforation, thrombosis, infection
- Electrolyte abnormalities: hyperkalemia, hypocalcemia
- Hypoglycemia
- Hypothermia
- Thrombocytopenia
- Infection/sepsis
- Necrotizing enterocolitis

- Mortality: <0.5% in modern practice

Post-Exchange Management

- Recheck bilirubin at 4-6 hours
- Continue phototherapy if indicated
- Monitor for rebound hyperbilirubinemia
- Restart feeding when stable
- Monitor vital signs and temperature
- Watch for complications

Kernicterus (Bilirubin Encephalopathy)

Pathophysiology

- Unconjugated bilirubin crosses blood-brain barrier
- Enters neurons and glia
- Binds to mitochondria and membranes
- Inhibits oxidative metabolism
- Causes neuronal death
- Particularly affects basal ganglia, brainstem, cerebellum

Risk Factors for Bilirubin Neurotoxicity

- Unconjugated hyperbilirubinemia >25-30 mg/dL
- Prematurity (<35 weeks)
- Hemolytic disease
- Acidosis (increases bilirubin crossing BBB)
- Sepsis/infection
- Hypoglycemia
- Hypothermia
- Isoimmune hemolytic disease
- Hypoalbuminemia
- Albumin-bilirubin binding capacity exceeded

Acute Phase (First Week)

- Lethargy, poor feeding
- Hypotonia or hypertonia
- Fever
- High-pitched cry
- Vomiting

- Seizures
- Opisthotonus (severe)
- May resolve or progress

Chronic Phase (After First Week)

- Choreoathetoid cerebral palsy
- Upward gaze limitation
- Hearing loss (auditory neuropathy)
- Enamel dysplasia of teeth
- Bilirubin staining of basal ganglia on MRI
- Intellectual disability
- Behavioral problems

Diagnosis

- Clinical presentation
- Elevated unconjugated bilirubin
- MRI: T2 hyperintensity in globus pallidus, subthalamic nuclei
- Auditory brainstem response (ABR): abnormal

- Neurological examination

Prevention

- Aggressive phototherapy
- Exchange transfusion when indicated
- Early recognition and treatment of jaundice
- Universal screening
- Risk stratification
- Follow-up after discharge

Management of Acute Kernicterus

- Intensive phototherapy
- Exchange transfusion
- Supportive care
- Seizure management
- Temperature regulation
- Fluid and electrolyte management

Long-Term Management

- Physical therapy
- Speech therapy
- Hearing aids or cochlear implants
- Educational support
- Family counseling
- Prognosis: variable, depends on severity

Breastfeeding and Jaundice

Breast Milk Jaundice

Pathophysiology:

- Inadequate milk transfer
- Poor breastfeeding technique
- Infrequent feeds
- Low caloric intake
- Increased enterohepatic circulation
- Dehydration

Risk Factors:

- Maternal inexperience
- Infant prematurity

- Tongue-tie
- Maternal breast anatomy issues
- Inadequate lactation support

Clinical Features:

- Jaundice peaks at 4-7 days
- Bilirubin 15-25 mg/dL typically
- Infant appears well
- Poor feeding or weight loss
- Inadequate stooling

Prevention:

- Early and frequent breastfeeding (8-12 times/day)
- Proper latch and positioning
- Assessment of milk transfer
- Lactation consultation
- Supplementation if needed
- Avoid pacifiers initially

Management:

- Increase breastfeeding frequency
- Optimize breastfeeding technique
- Lactation support

- Monitor weight and hydration
- Supplement with expressed breast milk or formula if needed
- Phototherapy if bilirubin elevated

Breast Milk-Induced Jaundice

Pathophysiology:

- Component in breast milk (possibly lipase)
- Increases intestinal bilirubin reabsorption
- Occurs despite adequate milk intake
- Rare

Clinical Features:

- Jaundice persists beyond 2 weeks
- Infant feeding well, gaining weight
- Bilirubin 10-20 mg/dL
- Elevated unconjugated bilirubin

Management:

- Continue breastfeeding
- Monitor bilirubin
- Phototherapy if indicated
- Temporary formula supplementation if bilirubin very ele-

vated

- Usually resolves by 3 months

Promoting Successful Breastfeeding

- Early skin-to-skin contact
- First feed within 1 hour
- Frequent feeds (8-12 times/day)
- Assess latch and positioning
- Monitor for adequate milk transfer
- Lactation support
- Monitor infant weight and hydration
- Educate about normal newborn behavior
- Address maternal concerns

Management of Hyperbilirubinemia: Summary Algorithm

Step 1: Identify Risk

- Assess gestational age, medical status

- Identify hemolytic disease risk
- Determine risk category (low, medium, high)

Step 2: Screen for Hyperbilirubinemia

- Measure bilirubin (TcB or STB) before discharge
- Plot on age-specific nomogram
- Determine if phototherapy indicated

Step 3: Initiate Phototherapy if Indicated

- Place infant under phototherapy lights
- Recheck bilirubin every 4-6 hours
- Ensure adequate feeding
- Monitor hydration and temperature

Step 4: Escalate Therapy if Needed

- Intensive phototherapy if rapid rise
- Exchange transfusion if approaching threshold
- Treat underlying cause

Step 5: Discontinue and Follow-Up

- Discontinue phototherapy when safe
- Schedule follow-up within 24-48 hours
- Assess feeding and hydration
- Recheck bilirubin
- Provide education about jaundice

Special Populations

Preterm Infants

- Lower phototherapy thresholds
- Higher risk of bilirubin neurotoxicity
- More frequent monitoring
- May need phototherapy longer
- Consider albumin level when assessing risk

Late Preterm Infants (34-36 Weeks)

- Increased risk of severe hyperbilirubinemia
- Lower phototherapy thresholds

- Close follow-up essential
- Consider early discharge precautions

Infants with Hemolytic Disease

- Aggressive phototherapy
- Lower exchange transfusion thresholds
- May need exchange transfusion at birth
- Close monitoring essential
- Consider intrauterine transfusion if severe

Infants with G6PD Deficiency

- Increased hemolysis with triggers
- Higher bilirubin production
- Lower phototherapy thresholds
- Avoid triggers: fava beans, sulfonamides, aspirin
- Screen in high-risk populations

Discharge Planning and Follow-Up

Pre-Discharge Assessment

- Bilirubin level and trajectory
- Feeding assessment (breast or bottle)
- Weight loss/gain
- Hydration status
- Risk factors for severe hyperbilirubinemia
- Parent education and understanding

Follow-Up Timing

- Low risk: 24-72 hours after discharge
- Medium risk: 24-48 hours after discharge
- High risk: within 24 hours after discharge
- Earlier if bilirubin near phototherapy threshold

Follow-Up Assessment

- Clinical examination
- Bilirubin level (TcB or STB)
- Feeding assessment
- Weight and hydration

- Parental concerns
- Signs of bilirubin encephalopathy

Parent Education

- Signs and symptoms of jaundice
- Importance of feeding
- When to seek medical attention
- Reassurance if physiologic jaundice
- Contact information for questions

Key Takeaways

Neonatal jaundice and hemolytic disease require:

- Universal screening before discharge
- Risk stratification and nomogram-based management
- Appropriate phototherapy initiation
- Exchange transfusion when indicated
- Prevention and early recognition of kernicterus
- Support for breastfeeding
- Close follow-up after discharge

- Family education and reassurance
- Prevention of bilirubin neurotoxicity

Systematic approach to hyperbilirubinemia management prevents serious complications and ensures optimal outcomes for neonates.

Chapter Fifteen

NEONATAL SKIN AND SOFT TISSUE DISORDERS

Neonatal Skin: Anatomy and Physiology

Structural Characteristics

Epidermis:

- Thinner than adult skin (0.05 mm vs. 0.1 mm)
- Reduced number of cell layers
- Immature barrier function
- Increased transepidermal water loss (TEWL)

- Increased percutaneous absorption

Dermis:

- Reduced collagen and elastin
- Decreased dermal-epidermal adhesion
- Increased fragility
- Reduced tensile strength

Subcutaneous Tissue:

- Increased subcutaneous fat
- Important for temperature regulation
- Brown adipose tissue for non-shivering thermogenesis

Physiologic Differences

- pH neutral to slightly alkaline at birth
- Colonization by flora begins immediately
- Skin flora establishment by 24-48 hours
- Barrier function matures over first 2-4 weeks
- Increased susceptibility to infection
- Increased percutaneous absorption of topical agents

Clinical Implications

- Fragile, easily traumatized
- Prone to infection
- Limited ability to thermoregulate
- Sensitive to irritants and allergens
- Careful handling and gentle care essential

Common Benign Neonatal Skin Conditions

Vernix Caseosa

Description:

- White, cheese-like coating on skin at birth
- Mixture of sebum, lanugo, and desquamated epithelial cells
- Protective and moisturizing

Management:

- Leave in place if possible
- Gently wipe away if needed
- Do not scrub or vigorously remove
- Provides natural moisturization
- Absorbs over first 24-48 hours

Lanugo

Description:

- Fine, downy hair covering fetal skin
- Present especially on preterm infants
- More prominent on face, shoulders, back

Management:

- Normal finding
- Sheds over first 1-2 weeks
- No treatment needed
- Reassure parents

Milia

Description:

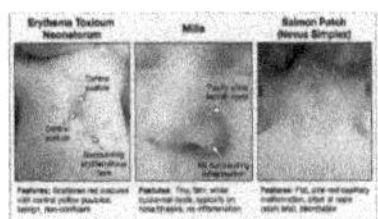

- Tiny white papules on nose, cheeks, forehead
- Blocked sebaceous glands
- Appear 2-3 days after birth
- 40% of newborns affected

Management:

- Benign, self-limited

- Resolve spontaneously by 2-4 weeks
- No treatment needed
- Do not squeeze or manipulate
- Reassure parents

Erythema Toxicum Neonatorum

Description:

- Benign rash appearing 24-72 hours after birth
- Red macules with central pustule
- Resembles flea bites
- Most common neonatal rash (70% of term infants)
- More common in term than preterm

Pathophysiology:

- Sterile pustules
- Eosinophilic infiltration
- Etiology unknown
- Not infectious

Clinical Features:

- Scattered red papules with central pustule
- Primarily on trunk and proximal extremities

- Face and palms/soles spared
- May be pruritic
- Appears and disappears over hours to days

Diagnosis:

- Clinical appearance
- Wright stain of pustule: eosinophils
- Culture negative
- No systemic symptoms

Management:

- Reassurance
- No treatment needed
- Resolves spontaneously within days
- Avoid unnecessary antibiotics

Neonatal Acne

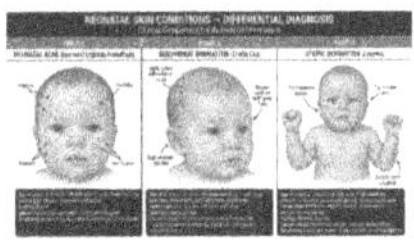

Description:

- Comedones and papules on face
- Appears 2-4 weeks after birth

- Related to maternal androgens
- More common in males

Management:

- Self-limited, resolves by 3-4 months
- Gentle washing with mild soap
- Avoid irritating products
- Topical benzoyl peroxide if severe
- Reassure parents

Seborrheic Dermatitis

Description:

- Cradle cap: scaling, crusting on scalp
- Yellow, greasy scale
- May extend to face and neck
- Common in first weeks to months

Management:

- Gentle shampooing with mild soap
- Soft brush to remove scales
- Moisturizing lotion
- Topical hydrocortisone if severe

- Usually self-limited

Transient Neonatal Pustulosis

Description:

- Sterile pustules on palms and soles
- Appear within first 24-48 hours
- More common in African American infants
- Benign, self-limited

Management:

- No treatment needed
- Resolves within 1-2 weeks
- Reassure parents

Birthmarks and Vascular Lesions

Salmon Patch (Nevus Simplex)

Description:

- Pink to red macule
- Most common birthmark (30-40% of infants)
- Located on eyelids, glabella, nape of neck

- Blanches with pressure
- Fades with crying or exertion

Pathophysiology:

- Dilated capillaries
- Not true hemangioma
- Benign vascular malformation

Clinical Course:

- Fade significantly by 1-2 years
- Nape lesions may persist longer
- No treatment needed

Management:

- Reassurance
- No treatment necessary
- Cosmetic concern only
- Laser therapy if persistent cosmetic concern

Port-Wine Stain (Nevus Flammeus)

Description:

- Dark red to purple macule
- Typically on face (V1, V2 distribution)

- Present at birth
- Darkens and thickens with age
- 3 per 1,000 births

Pathophysiology:

- Capillary malformation
- Progressive ectasia of vessels
- Does not blanch with pressure
- Permanent lesion

Associated Conditions:

- Sturge-Weber syndrome: port-wine stain + leptomeningeal angiomatosis
- Risk of seizures, stroke, glaucoma
- Requires ophthalmologic evaluation

Management:

- Referral to pediatric dermatology
- Pulsed dye laser therapy: most effective
- Multiple treatments often needed
- Earlier treatment better results
- Genetic counseling if syndromic

Hemangioma

Description:

- Benign vascular tumor
- Most common soft tissue tumor in infants
- Proliferating endothelial cells
- May be present at birth or appear in first weeks

Types:

Superficial Hemangioma:

- Bright red, raised lesion
- "Strawberry" appearance
- Blanches with pressure
- Typically on head/neck

Deep Hemangioma:

- Blue or purple color
- Subcutaneous mass
- Less blanching
- May not be visible at birth

Mixed Hemangioma:

- Combination of superficial and deep

Clinical Course:

- Rapid growth phase: first 6-12 months

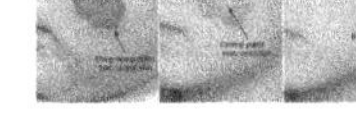

- Plateau phase: 1-3 years
- Involution phase: 3-7 years
- 90% involute by age 9 years

Complications:

- Obstruction (airway, vision)
- Ulceration and bleeding
- Infection
- Disfigurement
- PHACES syndrome (posterior fossa malformations, hemangiomas, arterial anomalies, cardiac defects, eye abnormalities, sternal cleft)

Diagnosis:

- Clinical appearance
- Ultrasound or MRI if diagnosis uncertain
- Assess for complications

Management:

Observation:

- Most hemangiomas involute spontaneously
- Regular monitoring
- Avoid trauma

Treatment Indicated If:

- Airway compromise
- Vision obstruction
- Ulceration with bleeding
- Infection
- Significant cosmetic concern
- Rapidly enlarging

Treatment Options:

- Topical timolol: first-line for superficial lesions
- Systemic propranolol: 2-3 mg/kg/day divided
  - Effective for large or complicated hemangiomas
  - Monitor heart rate, blood pressure, glucose
  - Discontinue gradually
- Corticosteroids: systemic or intralesional
- Pulsed dye laser
- Surgical excision if indicated
- Combination therapy for resistant lesions

Infectious Skin Conditions

Neonatal Herpes Simplex Virus (HSV) Infection

Pathophysiology:

- Vertical transmission from mother
- 30-50% transmission risk with primary infection
- 3-5% transmission risk with recurrent infection
- Typically HSV-2, can be HSV-1

Risk Factors:

- Maternal primary HSV infection at delivery
- Maternal recurrent infection with ruptured membranes
- Prematurity
- Prolonged rupture of membranes
- Fetal monitoring with scalp electrodes

Clinical Presentation:

Disseminated Disease (25%):

- Multiple organ involvement
- Sepsis-like picture
- Hepatitis, encephalitis, pneumonitis
- High mortality if untreated

CNS Disease (30%):

- Meningitis or encephalitis

- Seizures
- Fever
- Altered consciousness

Skin/Eye/Mouth (SEM) Disease (45%):

- Vesicular rash: grouped vesicles on erythematous base
- Typically appears 5-14 days after birth
- Scalp, buttocks, genitalia common sites
- Conjunctivitis, keratitis
- Oral ulcers
- May progress to disseminated disease

Diagnosis:

- PCR of vesicular fluid (most sensitive)
- Viral culture
- Tzanck smear: multinucleated giant cells
- Direct fluorescent antibody testing
- Serology less useful acutely

Management:

- Acyclovir: 10-15 mg/kg IV every 8 hours
- Duration: 10-14 days
- Treat empirically if suspected

- Do not delay treatment
- Supportive care
- Ophthalmologic evaluation
- Long-term neurodevelopmental follow-up

Prevention:

- Maternal antiviral suppression if history of HSV
- Cesarean delivery if active lesions at delivery
- Careful monitoring if vaginal delivery despite HSV history

Congenital Varicella

Pathophysiology:

- Maternal varicella in first/early second trimester
- Fetal infection via hematogenous spread
- Rare (1-2% risk before 20 weeks)

Clinical Features:

- Skin scarring in dermatomal distribution
- Eye abnormalities: cataracts, chorioretinitis
- Limb hypoplasia
- Microcephaly
- Growth restriction

- Intellectual disability

Management:

- Supportive care
- Ophthalmologic evaluation
- Neurodevelopmental assessment
- Genetic counseling

Neonatal Candidiasis

Pathophysiology:

- Vertical transmission from maternal vaginal colonization
- Ascending infection or direct contact during delivery
- Risk factors: prematurity, prolonged rupture of membranes, maternal antibiotic use

Clinical Presentation:

Oral Thrush:

- White patches on tongue, palate, buccal mucosa
- Cannot be wiped off (unlike milk)
- May be asymptomatic or cause feeding difficulty
- Appears 7-10 days after birth

Diaper Dermatitis:

- Erythematous rash in diaper area

- Satellite lesions
- Pruritic
- Responds to antifungal treatment

Invasive Candidiasis:

- Bloodstream infection
- Sepsis presentation
- Risk factors: central lines, prolonged antibiotics, prematurity
- High mortality

Diagnosis:

- Clinical appearance
- KOH preparation: pseudohyphae
- Culture: confirms diagnosis
- Blood culture if systemic infection suspected

Management:

Oral Thrush:

- Nystatin suspension: 100,000 units/mL, 1 mL to each side of mouth 4 times daily
- Fluconazole: 6 mg/kg/day for 7-14 days (more effective)
- Treat mother's nipples if breastfeeding
- Continue 2-3 days after resolution

Diaper Dermatitis:

- Topical antifungal: nystatin, clotrimazole, or miconazole
- Keep area dry
- Frequent diaper changes
- Barrier cream

Invasive Candidiasis:

- Fluconazole: 6-12 mg/kg/day IV or oral
- Duration: 2-3 weeks
- Consider amphotericin B for resistant organisms
- Remove central lines if possible

Impetigo and Bacterial Skin Infections

Neonatal Impetigo

Pathophysiology:

- Bacterial infection of skin
- Staphylococcus aureus or Group A Streptococcus (GAS)
- Transmission from maternal flora or healthcare workers
- Enters through breaks in skin

Clinical Features:

- Vesicles or pustules
- Rapidly evolve to honey-crusted lesions
- Non-bullous form most common
- Typically on face, neck, diaper area
- May be pruritic
- Regional lymphadenopathy

Diagnosis:

- Culture of lesion
- Gram stain: cocci in clusters (staph) or chains (strep)
- Clinical appearance

Management:

- Topical antibiotics: mupirocin ointment
- Applied 2-3 times daily for 7-10 days
- Systemic antibiotics if:
    - Widespread involvement
    - Signs of systemic infection
    - Immunocompromised
    - Streptococcal infection (risk of post-streptococcal sequelae)
- Dicloxacillin or cephalexin: 25-50 mg/kg/day divided

- Or clindamycin if MRSA suspected
- Infection control measures
- Avoid spread to other infants

Omphalitis (Umbilical Cord Stump Infection)

Pathophysiology:

- Infection of umbilical cord stump
- Bacterial colonization
- Risk factors: poor umbilical hygiene, delayed cord separation
- Common organisms: S. aureus, GAS, E. coli, Klebsiella

Clinical Features:

- Erythema, edema, purulence around umbilicus
- Foul-smelling drainage
- Fever
- Systemic signs: lethargy, poor feeding
- May progress to sepsis
- Umbilical granuloma (benign, red nodule at cord site)

Diagnosis:

- Clinical appearance
- Culture of drainage

- CBC: elevated WBC
- Blood culture if systemic symptoms

Management:

Prevention:

- Dry umbilical cord care
- Alcohol or chlorhexidine cleansing
- Keep cord dry and exposed
- Avoid tight diapers
- Monitor for signs of infection

Treatment:

- Topical antibiotics: mupirocin or bacitracin
- Systemic antibiotics if:
    - Signs of systemic infection
    - Cellulitis extending beyond umbilicus
    - Fever
    - Sepsis
- Broad-spectrum: ampicillin + gentamicin
- Duration: 7-10 days
- Supportive care
- Close monitoring

- Hospitalization if systemic infection

Diaper Dermatitis

Pathophysiology

- Irritant contact dermatitis most common
- Prolonged contact with urine and feces
- Ammonia production from bacterial urease
- Maceration and alkaline environment
- Friction and moisture

Types

Irritant Diaper Dermatitis:

- Most common form (80%)
- Erythematous patches and plaques
- Spares skin folds
- Itching and discomfort
- Caused by moisture, friction, irritants

Allergic Contact Dermatitis:

- Reaction to diaper material, wipes, or products

- Erythema, edema, vesicles
- Involves skin folds
- Pruritic

Candida Diaper Dermatitis:

- Secondary to Candida colonization
- Bright red erythema
- Satellite lesions
- Maceration
- Responds to antifungal therapy

Management

Prevention:

- Frequent diaper changes
- Keep skin dry
- Avoid excessive moisture
- Use soft, breathable diapers
- Gentle cleansing
- Barrier creams (zinc oxide, petrolatum)

Treatment:

- Frequent diaper changes

- Dry thoroughly after each change
- Barrier cream at each change
- Air exposure when possible
- Avoid irritants and allergens
- Antifungal cream if Candida suspected
- Topical hydrocortisone if severe inflammation
- Avoid plastic pants

Epidermolysis Bullosa (EB)

Pathophysiology

- Genetic disorder of skin fragility
- Defects in structural proteins
- Blistering at dermal-epidermal junction
- Autosomal dominant or recessive inheritance

Types

Epidermolysis Bullosa Simplex (EBS):

- Intraepidermal blistering

- Autosomal dominant
- Mutations in keratin genes (KRT5, KRT14)
- Mild form: blisters on hands, feet, friction areas
- Severe form: extensive blistering, erosions
- Healing without scarring

Junctional Epidermolysis Bullosa (JEB):

- Blistering at dermal-epidermal junction
- Autosomal recessive
- Mutations in genes encoding hemidesmosomes
- Severe form: lethal, extensive blistering, sepsis risk
- Mild form: localized blistering, better prognosis

Dystrophic Epidermolysis Bullosa (DEB):

- Subepidermal blistering
- Autosomal dominant or recessive
- Mutations in COL7A1 (collagen VII)
- Recessive form more severe
- Extensive scarring and contractures
- Risk of squamous cell carcinoma

Clinical Presentation

- Blistering and erosions at birth or with minor trauma
- Mucosal involvement in severe forms
- Scarring in dystrophic forms
- Pain from erosions
- Infection risk
- Feeding difficulties if oral involvement

Diagnosis

- Clinical appearance
- Skin biopsy: electron microscopy, immunofluorescence
- Genetic testing: confirms diagnosis, guides prognosis

Management

- Gentle handling to prevent trauma
- Avoid adhesive dressings
- Non-adherent dressings (non-stick gauze, silicone-based)
- Topical antibiotics
- Pain management
- Nutritional support

- Ophthalmologic evaluation if ocular involvement
- Genetic counseling
- Multidisciplinary team approach
- Prognosis depends on type and severity

Congenital Dermatologic Conditions

Ichthyosis

Description:

- Disorder of keratinization
- Dry, scaly skin
- Multiple genetic forms
- Autosomal recessive or dominant

Clinical Features:

- Collodion baby: waxy, translucent membrane at birth
- Severe scaling and dryness
- Hyperkeratosis
- May have systemic involvement

Management:

- Emollients and moisturizers

- Gentle cleansing
- Avoid irritants
- Treat infections
- Genetic testing
- Long-term dermatologic management

Congenital Nevus

Description:

- Pigmented lesion present at birth
- Benign melanocytic proliferation
- Vary in size and appearance
- Risk of malignant transformation

Management:

- Photographic documentation
- Regular monitoring
- Genetic counseling
- Surgical removal if indicated
- Dermatologic follow-up

Aplasia Cutis

Description:

- Localized absence of skin
- Usually on scalp vertex
- May be associated with chromosomal abnormalities or maternal factors
- Ranges from small erosion to large defect

Management:

- Wound care
- Gentle cleaning and dressing
- Topical antibiotics
- Surgical closure if large
- Monitor for infection
- Genetic evaluation if syndromic

Neonatal Acne Rosacea and Seborrheic Conditions

Neonatal Acne Rosacea

Description:

- Facial erythema, telangiectasia, papules
- Related to maternal androgens

- Appears weeks to months after birth
- More common in males
- Benign, self-limited

Management:

- Gentle facial cleansing
- Avoid irritants
- Topical benzoyl peroxide if needed
- Reassurance
- Resolves by 3-4 months

Seborrheic Dermatitis

Description:

- Cradle cap most common manifestation
- Yellow, greasy scaling on scalp
- May extend to face, neck, trunk
- Related to Malassezia colonization
- Benign, self-limited

Management:

- Gentle shampooing
- Soft brush to remove scales

- Moisturizing lotion
- Topical hydrocortisone if severe
- Antifungal shampoo if needed
- Usually resolves by 3-6 months

Skin Care and Prevention of Complications

Basic Neonatal Skin Care

Bathing:

- First bath after temperature stabilization
- Lukewarm water
- Mild, fragrance-free cleanser
- Gentle technique
- Pat dry thoroughly
- Avoid excessive bathing (dries skin)

Moisturization:

- Apply emollient after bathing
- Plain petrolatum or fragrance-free lotion
- Reduces transepidermal water loss
- Improves barrier function

- Particularly important in preterm infants

Umbilical Cord Care:

- Keep cord clean and dry
- Alcohol or chlorhexidine cleansing
- Avoid covering with diaper
- Monitor for signs of infection
- Cord separation typically 7-14 days

Diaper Care:

- Frequent changes (8-12 per day)
- Gentle cleansing with water or mild wipes
- Thorough drying
- Barrier cream at each change
- Air exposure when possible

Nail Care:

- Trim nails short to prevent scratching
- Use soft nail file
- Avoid cutting skin
- Consider soft mittens to prevent scratching

Prevention of Infections

- Hand hygiene before handling infant
- Avoid exposure to ill individuals
- Keep umbilical cord clean and dry
- Monitor for signs of infection
- Prompt treatment of any infections
- Avoid unnecessary invasive procedures

Temperature Regulation

- Maintain neutral thermal environment
- Skin-to-skin contact
- Appropriate clothing and bedding
- Avoid excessive heat exposure
- Monitor temperature regularly

Sun Protection

- Avoid direct sun exposure first 6 months
- Use protective clothing
- Sunscreen SPF 30+ after 6 months
- Seek shade during peak sun hours

Key Takeaways

Neonatal skin and soft tissue disorders require:

- Understanding of neonatal skin physiology
- Recognition of benign vs. pathologic conditions
- Appropriate diagnostic approach
- Evidence-based management
- Prevention of complications
- Gentle skin care practices
- Family education and reassurance
- Specialist referral when indicated
- Long-term follow-up for chronic conditions

Early recognition and appropriate management of skin conditions optimize neonatal outcomes and prevent serious complications.

Chapter Sixteen

HEMATOLOGIC DISORDERS AND TRANSFUSION MEDICINE

Neonatal Hematology: Overview

Normal Neonatal Blood Values

Hemoglobin and Hematocrit:

- Hemoglobin: 13.5-20 g/dL (term), 13-17 g/dL (preterm)
- Hematocrit: 41-65% (term), 39-59% (preterm)

- Higher than adults due to intrauterine hypoxia adaptation
- Decline over first 8-12 weeks (physiologic anemia)

White Blood Cells:

- WBC: 5,000-21,000/μL
- Higher than adults
- Immature forms common
- Neutrophils: 45-80%
- Lymphocytes: 20-40%
- Monocytes: 3-10%

Platelets:

- 150,000-400,000/μL
- Similar to adults
- Functional differences in neonates

Red Blood Cell Indices:

- MCV: 95-120 fL (higher than adults)
- MCH: 32-37 pg
- MCHC: 32-36 g/dL

Coagulation Parameters:

- PT: 12-21 seconds (prolonged vs. adults)
- aPTT: 30-60 seconds "could reach 90" (prolonged vs. adults)

- Thrombin time: 16-24 seconds (prolonged)
- Fibrinogen: 150-400 mg/dL (lower than adults)
- Factors II, VII, IX, X: 30-50% of adult values
- Factors V, VIII, XII: near adult values
- Protein C and S: 30-40% of adult values

Physiologic Changes

- Hemoglobin peaks at birth
- Declines over first 8-12 weeks (physiologic anemia)
- Reticulocyte count elevated initially, then decreases
- Fetal hemoglobin (HbF) gradually replaced by adult hemoglobin (HbA)
- WBC counts decrease gradually over first weeks
- Coagulation factors increase toward adult values

Anemia in Neonates

Classification

Acute Blood Loss:

- Hemorrhage during delivery
- Placental abruption
- Cord laceration
- Fetal-maternal hemorrhage
- Twin-twin transfusion syndrome

Chronic Blood Loss:

- Intrauterine growth restriction
- Chronic fetal-maternal hemorrhage
- Placental insufficiency

Hemolysis:

- Isoimmune hemolytic disease (ABO, Rh, other blood groups)

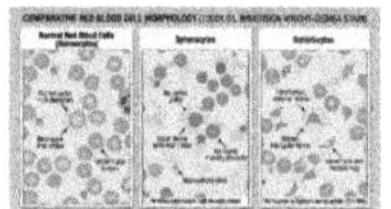

- Non-immune hemolysis (infection, G6PD deficiency)
- Microangiopathic hemolytic anemia

Decreased RBC Production:

- Prematurity (decreased EPO response)
- Infection/sepsis
- Congenital infections (TORCH)
- Diamond-Blackfan anemia
- Transient erythroblastopenia of infancy

- Bone marrow suppression

Clinical Presentation

- Pallor
- Tachycardia
- Tachypnea
- Poor feeding
- Lethargy
- Jaundice (if hemolysis)
- Hepatosplenomegaly
- Edema or ascites (if severe)
- Shock (severe acute anemia)

Diagnosis

- Hemoglobin and hematocrit
- Reticulocyte count
- Blood smear morphology
- Direct antiglobulin test (DAT/Coombs)
- Bilirubin level

- Peripheral blood smear
- Assess for bleeding sources
- Coagulation studies if indicated

Management

Acute Blood Loss:

- IV fluids: 0.9% saline 10-20 mL/kg bolus
- Oxygen and ventilation support
- Packed RBC transfusion if hemodynamically unstable
- Identify and control bleeding source
- Monitor vital signs and perfusion
- Serial hemoglobin checks

Hemolytic Anemia:

- Phototherapy
- Exchange transfusion if indicated
- Treat underlying cause
- Monitor bilirubin and hemoglobin
- Supportive care

Decreased RBC Production:

- Supportive care

- Treat underlying cause
- Transfusion if symptomatic or severe
- EPO for prematurity-related anemia (controversial)
- Monitor for recovery

Transfusion Indications:" depends on clinical context , gestational age , post natal age""follow your local protocol"

- Symptomatic anemia (tachycardia, tachypnea, poor perfusion)
- Hemoglobin <7 g/dL
- Hemoglobin <10 g/dL with respiratory support
- Hemoglobin <12 g/dL with severe cardiopulmonary disease
- Acute blood loss >15% blood volume
- Ongoing bleeding

Polycythemia

Brief Review

- Hemoglobin >20 g/dL or hematocrit >65%
- Risk factors: IUGR, maternal diabetes, delayed cord clamping, twin-twin transfusion

- Symptoms: plethora, poor feeding, hypoglycemia, seizures
- Management: partial exchange transfusion if symptomatic
- Monitor for complications: thrombosis, NEC, pulmonary hemorrhage

Thrombocytopenia

Classification

Decreased Production:

- Bone marrow suppression (sepsis, medications)
- Congenital infections (TORCH)
- Genetic disorders (TAR syndrome, Fanconi anemia)
- Prematurity (mild thrombocytopenia common)

Increased Destruction:

- Immune: maternal ITP, neonatal alloimmunization (NAIT)
- Non-immune: sepsis, DIC, hemolytic disease
- Microangiopathic: thrombotic microangiopathy

Sequestration:

- Splenomegaly
- Hemangioma (Kasabach-Merritt syndrome)

Dilutional:

- Massive transfusion
- Exchange transfusion

Clinical Presentation

- Often asymptomatic
- Petechiae and purpura
- Bleeding from puncture sites
- Gastrointestinal bleeding
- Intracranial hemorrhage (severe)
- Mucosal bleeding

Diagnosis

- Platelet count <150,000/μL
- Peripheral blood smear
- Coagulation studies (PT, aPTT, fibrinogen)
- D-dimer
- Sepsis workup if indicated
- Maternal ITP history

- Maternal platelet count
- DAT if hemolytic disease

Management

Immune Thrombocytopenia (Maternal ITP):

- Platelet count usually 50,000-100,000/μL
- Risk of intracranial hemorrhage
- Avoid scalp electrodes, fetal scalp sampling, forceps delivery
- Platelet transfusion if:
    - Platelet count <30,000/μL
    - Active bleeding
    - Invasive procedures planned
- IVIG: 0.5-1 g/kg IV over 2-4 hours
- Corticosteroids "controversial"
- Close monitoring
- Usually resolves by 1-2 weeks

Neonatal Alloimmunization (NAIT):

- Maternal alloantibodies against fetal platelet antigen
- Severe thrombocytopenia (often <20,000/μL)
- Risk of intracranial hemorrhage

- Diagnosis: maternal serum antibodies against fetal platelet antigen
- Management:
    - HPA-matched platelets if available
    - Maternal platelets (washed to remove plasma)
    - IVIG
    - Corticosteroids
    - Avoid NSAIDs
    - Transfuse prophylactically if <30,000/μL

Sepsis-Related Thrombocytopenia:

- Often part of DIC
- Treat underlying infection
- Platelet transfusion if:
    - Platelet count <50,000/μL and bleeding
    - Platelet count <30,000/μL
    - Invasive procedures
- Treat coagulopathy

Kasabach-Merritt Syndrome:

- Hemangioma with consumption coagulopathy
- Severe thrombocytopenia

- Bleeding risk
- Management:
  - Propranolol or corticosteroids for hemangioma
  - Platelet transfusion if bleeding
  - Fresh frozen plasma if coagulopathy
  - Avoid trauma to lesion

Coagulation Disorders

Vitamin K Deficiency Bleeding (VKDB)

Pathophysiology:

- Deficiency of vitamin K-dependent factors (II, VII, IX, X)
- Immature gut flora unable to synthesize vitamin K
- Limited placental transfer
- Neonatal factors naturally lower

Risk Factors:

- Lack of prophylactic vitamin K
- Exclusive breastfeeding (low vitamin K in breast milk)
- Malabsorption
- Antibiotic use (destroys gut flora)

- Maternal anticonvulsant use

Clinical Presentation:

Early VKDB (24-48 hours):

- Cephalohematoma
- Intracranial hemorrhage
- GI bleeding
- Skin bleeding

Classic VKDB (2-7 days):

- GI bleeding (most common)
- Melena
- Hematemesis
- Jaundice

Late VKDB (2-12 weeks):

- Intracranial hemorrhage (most common)
- GI bleeding
- Skin bleeding
- Associated with exclusive breastfeeding

Diagnosis:

- Prolonged PT and aPTT
- Normal fibrinogen
- Normal platelet count

- Normal thrombin time
- Corrects with vitamin K administration

Management:

- Vitamin K1 (phytonadione): 1 mg IV/IM
- Repeat dose if no response
- Fresh frozen plasma if active bleeding and vitamin K given
- Prothrombin complex concentrate alternative
- Supportive care
- Identify and treat underlying cause

Prevention:

- Vitamin K prophylaxis at birth: 1 mg IM
- More effective than oral route
- Single dose provides protection

Disseminated Intravascular Coagulation (DIC)

Pathophysiology:

- Activation of coagulation cascade
- Consumption of platelets and clotting factors
- Formation of microthrombi
- Tissue damage and bleeding

Risk Factors:

- Sepsis (most common)
- Severe asphyxia
- Massive hemolysis
- Placental abruption
- Severe respiratory distress
- Severe liver disease
- Transfusion reaction

Clinical Presentation:

- Bleeding from multiple sites
- Petechiae and purpura
- GI bleeding
- Pulmonary hemorrhage
- Intracranial hemorrhage
- Shock
- Organ dysfunction
- Acrocyanosis, gangrene (severe)

Diagnosis:

- Prolonged PT and aPTT
- Thrombocytopenia

- Low fibrinogen (<100 mg/dL)
- Elevated D-dimer
- Elevated fibrin degradation products
- Schistocytes on blood smear
- Bleeding manifestations

Management:

- Treat underlying cause (antibiotics for sepsis)
- Supportive care
- Platelet transfusion: target >50,000/μL
- Fresh frozen plasma: 10-15 mL/kg
- Cryoprecipitate: 1 unit/kg if fibrinogen <100 mg/dL
- Prothrombin complex concentrate if available
- Avoid further triggering events
- Monitor coagulation parameters
- Serial hemoglobin checks
- Organ support as needed

Hemophilia

Hemophilia A (Factor VIII Deficiency):

- X-linked recessive

- Rare presentation in neonates (usually diagnosed later): "typically you can pick it up whenever baby experienced a swelling after IM injection , notably after vitamin k injection post delivery"
- Risk of bleeding with trauma or invasive procedures
- Diagnosis: low factor VIII level
- Management: factor VIII replacement

Hemophilia B (Factor IX Deficiency – Christmas Disease):

- X-linked recessive
- Similar to hemophilia A
- Diagnosis: low factor IX level
- Management: factor IX replacement

Management in Neonatal Period:

- Avoid invasive procedures if possible
- Use gentle technique if procedures necessary
- Factor replacement if bleeding occurs
- Genetic counseling
- Long-term hematology management

Neonatal Blood Products Transfusion

Indications for Transfusion

Packed Red Blood Cells:

- Symptomatic anemia
- Hemoglobin <7 g/dL (stable infant)
- Hemoglobin <10 g/dL (with respiratory support)
- Hemoglobin <12 g/dL (severe cardiopulmonary disease)
- Acute blood loss >15% blood volume
- Ongoing bleeding
- Severe hemolytic disease

Whole Blood:

- Massive hemorrhage requiring >50% blood volume replacement
- Rare in modern practice
- Fresh whole blood preferred if available

Fresh Frozen Plasma:

- Coagulation factor deficiency
- DIC
- Vitamin K deficiency bleeding (with vitamin K)
- Massive transfusion

- Dose: 10-15 mL/kg
- Thaws at 37°C, use within 30 minutes

Platelets:

- Platelet count <50,000/μL and bleeding
- Platelet count <30,000/μL (prophylactic)
- Invasive procedures with thrombocytopenia
- Dose: 10 mL/kg or 1 unit per kg
- Transfuse over 15-30 minutes

Cryoprecipitate:

- Fibrinogen <100 mg/dL
- DIC with bleeding
- Dose: 1 unit/kg
- Contains fibrinogen, factor VIII, von Willebrand factor, fibronectin

Blood Product Selection

Type and Crossmatch:

- Type O negative blood preferred for emergency transfusion
- Type-specific blood if available
- Crossmatched blood preferred

- Direct antiglobulin test (DAT) negative blood for HDN

CMV Status:

- CMV-negative blood for preterm infants <32 weeks
- CMV-negative for immunocompromised infants
- Leukoreduction alternative to CMV testing

Irradiation:

- Irradiated blood for:
  - Immunocompromised infants
  - Intrauterine transfusion recipients
  - Exchange transfusion (controversial)
- Prevents transfusion-associated graft-versus-host disease (TA-GVHD)

Age of Blood:

- Fresh blood preferred for massive transfusion
- Avoid blood >7 days old if possible
- Consider 2,3-DPG levels (lower in older blood)

Transfusion Technique

Vascular Access:

- Peripheral IV line acceptable
- Central line preferred for large volumes

- Umbilical venous catheter for emergency transfusion

Administration:

- Use blood warmer (avoid hypothermia)
- Use 18-20 gauge needle or IV catheter
- Infuse over 15-30 minutes (slower for cardiac disease)
- Monitor vital signs throughout
- Have resuscitation equipment available

Monitoring:

- Vital signs before, during, after transfusion
- Assess for transfusion reaction
- Monitor for volume overload
- Serial hemoglobin/hematocrit
- Reassess clinical status

Transfusion Reactions

Acute Hemolytic Reaction:

- Incompatible blood
- Fever, chills, hemoglobinuria
- Hemolysis, jaundice
- Shock, renal failure

- Management: stop transfusion, supportive care, fluids

Febrile Reaction:

- Fever during or after transfusion
- Common in preterm infants
- Usually benign
- Management: slow infusion rate, antipyretics

Allergic Reaction:

- Urticaria, pruritus
- Usually mild
- Management: slow infusion, antihistamines
- Severe: stop transfusion, treat anaphylaxis

Transfusion-Associated Circulatory Overload (TACO):

- Fluid overload
- Pulmonary edema, respiratory distress
- Hypertension
- Risk factors: cardiac disease, renal failure
- Management: slow infusion rate, diuretics, oxygen

Transfusion-Associated Acute Lung Injury (TRALI):

- Acute respiratory distress 1-6 hours post-transfusion
- Fever, hypoxemia, pulmonary edema

- Rare in neonates
- Management: oxygen, ventilation support, supportive care

Transfusion-Associated Graft-versus-Host Disease (TA-GVHD):

- Donor T cells attack host tissues
- Rash, diarrhea, hepatitis, cytopenias
- Usually fatal if develops
- Prevention: irradiate blood

Exchange Transfusion

Brief Review

- Indications: severe hyperbilirubinemia, hemolytic disease
- Removes bilirubin (85%) and RBCs
- Double volume exchange: 160-180 mL/kg
- Umbilical venous catheter placement
- Risks: electrolyte abnormalities, infection, cardiac arrhythmias
- Complications: thrombosis, perforation, NEC

Erythropoietin (EPO) and Anemia of Prematurity

Pathophysiology

- Decreased EPO response to anemia
- Relative EPO deficiency
- Blunted erythropoiesis
- Multiple phlebotomies for laboratory testing
- Shortened RBC lifespan
- Results in hemoglobin decline over first 8-12 weeks

Clinical Significance

- "Physiologic anemia" of prematurity
- Usually requires transfusion by 4-8 weeks
- Associated with poor growth and neurodevelopmental outcomes
- Chronic hypoxia may occur

EPO Therapy

Indications:

- Hemoglobin <10 g/dL in preterm infant "persistent , not responding to transfusions"

- Ongoing transfusion requirements
- Contraindication to transfusion
- Maternal preference
- "Some clinicians advocate its use in HIE"

Dosing:

- Recombinant EPO (rEPO): 400-600 units/kg 2-3 times weekly
- Or darbepoetin alfa (longer half-life)
- IV or SC administration
- Requires iron supplementation

Efficacy:

- Reduces transfusion requirements by 30-50%
- Takes 1-2 weeks to show effect
- Requires adequate iron stores
- Response variable among infants

Risks:

- Hypertension
- Thrombosis
- Retinopathy of prematurity (controversial)
- Increased infection risk

- Cost

Current Use:

- Not routinely recommended
- Consider in specific situations
- Requires careful monitoring
- Iron supplementation essential

Iron Metabolism and Supplementation

Iron Status in Neonates

- Higher iron stores at birth (from maternal transfer)
- Preterm infants have lower iron stores
- Iron stores adequate for first 2-3 months
- After 3 months, exogenous iron needed

Iron Supplementation

Indications:

- Preterm infants: start at 2-4 weeks
- Term infants: start at 4-6 months
- Exclusive formula feeding (iron-fortified formula)

- Exclusive breastfeeding (breast milk low in iron)
- EPO therapy

Dosing:

- Elemental iron: 2-4 mg/kg/day
- Ferrous sulfate: 6-12 mg/kg/day (contains 20% elemental iron)
- Divide into once or twice daily dosing
- Give with vitamin C for better absorption
- Separate from calcium, phosphate, zinc

Monitoring:

- Hemoglobin and hematocrit
- Ferritin levels
- Assess for iron overload
- Monitor for constipation (common side effect)

Hemoglobinopathies in Neonates

Sickle Cell Disease

Newborn Screening:

- Hemoglobin electrophoresis on dried blood spot

- Part of universal newborn screening
- Identifies HbS and HbC
- Early identification allows intervention

Clinical Presentation in Neonates:

- Usually asymptomatic (HbF protective)
- First symptoms typically 3-6 months
- Dactylitis (hand-foot syndrome)
- Painful vaso-occlusive crises
- Acute chest syndrome
- Splenic sequestration
- Stroke risk

Neonatal Management:

- Confirmation of diagnosis
- Genetic counseling
- Family education
- Penicillin prophylaxis: 125 mg PO BID starting 2 months
- Folic acid supplementation
- Immunizations (pneumococcal, meningococcal)
- Pain management

- Hydration
- Hematology referral

Long-term Outcomes:

- Highly variable
- Organ involvement over time
- Stroke risk 5-15% by age 18
- Bone marrow transplantation option
- Gene therapy emerging

Thalassemia

Neonatal Presentation:

- Usually asymptomatic at birth
- HbF protective initially
- Symptoms develop after 3-6 months
- Severe anemia
- Hepatosplenomegaly
- Growth retardation
- Bone deformities

Newborn Screening:

- Hemoglobin electrophoresis

- Elevated HbA2 and HbF
- Microcytic, hypochromic anemia

Neonatal Management:

- Confirmation of diagnosis
- Genetic counseling
- Family education
- Transfusion protocol
- Iron chelation
- Folic acid supplementation
- Hematology referral

Key Takeaways

Neonatal hematologic disorders and transfusion medicine require:

- Understanding of normal neonatal hematology
- Recognition of pathologic values and conditions
- Appropriate diagnostic approach
- Evidence-based transfusion practice
- Careful monitoring during transfusions
- Prevention of transfusion complications

- Management of coagulation disorders
- Long-term follow-up for hemoglobinopathies
- Family education and genetic counseling
- Multidisciplinary team approach

Optimal hematologic management and judicious transfusion practice improve neonatal outcomes and reduce morbidity and mortality.

Chapter Seventeen

CARDIOVASCULAR DISORDERS IN NEONATES

Introduction: Why Cardiac Problems Matter in the First Days of Life

If you're managing a newborn with cardiovascular compromise, you're dealing with one of the most time-sensitive challenges in neonatology. The difference between recognizing a cardiac problem early and missing it can be the difference between a good outcome and a catastrophic one. The heart is working "overtime" in those first hours and days—transitioning from fetal circulation, adapting to breathing air, and managing the demands of extrauterine life. When things go wrong, they can deteriorate rapidly.

In this chapter, we're not diving into exhaustive cardiac physiology or rare congenital lesions. Instead, we're focusing on what you need to recognize and manage at the bedside"Clinically-Oriented-Approach". We're talking about the conditions that will actually cross your path, the ones that demand immediate action, and the ones where your clinical judgment makes the difference between life and death.

The cardinal rule: If a baby looks sick and you can't explain it with respiratory disease, infection, or metabolic problems, think cardiac. Your index of suspicion needs to be high.

Understanding the Transition: Normal Versus Abnormal

What's Supposed to Happen

Fetal circulation is fundamentally different from postnatal circulation. In utero, the baby doesn't breathe, so the lungs are fluid-filled and high-resistance. Blood bypasses the lungs through the ductus venosus, foramen ovale, and ductus arteriosus. The placenta does the work of gas exchange.

When that baby takes its first breath, everything changes—and it has to change quickly. Pulmonary vascular resistance drops dramatically as the lungs expand. The foramen ovale functionally closes as left atrial pressure exceeds right atrial pressure. The ductus arteriosus begins to close. Within hours to days, these transitions should be complete.

When It Goes Wrong

Cardiovascular problems in neonates fall into several categories:

1. Failure of normal transition (persistent pulmonary hypertension, patent ductus arteriosus)

2. Congenital heart defects (some present immediately, others take days to manifest)

3. Acquired problems (myocarditis, arrhythmias, shock states)

4. Structural issues (cardiomyopathy, pericardial effusion)

Your job is to recognize which category you're dealing with and act accordingly.

Recognition: The Clinical Red Flags

What You're Looking For

Don't wait for a perfect clinical picture. If you see "ANY combination" of these signs, you need to think cardiac:

Respiratory Distress That Doesn't Match the Chest X-ray

- The baby is working hard to breathe, but the lungs look relatively clear

- Or the baby has pulmonary edema but minimal respiratory effort (that's a bad sign—means the heart is failing)

- Tachypnea out of proportion to oxygen needs

Poor Perfusion

- Delayed capillary refill time(>2 seconds)

- Weak or thready pulses
- Cold extremities
- Mottled skin
- Low blood pressure target for age

Cyanosis

- Central cyanosis (tongue, lips, trunk) that doesn't improve with oxygen
- This is your red flag for right-to-left shunting

Hepatomegaly

- Liver edge >2 cm below costal margin"measuring liver span is challenging"
- Suggests right heart failure or severe left heart failure

Murmurs or Abnormal Heart Sounds

- Not all murmurs are benign
- A continuous murmur suggests PDA
- A single loud S2 suggests pulmonary hypertension
- Gallop rhythm (S3) suggests heart failure

Metabolic Acidosis Out of Proportion

- Lactic acidosis with normal glucose and oxygen
- Suggests tissue hypoperfusion from cardiogenic shock

Feeding Intolerance

- Baby won't feed or tires quickly
- Excessive sweating during feeds
- This is heart failure until proven otherwise

The Baby Just Looks Sick

- Lethargy, poor tone, weak cry
- Trust your gut. If something feels wrong, it probably is.

What to Do Immediately

Your First Actions (Do These at the moment)

1. Get Oxygen On Board
   - Place on pulse oximetry and continuous monitoring
   - Provide supplemental oxygen if SpO_2 <90%
   - Remember: oxygen is a pulmonary vasodilator—if the baby improves dramatically with oxygen, you're likely dealing with pulmonary hypertension
2. Establish IV Access
   - You'll need this for medications and fluids
   - Don't delay—get a line in
3. Get a Blood Gas
   - Arterial or capillary

- You need to know: pH, pCO_2, pO_2, lactate, base deficit
- Metabolic acidosis with normal pO_2 = "shock"

4. Check Blood Pressure
    - Use appropriate cuff size (bladder encircles 80% of arm)
    - The gold standard of monitoring is through "Invasive arterial line transducer"
    - Hypotension in a sick baby is a LATE finding—don't wait for it
    - Normal systolic BP roughly = 50 + (weight in kg × 2)
5. Assess Perfusion
    - Capillary refill
    - Pulse quality (central and peripheral)
    - Skin temperature gradient (cold extremities = poor perfusion)
    - Urine output
6. Get a Chest X-Ray
    - Look for pulmonary edema, cardiomegaly, pneumothorax
    - Compare to respiratory findings
7. Call for Help
    - Don't manage this alone
    - Get pediatric cardiology or transport team involved early

- Don't wait until the baby is crashing

Diagnostic Approach: Making Sense of the Data

The Echocardiogram: Your Most Useful Tool

If you suspect a cardiac problem, get an echo done. Period. Don't wait for other tests.

What the echo tells you:

- Cardiac structure (are there obvious defects?)
- Cardiac function (is the heart squeezing well?)
- Shunt direction (is blood going the right way?)
- Pulmonary artery pressure (is there hypertension?)
- Pericardial effusion
- Ductus arteriosus size and direction of flow

The bedside echo is your friend. Even if you're not a cardiologist, a good bedside echo can answer critical questions:

- Is the heart function depressed?
- Is there a large PDA?
- Is there pulmonary hypertension?
- Is there a pericardial effusion?

If you don't have echo capability, transfer the baby. This is not something to guess about.

ECG"EKG": Quick and Informative

Get an ECG if:

- You suspect an arrhythmia (irregular heart rate, very fast or very slow)
- You suspect myocarditis (sick baby with cardiac signs)
- You're evaluating for structural defects

What to look for:

- Rate: Is it reasonable for age? (Normal: 100-160 bpm)
- Rhythm: Regular or irregular?
- Axis: Is it normal for age?
- ST changes or T wave abnormalities suggesting ischemia"remember that T wave is normally showed a positive deflection in the first week of life then becomes negative afterwards during the entire neonatal period and mostly beyond in infancy"

Troponin and BNP

These can be helpful but don't drive management alone.

- Troponin: Elevated in myocarditis, hypoxia, or severe heart failure

- BNP"B-type Natriuretic Peptide": Elevated in heart failure

They're useful for confirming your clinical suspicion, not for ruling things in or out.

Lactate

If your baby has metabolic acidosis with elevated lactate, you're dealing with tissue hypoperfusion. This is cardiogenic shock until proven otherwise. It demands immediate intervention.

Common Conditions: Recognition and Management

1. PATENT DUCTUS ARTERIOSUS (PDA)

What's Happening: The ductus arteriosus fails to close, allowing blood to shunt left-to-right from the aorta to the pulmonary artery. In premature infants, this is common. In term infants, it's usually clinically insignificant. But when it matters, it matters a lot.

When It Matters:

- Premature infants (especially <28 weeks)
- Babies with respiratory distress syndrome
- Babies with sepsis
- Babies receiving indomethacin or ibuprofen (which can paradoxically worsen PDA by reducing renal blood flow)

Recognition:

- Continuous "machinery" murmur (or at least a continuous

component)

- Wide pulse pressure (bounding pulses)
- Hyperactive precordium
- Pulmonary edema on CXR
- Left heart volume overload on echo
- Large LA:Ao ratio on echo

The Mistake Many Clinicians Make: Thinking a PDA murmur means the baby needs treatment. Most PDAs in term infants are benign. You treat based on clinical impact, not the presence of a murmur.

What to Do:

Immediate management:

- Fluid restriction (typically 120-140 mL/kg/day)
- Diuretics if pulmonary edema (furosemide 1 mg/kg IV)
- Maintain adequate oxygenation and ventilation
- Avoid excessive fluid administration

Pharmacologic closure (if clinically significant):

- Indomethacin: 0.1 mg/kg IV every 12-24 hours × 3 doses
    - Avoid if: active infection, NEC, thrombocytopenia <50k, bleeding
    - Success rate ~70%
- Ibuprofen: 10 mg/kg loading, then 5 mg/kg at 24 and 48 hours

- Similar efficacy to indomethacin, possibly fewer renal effects
- Still avoid in active infection, NEC

Acetaminophen is emerging as a first line : 15mg/kg/dose every 6 hours for 5-7 days

Surgical closure:

- Reserved for failed medical management or contraindications to medical therapy
- Ligation or catheter-based closure

When to Escalate:

- If the baby requires increasing oxygen despite PDA treatment
- If pulmonary edema worsens
- If renal function deteriorates
- If the baby develops NEC (stop medical therapy immediately)

2. PERSISTENT PULMONARY HYPERTENSION OF THE NEWBORN (PPHN)

What's Happening: Pulmonary vascular resistance fails to drop after birth. Blood shunts right-to-left through fetal channels (foramen ovale, ductus arteriosus), causing severe hypoxemia that doesn't respond to oxygen.

Risk Factors:

- Meconium aspiration syndrome
- Sepsis/chorioamnionitis
- Maternal diabetes
- Maternal NSAID use
- Congenital diaphragmatic hernia
- Idiopathic (sometimes no clear cause)

Recognition:

- Central cyanosis that doesn't respond to high-flow oxygen—this is your key sign
- Severe tachypnea and respiratory distress
- Hypoxemia with normal or low pCO_2
- Right-to-left shunting on echo (bubble study positive)
- Elevated right atrial pressure
- RV hypertrophy on echo
- Labile oxygen saturations (drops with handling, improves with sedation)

The Critical Insight: If a baby is cyanotic and oxygen doesn't help, you're thinking PPHN. The baby's lungs are fine—it's the pulmonary vessels that won't relax.

What to Do:

Immediate stabilization:

- Avoid stimulation (handling causes desaturation)

- Keep baby warm and calm
- Adequate sedation (morphine or fentanyl)
- Mechanical ventilation if needed
- Maintain adequate oxygenation and ventilation (pCO_2 35-45)

Pulmonary vasodilation:

- Inhaled nitric oxide (iNO): 20 ppm initially
  - Gold standard for PPHN
  - Dilates pulmonary vessels, reduces shunting
  - Response usually seen within 30 minutes
  - Taper slowly to avoid rebound
- Sildenafil: 0.5-2 mg/kg IV or PO
  - Phosphodiesterase-5 inhibitor
  - Useful when iNO unavailable or for chronic PPHN
- Milrinone: 0.25-0.75 mcg/kg/min IV
  - Inotrope and pulmonary vasodilator
  - Useful for RV failure
  - Avoid if there is significant hypotension

Systemic support:

- Maintain adequate blood pressure (dopamine or dobutamine if hypotensive)

- Correct metabolic acidosis (which worsens pulmonary vasoconstriction)
- Avoid hypothermia

ECMO:

- If refractory to maximum medical management
- This is a rescue therapy—transfer to ECMO center immediately if available

When to Escalate:

- If SpO_2 remains <85% despite high-flow oxygen and ventilation
- If iNO is unavailable, transfer immediately
- If the baby develops shock or severe acidosis
- If you see signs of right heart failure (rising CVP, hepatomegaly)

3. CONGENITAL HEART DEFECTS: The Ones You Need to Recognize

<u>Cyanotic Defects (Right-to-Left Shunt)</u>

Transposition of the Great Arteries (TGA):

- Aorta arises from RV, pulmonary artery from LV (backwards)

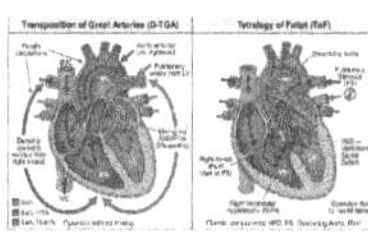

- Presents with severe cyanosis in first hours/days
- CXR shows "egg on string" appearance
- Echo shows aorta anterior to PA
- EMERGENCY: Start prostaglandin E1 (PGE1) 0.05-0.1 mcg/kg/min IV to keep ductus arteriosus open
- Balloon atrial septostomy (Rashkind procedure) at catheterization
- Definitive treatment: Arterial switch operation

Tetralogy of Fallot (TOF):

- VSD, RV outflow obstruction, RV hypertrophy, overriding aorta
- Presents with cyanosis (blue baby)
- May have "tet spells" (sudden severe cyanosis from increased RV outflow obstruction)
- Management: Prostaglandin E1 to keep PDA open, beta-blockers for spells, definitive surgical repair

Tricuspid Atresia:

- No tricuspid valve, ASD and PDA required for survival
- Severe cyanosis
- EMERGENCY: Start PGE1 immediately
- Staged surgical repair (Fontan procedure)

Acyanotic Defects (Left-to-Right Shunt)

Ventricular Septal Defect (VSD):

- Most common congenital heart defect
- Small defects: asymptomatic, incidental murmur
- Large defects: heart failure, pulmonary edema
- Management: Fluid restriction, diuretics, ACE inhibitors if needed
- Most small VSDs close spontaneously

Atrial Septal Defect (ASD):

- Usually well-tolerated in infancy
- May present later with exercise intolerance
- Often detected incidentally on echo
- Usually no acute management needed

Patent Foramen Ovale (PFO):

- Normal variant in many people
- Clinically insignificant in infancy
- Don't treat it "Needs follow up with cardiologist later on"

Coarctation of the Aorta:

- Narrowing of descending aorta
- May present with shock or differential BP between upper and lower extremities

- Lower extremity pulses weak or absent
- Start PGE1 to keep PDA open (maintains lower body perfusion)
- Definitive treatment: Surgical repair

The Key Point About Congenital Defects: If you suspect a structural heart defect, get an echo immediately. Don't guess. Don't wait. The echo will tell you what you're dealing with and what needs to happen next.

4. CARDIOGENIC SHOCK

What's Happening: The heart can't pump enough blood to meet the body's needs. This can result from poor contractility, arrhythmia, excessive afterload, or other causes.

Recognition:

- Poor perfusion (delayed cap refill, weak pulses, cool extremities)
- Hypotension (late sign—don't wait for this)
- Metabolic acidosis with elevated lactate
- Oliguria (<1 mL/kg/hr)
- Altered mental status
- Pulmonary edema
- Hepatomegaly

Causes in Neonates:

- Myocarditis (viral, bacterial)
- Severe sepsis
- Cardiomyopathy
- Severe anemia
- Severe arrhythmia
- Tamponade (pericardial effusion)

What to Do:

Immediate:

- Establish IV access (central line preferred)
- Aggressive fluid resuscitation: 10-20 mL/kg normal saline bolus over 5-10 minutes
- Assess response: improved perfusion, higher BP, better urine output
- If no response or worsening, hold further fluids

Inotropic support:"The First choice of these medications is guaranteed by clinical context"

- Epinephrine , and or Norepinephrine both of almost same dosages 0.1-1 mcg/kg/m "potent vasopressors"
- Vasopressin "0.01-0.1 unit/kg/h "reserved for intractable hypotension , not responding to vasopressors"
- Dopamine: 5-20 mcg/kg/min
    - At low doses: renal vasodilation

    - At higher doses: inotropy and systemic vasoconstriction
- Dobutamine: 5-20 mcg/kg/min
    - Inotrope with less vasoconstriction
    - Good for cardiogenic shock with adequate BP
- Milrinone: 0.25-0.75 mcg/kg/min
    - Inotrope + pulmonary/systemic vasodilator
    - Avoid in conditions with "low peripheral resistance " "as in septic shock"
    - Good for right heart failure or pulmonary hypertension

Address underlying cause:

- Antibiotics if sepsis
- Specific treatment if myocarditis
- Drain pericardial effusion if tamponade
- Treat arrhythmia if present

Supportive care:

- Maintain oxygenation and ventilation
- Correct metabolic acidosis
- Maintain normothermia
- Monitor urine output closely

When to Escalate:

- If shock worsens despite two inotropes
- If lactate continues rising
- If urine output remains <0.5 mL/kg/hr
- Consider ECMO if available

5. ARRHYTHMIAS

Supraventricular Tachycardia (SVT):

- Heart rate >220 bpm
- Usually regular rhythm
- Often secondary to accessory pathway (Wolff-Parkinson-White)
- Recognition: Suddenly fast heart rate, may have poor perfusion if sustained
- Management:
    - Traditionally "Ice to face" (vagal maneuver) only try it if you have no facility.
    - Adenosine 0.1 mg/kg IV push (max 6 mg) if IV access available
    - Synchronized cardioversion (0.5-1 J/kg) if unstable
    - Propranolol or digoxin for chronic management"prescribed by cardiologist"

Bradycardia:

- Heart rate <100 bpm
- Often secondary to hypoxia, hypothermia, increased ICP, or heart block
- Management: Treat underlying cause
    - Oxygen and ventilation if hypoxic
    - Rewarm if hypothermic
    - Atropine 0.02 mg/kg IV if no response to above
    - Pacing if complete heart block

Premature Atrial or Ventricular Contractions:

- Usually benign
- Disappear with maturation
- No treatment needed unless frequent and causing symptoms

Common Pitfalls and Mistakes

Mistake #1: Assuming a Murmur Means Disease – Many newborns have innocent murmurs. A PDA murmur doesn't mean the baby needs treatment. Clinical context matters.

Mistake #2: Missing Cyanosis Because You're Focused on Respiratory Disease – If the baby is cyanotic and the lungs look relatively clear, think cardiac. Don't assume it's all respiratory.

Mistake #3: Delaying Echocardiography – If you suspect a cardiac problem, get an echo. Don't wait for other tests. The echo is your diagnostic tool.

Mistake #4: Treating PDA Aggressively in Term Infants – Most PDAs in term infants are hemodynamically insignificant. Treat the baby, not the murmur.

Mistake #5: Not Starting Prostaglandin E1 Early in Suspected Ductus-Dependent Lesions – If you suspect TGA, critical aortic stenosis, or other ductus-dependent lesion, start PGE1 immediately. Don't wait for confirmation. Every minute counts.

Mistake #6: Attributing All Shock to Sepsis – Not all shocked babies have infection. Consider cardiogenic shock, especially if the baby has signs of heart failure or metabolic acidosis out of proportion.

Mistake #7: Giving Excessive Fluids in Heart Failure – Fluid overload worsens pulmonary edema and heart failure. Use diuretics and fluid restriction, not more fluids.

When to Escalate Care

Don't hesitate to escalate if:

- Severe cyanosis not responding to oxygen: Think PPHN or cyanotic heart defect. Consider transfer to a facility with iNO and ECMO capability.
- Shock that doesn't respond to initial resuscitation: Get inotropes started and consider transfer for advanced support.
- Suspected ductus-dependent lesion: Transfer to cardiac center for intervention.
- Severe arrhythmia: Get cardiology involved immediately.

- Signs of pericardial tamponade: Drain immediately or transfer.
- Myocarditis with declining function: Consider transfer for possible ECMO.

The Bottom Line: If you're uncertain, escalate. These babies deteriorate quickly, and having advanced support available is critical.

Key Clinical Pearls

1. Trust your gut. If a baby looks sick and you can't explain it with lungs or infection, think cardiac.
2. Cyanosis that doesn't improve with oxygen = cardiac problem until proven otherwise. This is your red flag.
3. Get an echo early. It's your most useful diagnostic tool. Don't manage cardiac problems without it.
4. Prostaglandin E1 is your friend in suspected ductus-dependent lesions. Start it early. It's hard to hurt with PGE1.
5. Poor perfusion is a sign of shock. Don't wait for hypotension. Act on cool extremities, delayed cap refill, and oliguria.
6. Metabolic acidosis with elevated lactate = tissue hypoperfusion. This is cardiogenic shock until proven otherwise.
7. Treat the baby, not the murmur. Many murmurs are innocent. Clinical context determines management.
8. Pulmonary edema + normal lung sounds = heart failure until

proven otherwise.

9. Hepatomegaly in a sick baby = heart failure or shock. Investigate immediately.

10. When in doubt, transfer. Cardiac emergencies move fast. Having the right level of care available early makes a difference.

Summary

Cardiovascular problems in neonates demand your highest index of suspicion and fastest action. The key is recognizing when a baby is sick from a cardiac cause rather than attributing everything to respiratory disease or infection.

Your tools are simple: clinical assessment, oxygen response, echocardiography, and basic labs. Your actions are decisive: oxygen, IV access, fluid management, inotropes, and early escalation when needed.

Remember: these babies don't have time for you to be uncertain. If you suspect a cardiac problem, act on it. Get help. Get an echo. Start treatment. Transfer if needed. The babies who do well are the ones whose problems are recognized early and managed aggressively from the start.

Chapter Eighteen

GASTROINTESTINAL DISORDERS IN NEONATES

Introduction: The GI Tract as Your Window into Neonatal Health

If a baby isn't feeding well, isn't defecate normally, or has a distended abdomen, you need to pay attention. The gastrointestinal tract tells you things about what's happening systemically—it's not just about digestion and nutrition, though those matter enormously. A baby with feeding intolerance might be septic. A baby with bilious vomiting might have a surgical emergency. A baby with bloody stools might be developing necrotizing enterocolitis, one of the most devastating complications of neonatal care.

In this chapter, we're focusing on the GI problems you'll actually encounter at the bedside. We're not going deep into rare anatomic anomalies or obscure metabolic disorders. We're talking about the conditions that will test your clinical judgment, demand quick decision-making, and require you to know when to feed, when to hold feeds, and when to call the surgeon.

The cardinal rule: Any change in feeding tolerance, any abdominal distension, any vomiting or stool changes requires investigation. Don't assume it's normal. Don't assume it will resolve. Investigate.

Understanding Normal Neonatal GI Function

What Should Be Happening

In the first hours and days of life, the neonatal GI tract is establishing itself. Meconium should pass within the first 24-48 hours. Feeding should progress gradually. Stools should transition from meconium (black, sticky) to transitional stools (greenish-brown) to milk stools (yellow, seedy in breastfed infants; tan and paste-like in formula-fed).

Abdominal distension should be minimal. Residual gastric volumes should be small or absent. The baby should show hunger cues and coordinate sucking, swallowing, and breathing.

When It's Not Normal

You need to recognize the warning signs early:

- Feeding intolerance: Large residual volumes, vomiting, poor intake

- Abdominal distension: Tight, shiny abdomen; visible veins
- Abnormal stools: Bloody, mucoid, absent, or explosive
- Bilious vomiting: Any green vomit is abnormal and needs investigation
- Abdominal tenderness: Baby pulls away, cries with palpation
- Signs of systemic illness: Lethargy, temperature instability, poor perfusion

Recognition: Reading the Signs

What You're Looking For

Feeding Intolerance:

- Residual volumes >50% of previous feeding volume
- Vomiting or spitting up more than expected
- Abdominal distension before or after feeds
- Baby refuses to feed or falls asleep immediately
- Excessive gas or stooling

Abdominal Examination Red Flags:

- Distension that's tense or rigid (not just soft fullness)
- Visible peristalsis or loops of bowel

- Abdominal wall erythema or discoloration (suggests underlying inflammation or perforation)
- Tenderness with palpation
- Absent or hyperactive bowel sounds
- Hepatomegaly or splenomegaly
- Palpable mass

Vomiting Characteristics:

- Bilious (green): Always abnormal—suggests obstruction or ileus
- Projectile: Suggests pyloric stenosis (though rare in first days)
- Bloody or coffee-ground: Suggests GI bleeding or NEC
- Frequency: Occasional spit-up is normal; frequent vomiting is not

Stool Changes:

- Bloody stools: Can be swallowed maternal blood (Apt test), cow's milk protein allergy, or NEC
- Mucoid stools: Suggests inflammation
- Absent stools: In first 48 hours, normal; after that, concerning
- Explosive diarrhea: Suggests infection or food intolerance

Systemic Signs:

- Lethargy or poor tone

- Temperature instability (hypothermia especially concerning)
- Tachycardia or bradycardia
- Poor perfusion
- Metabolic acidosis

The Mistake Many Clinicians Make: Assuming that feeding intolerance is benign. It's not. Feeding intolerance is often the first sign of something serious—sepsis, NEC, obstruction, or other surgical pathology.

What to Do Immediately

Your First Actions (Do These at the moment)

1. Stop Feeds – Don't continue pushing feeds into a baby with feeding intolerance. Get an IV line for fluids and hold feeds pending investigation.

2. Assess Hydration and Perfusion

- Capillary refill
- Urine output
- Skin turgor
- Mucous membranes
- Blood pressure

3. Get Labs
    - CBC (infection, anemia)
    - CRP or procalcitonin (inflammation/infection)
    - Blood culture (if sepsis suspected)
    - Electrolytes (dehydration, imbalance)
    - Blood gas (metabolic acidosis suggests tissue damage)
    - Lactate (elevated in shock or NEC)
    - Glucose (hypoglycemia can cause poor feeding)
4. Get Abdominal Imaging
    - Abdominal X-ray (supine and left lateral decubitus or cross-table):
        - Look for: pneumatosis (air in bowel wall—NEC), free air (perforation), dilated loops, air-fluid levels
        - Pneumatosis is the most specific sign of NEC
        - Free air is a surgical emergency
    - Abdominal ultrasound: Can assess for obstruction, assess bowel wall thickness, evaluate for free fluid
5. Establish IV Access and Fluid Support
    - Normal saline or lactated Ringer's
    - Maintenance fluids initially
    - Hold feeds until you understand what's happening

6. Keep Baby NPO (Nothing by Mouth)
    - Nothing oral, nothing via tube
    - This gives the GI tract a rest and prevents further injury if there's inflammation
7. Consider Antibiotics
    - If sepsis is suspected, start empiric antibiotics after blood culture
    - Don't wait for confirmation
8. Call for Help
    - If you suspect NEC, surgical pathology, or severe illness, get senior support and surgical consultation
    - Don't manage this alone

Diagnostic Approach: Making Sense of the Data

Imaging Interpretation

Abdominal X-ray:

Normal findings:

- Gas throughout the bowel
- No free air
- No dilated loops
- Bowel wall thickness normal

Abnormal findings requiring action:

- Pneumatosis intestinalis: Air in the bowel wall (appears as linear lucency along bowel wall). This is NEC until proven otherwise.
- Free air (pneumoperitoneum): Air outside the bowel (appears as lucency under diaphragm on upright film or along liver edge on decubitus). This is perforation—surgical emergency.
- Dilated bowel loops: Suggests obstruction or ileus
- Air-fluid levels: Suggests obstruction
- Bowel wall edema: Thickened bowel wall suggests inflammation
- Ascites: Free fluid in abdomen suggests perforation or severe inflammation

Ultrasound:

- Can assess bowel wall thickness (normal <2 mm)
- Can look for free fluid
- Can assess for obstruction
- Can evaluate for pyloric stenosis if suspected
- More sensitive than X-ray for early NEC changes
- Recently "Point-Of-Care-UltraSound" promising to tackle the disease early

Clinical Scoring Systems

Modified Bell's Staging for NEC:

- Helps standardize severity and guide management
- Stage I (suspected): feeding intolerance, abdominal distension, mild metabolic acidosis
- Stage II (definite): pneumatosis on imaging, mild systemic signs
- Stage III (advanced): perforation, severe systemic illness, shock

Common Conditions: Recognition and Management

1. NECROTIZING ENTEROCOLITIS (NEC)

What's Happening: NEC is inflammation and necrosis of the bowel, typically affecting premature infants. The exact cause isn't fully understood, but it involves intestinal immaturity, abnormal bacterial colonization, feeding practices, and often a triggering event (hypoxia, sepsis, PDA).

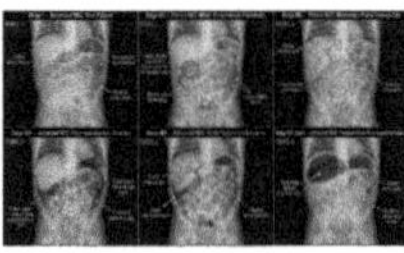

Risk Factors:

- Prematurity (especially <32 weeks)

- Low birth weight
- Hypoxia or shock
- Sepsis
- Rapid advancement of feeds
- Cow's milk formula (breast milk is protective)
- Patent ductus arteriosus

Recognition:

- Classic triad: Feeding intolerance + abdominal distension + bloody stools
- But not all babies present with all three
- Lethargy, temperature instability, poor perfusion (signs of systemic illness)
- Metabolic acidosis, elevated lactate
- Thrombocytopenia (platelets drop as disease progresses)
- Pneumatosis on imaging (most specific finding)

The Critical Insight: NEC is a progressive disease. Early recognition is everything. A baby with feeding intolerance and pneumatosis on X-ray is at risk of progressing to perforation and death if not managed aggressively.

What to Do:

Immediate:

- NPO (nothing by mouth)

- IV fluids (maintenance + replace losses)
- Nasogastric tube to suction (decompress bowel)
- Broad-spectrum antibiotics (ampicillin + gentamicin + metronidazole to cover gram-positive, gram-negative, and anaerobes)
- Continuous monitoring
- Serial abdominal exams (every 2-4 hours)
- Serial abdominal X-rays (to detect progression, free air)

Supportive care:

- Correct metabolic acidosis
- Maintain blood pressure (inotropes if needed)
- Correct coagulopathy (platelets, FFP if bleeding)
- Maintain oxygenation and ventilation
- NPO period: typically 7-10 days minimum

Feeding restart:

- After signs of inflammation resolve (normal exam, normal labs, normal imaging)
- Start with trophic feeds (10-20 mL/kg/day)
- Advance slowly (10-20 mL/kg/day increments)
- Use breast milk if possible (more protective than formula)
- Watch for recurrence

Surgical intervention:

- Indicated if: perforation (free air), clinical deterioration despite maximal medical management, abdominal wall erythema, palpable mass
- Procedures: Drain placement, resection of necrotic bowel, ostomy
- Don't delay surgery if baby is deteriorating

When to Escalate:

- If free air appears on imaging (surgical emergency)
- If baby deteriorates despite antibiotics and support
- If platelets drop rapidly (suggests worsening disease)
- If you see abdominal wall erythema or discoloration
- If lactate continues rising

2. GASTROESOPHAGEAL REFLUX

What's Happening: Acid from the stomach refluxes into the esophagus. In newborns, this is usually physiologic and improves with maturation.

Recognition:

- Spitting up or vomiting after feeds
- Irritability during or after feeds
- Arching back (suggests discomfort)

- Poor feeding or refusing feeds
- Hoarseness or stridor (if severe)
- Aspiration risk (especially if neurologically impaired)

The Mistake Many Clinicians Make: Treating every baby who spits up. Most babies with physiologic reflux don't need medication—they just need time to mature.

What to Do:

- Positioning: Head of bed elevated 30 degrees
- Small, frequent feeds
- Burp frequently during feeds
- Allow 20-30 minutes after feeds before lying flat
- Thickened feeds (rice cereal) if formula-fed and reflux significant
- Medications (if truly problematic):
    - Ranitidine: 2 mg/kg PO twice daily (reduces acid)
    - Omeprazole: 0.7-3.5 mg/kg PO daily (stronger acid reduction)
    - Metoclopramide: 0.1 mg/kg PO three times daily (increases gastric motility)
- Most babies improve without medication by 12-18 months

3. PYLORIC STENOSIS

What's Happening: Hypertrophy of the pylorus causes gastric outlet obstruction. More common in males, typically present at 2-8 weeks (rarely can occur in newborn period).

Recognition:

- Projectile vomiting (vomit shoots across room)
- Hungry after vomiting (wants to feed again immediately)
- Weight loss or failure to gain
- Dehydration
- Hypochloremic hypokalemic metabolic alkalosis (from loss of gastric acid)
- Visible peristaltic waves
- Palpable "olive" (hypertrophied pylorus) in epigastrium

Diagnosis:

- Ultrasound: Gold standard
    - Pyloric muscle thickness >3-4 mm
    - Pyloric channel length >14-16 mm
    - Gastric outlet obstruction

What to Do:

- NPO
- IV fluids (correct dehydration and electrolyte abnormalities first)

- Nasogastric tube to suction
- Surgical consultation (pyloromyotomy)
- Critical: Correct alkalosis and hypokalemia BEFORE surgery (risk of cardiac arrhythmias)
- Surgery: Ramstedt pyloromyotomy (dividing muscle without opening mucosa)

4. INTESTINAL OBSTRUCTION

Meconium Ileus:

- Occurs in cystic fibrosis
- Meconium is thick and inspissated, causing obstruction
- Recognition: Abdominal distension, bilious vomiting, no meconium passage
- Imaging: Dilated bowel loops, air-fluid levels, "microcolon"
- Management: Contrast enema (therapeutic—Gastrografin breaks down meconium), surgery if fails

Meconium Plug Syndrome:

- Meconium plug lower in colon
- Similar presentation to meconium ileus but less severe
- Often resolves with osmotic laxatives or enema

Small Bowel Atresia:

- Complete absence of bowel segment
- Bilious vomiting, abdominal distension
- "Double bubble" sign on X-ray (duodenal atresia)
- Surgical repair needed

Hirschsprung Disease:

- Absence of ganglion cells (aganglionosis) in distal bowel
- Presents with failure to pass meconium in first 48 hours
- Abdominal distension
- Contrast enema shows transition zone
- Definitive diagnosis: rectal biopsy (shows absence of ganglion cells)
- Surgical resection of aganglionic segment

Recognition of Obstruction:

- Bilious vomiting (any green vomit is abnormal)
- Progressive abdominal distension
- Absent or minimal stooling
- Air-fluid levels on X-ray
- Dilated bowel loops
- History of maternal polyhydramnios (suggests in-utero obstruction)

What to Do:

- NPO
- IV fluids
- Nasogastric tube to suction
- Abdominal imaging (X-ray, ultrasound, contrast studies as indicated)
- Surgical consultation
- Surgery for complete obstruction or failed conservative management

5. FEEDING INTOLERANCE (Non-Surgical)

What's Happening: The baby's GI tract isn't tolerating feeds, but there's no surgical pathology. This can be due to immaturity, mild infection, or other systemic illness.

Recognition:

- Large residual volumes
- Mild abdominal distension
- Vomiting or spit-up
- Normal imaging (no pneumatosis, no free air, no obstruction)
- Normal labs (no severe infection, no severe acidosis)
- Baby otherwise stable

What to Do:

- Hold feeds temporarily (24-48 hours)
- IV fluids
- Investigate for underlying cause (sepsis, other illness)
- Treat any underlying condition
- Resume feeds slowly when baby is ready
- Consider trophic feeds (minimal volume, not for nutrition) initially
- Advance feeds gradually
- Monitor residuals and tolerance

When Feeding Intolerance is a Sign of Something Else:

- Sepsis: Feeding intolerance is often the first sign. Get cultures and start antibiotics.
- Heart failure: Babies with cardiac disease often have poor feeding. Consider echo.
- Metabolic disease: Hypoglycemia, hyperglycemia, or other metabolic derangement can cause poor feeding.
- Neurologic issues: Poor suck, aspiration risk.

6. BLOODY STOOLS

Differential Diagnosis:

Swallowed Maternal Blood:

- Most common cause of bloody stools in first days
- Baby may have blood in mouth from delivery
- APT test: Stool tested for fetal vs. maternal hemoglobin (distinguishes)
- No treatment needed

Cow's Milk Protein Allergy:

- Occurs in formula-fed infants
- Bloody or mucoid stools
- Vomiting, diarrhea
- Usually after several days of formula feeding
- Management: Switch to hydrolyzed formula or amino acid formula
- Usually resolves within 72 hours of diet change

Necrotizing Enterocolitis:

- Bloody stools + feeding intolerance + distension + pneumatosis
- Requires immediate intervention (see NEC section)

Anal Fissure:

- Bright red blood on stool surface
- Baby strains during bowel movement

- Usually from constipation
- Management: Stool softeners, increased fluids

Infectious Gastroenteritis:

- Bloody diarrhea, vomiting
- Fever, systemic signs
- Viral or bacterial
- Management: Supportive care, antibiotics if bacterial

What to Do:

- Assess volume of bleeding (spot vs. significant)
- Get Apt test if unsure about source
- Assess hydration and perfusion
- Imaging if concerned about NEC or other pathology
- Treat underlying cause

Common Pitfalls and Mistakes

Mistake #1: Ignoring Feeding Intolerance – Feeding intolerance is a sign that something is wrong. Investigate it. Don't assume it will resolve on its own.

Mistake #2: Continuing to Advance Feeds in a Baby with Feeding Intolerance – Stop feeds. Hold feeds. Give the GI tract a rest. Forcing feeds into an intolerant baby worsens inflammation and increases risk of NEC.

Mistake #3: Missing Bilious Vomiting – Any green vomit is abnormal. It suggests obstruction or ileus. Investigate immediately.

Mistake #4: Delaying Surgery in a Baby with Perforation – Free air on X-ray is a surgical emergency. Don't wait. Get the surgeon now.

Mistake #5: Not Considering Sepsis in a Baby with Feeding Intolerance – Feeding intolerance is often the first sign of sepsis. Get cultures and start antibiotics before you're sure.

Mistake #6: Treating Physiologic Reflux Aggressively – Most babies spit up. It's normal. Don't medicate every baby. Position changes and time usually solve it.

Mistake #7: Not Correcting Electrolytes Before Surgery in Pyloric Stenosis – These babies are alkalotic and hypokalemic. Surgery in this state risks cardiac arrhythmias. Correct first.

Mistake #8: Advancing Feeds Too Quickly After NEC – The bowel needs time to heal. Start with trophic feeds. Advance slowly. Watch for recurrence.

When to Escalate Care

Don't hesitate to escalate if:

- Free air on imaging: Surgical emergency. Get surgeon now.
- Pneumatosis on imaging: Probable NEC. Needs intensive management.
- Bilious vomiting: Needs imaging and possible surgery.
- Severe abdominal distension with systemic signs: Possible perforation or severe illness.
- Rapidly deteriorating baby: Shock, severe acidosis, declining

platelets.

- Suspected surgical pathology: Don't wait. Get surgical consultation early.
- Baby not improving with conservative management: Consider transfer to facility with surgical capability.

Key Clinical Pearls

1. Feeding intolerance is abnormal. Investigate it. Don't assume it's benign.
2. Bilious vomiting is never normal. Any green vomit demands investigation.
3. Pneumatosis on X-ray = NEC until proven otherwise. Act immediately.
4. Free air = surgery. Don't delay.
5. The baby's abdomen tells you a lot. Serial exams matter. Changes matter.
6. Metabolic acidosis with elevated lactate in a baby with GI symptoms = tissue damage. Act urgently.
7. Breast milk is protective. If possible, use breast milk for feeding.
8. Hold feeds when you're unsure. It's better to hold feeds temporarily than to push feeds into a baby with an acute abdomen.

9. Sepsis often presents as feeding intolerance. Get cultures and start antibiotics early.

10. Trust your gut. If a baby's abdomen doesn't look or feel right, investigate. Don't reassure yourself it's normal.

Summary

Gastrointestinal problems in neonates range from benign to life-threatening. Your job is recognizing which is which and acting accordingly. The key is high index of suspicion for serious pathology, early investigation, and willingness to hold feeds and call for help when needed.

Remember: the baby who does well with NEC is the one whose disease is caught early. The baby who survives an obstruction is the one who gets to surgery before perforation. The baby who tolerates feeds is the one whose underlying illness was identified and treated.

Your clinical judgment, combined with appropriate imaging and laboratory studies, will guide you. When in doubt, hold feeds, investigate, and escalate. These babies don't have time for you to be uncertain.

Chapter Nineteen

RENAL AND UROLOGIC DISORDERS IN NEONATES

Introduction: The Kidneys as "Guardians of Homeostasis"

If a baby isn't making urine, has abnormal urine output, or has electrolyte derangements you can't explain, you need to think about kidneys. The renal system in a newborn is immature—it's still developing its ability to concentrate urine, regulate electrolytes, and handle the demands of extrauterine life. This immaturity makes neonatal kidneys vulnerable, but it also means many problems are reversible if caught early.

In this chapter, we're focusing on the renal and urologic problems you'll encounter at the bedside. We're not going deep into rare genetic syndromes. We're talking about acute kidney injury, electrolyte disorders, urinary tract obstruction, and infection—the conditions that will test your ability to recognize renal dysfunction and manage it before it causes irreversible damage.

The cardinal rule: Urine output matters. Track it. Know what's normal. Act when it's abnormal. Normal urine output in a newborn is approximately 1-2 mL/kg/hour after the first 24-48 hours. Anything less is oliguria. Anything absent is anuria. Both demand investigation.

Understanding Normal Neonatal Renal Function

What Should Be Happening

In utero, the fetus produces urine but the kidneys aren't responsible for electrolyte regulation or fluid balance—the placenta handles that. At birth, everything changes. The kidneys suddenly have to maintain fluid balance, regulate electrolytes, and handle the metabolic waste from a functioning body.

Normal patterns:

- First 24 hours: Urine output may be minimal (oliguria is expected)
- Days 2-3: Output increases; most babies produce 1-2 mL/kg/hour by day 3-4
- Urine specific gravity: Initially high (concentrated), normalizes as fluid intake increases

- Urine electrolytes: Vary based on intake and renal function
- Creatinine: Maternal creatinine at birth (0.7-1.0 mg/dL); rises then falls as maternal creatinine clears
- BUN: Rises in first days as catabolism occurs

When It's Not Normal

You need to recognize red flags:

- Oliguria: <1 mL/kg/hour after first 48 hours
- Anuria: No urine output for >12-24 hours
- Abnormal urine color: Dark, tea-colored, or frankly bloody
- Electrolyte derangements: Hyperkalemia, hyponatremia, hypocalcemia
- Rising creatinine: Should fall after day 3-4, not rise
- Abnormal vital signs: Hypertension (rare in neonates but significant if present)
- Abdominal mass: Palpable kidney or bladder
- Signs of urinary obstruction: Abdominal distension, palpable mass

Recognition: Reading the Signs

What You're Looking For

Oliguria/Anuria:

- No wet diapers
- Careful measurement of urine output (don't guess)
- Dehydration or signs of shock
- Rising electrolytes and creatinine
- Metabolic acidosis

Hematuria:

- Gross hematuria (visible blood in urine)
- Microscopic hematuria (RBCs on urinalysis)
- Causes: Renal artery thrombosis, renal vein thrombosis, trauma, infection, coagulopathy, obstruction

Proteinuria:

- Protein on urinalysis
- Can be transient (dehydration, fever) or pathologic (kidney disease, infection)

Abnormal Electrolytes:

- Hyperkalemia: Muscle weakness, bradycardia, peaked T waves on ECG (dangerous)
- Hyponatremia: Lethargy, seizures, altered mental status
- Hypocalcemia: Jitteriness, seizures, tetany

Signs of Urinary Tract Infection:

- Fever or hypothermia
- Poor feeding
- Jaundice (especially conjugated)
- Sepsis
- Positive urine culture

Signs of Obstruction:

- Abdominal mass (enlarged kidney or distended bladder)
- Oliguria or anuria
- Hypertension
- Prenatal history of hydronephrosis

Systemic Signs of Renal Failure:

- Lethargy or poor tone
- Poor feeding
- Vomiting
- Respiratory distress (from pulmonary edema or metabolic acidosis)
- Seizures (from electrolyte derangement or uremia)

What to Do Immediately

Your First Actions (Do These at the moment)

1. Measure and Document Urine Output
    - Use accurate measurement (don't estimate)
    - Calculate mL/kg/hour
    - Track trends over time
    - If oliguria/anuria, investigate immediately
2. Get Labs
    - Serum: Creatinine, BUN, electrolytes (sodium, potassium, calcium, phosphate), glucose
    - Urine: Urinalysis, urine culture, urine electrolytes (sodium, potassium, osmolality)
    - Coagulation: PT, PTT, platelets (if hematuria)
    - Blood gas: Assess for metabolic acidosis
3. Check Blood Pressure
    - Hypertension in a neonate is rare but significant
    - Use appropriate cuff size
    - Normal systolic BP roughly = 50 + (weight in kg × 2)
4. Assess Hydration Status
    - Capillary refill
    - Skin turgor

- Mucous membranes
- Fontanelle (full vs. flat)
- Weight change

5. Abdominal Examination
   - Palpate for masses (enlarged kidney, distended bladder)
   - Assess for distension
   - Assess for tenderness
   - Assess for costovertebral angle tenderness
6. Imaging
   - Renal ultrasound: Gold standard for assessing kidney size, echogenicity, hydronephrosis, obstruction
   - Abdominal X-ray: Assess for calcifications, masses, bowel gas pattern
   - Voiding cystourethrogram (VCUG): If reflux or posterior urethral valves suspected
7. Establish IV Access
   - Will need for fluids and medications
   - Avoid extravasation (renal function already compromised)
8. Manage Fluid Status Carefully
   - If hypovolemic: Cautious fluid resuscitation (10 mL/kg normal saline over 20-30 minutes)
   - If euvolemic or hypervolemic: Fluid restriction

- Monitor response: improved urine output, improved perfusion
- Don't give excessive fluids to an oliguric baby

9. Address Electrolyte Abnormalities
    - Hyperkalemia: Calcium gluconate (cardiac membrane stabilizer), insulin + glucose, beta-agonists, diuretics, exchange transfusion if severe
    - Hyponatremia: Fluid restriction if dilutional; hypertonic saline if symptomatic
    - Hypocalcemia: Calcium gluconate IV

10. Call for Help
    - Get nephrology consultation if available
    - Consider transfer if dialysis needed

Diagnostic Approach: Making Sense of the Data

Differentiating Prerenal from Intrinsic Renal Disease

Prerenal Azotemia (Most Common):

- Kidney function is normal; problem is perfusion
- Causes: Dehydration, shock, poor cardiac output
- Labs: BUN/Cr ratio >20:1, urine sodium <20 mEq/L, urine osmolality >400 mOsm/kg

- Management: Restore perfusion (fluids, inotropes)
- Usually reversible

Intrinsic Renal Disease:

- Kidney tissue is damaged
- Causes: Acute tubular necrosis, glomerulonephritis, hemolytic uremic syndrome, obstruction
- Labs: BUN/Cr ratio <20:1, urine sodium >40 mEq/L, urine osmolality <350 mOsm/kg
- Management: Depends on cause
- May be irreversible

Postrenal (Obstruction):

- Urine produced but can't drain
- Causes: Posterior urethral valves, ureteropelvic junction obstruction, vesicoureteral reflux with obstruction
- Labs: Similar to intrinsic disease
- Imaging: Shows hydronephrosis, dilated ureters
- Management: Relieve obstruction (catheter, surgery)

Ultrasound Interpretation

Normal findings:

- Kidney size appropriate for age

- Normal echogenicity (not too bright)
- No hydronephrosis
- Normal bladder

Abnormal findings:

- Hydronephrosis: Dilated renal pelvis and/or calyces (suggests obstruction)
- Increased echogenicity: Suggests kidney disease, infection, or infiltration
- Decreased echogenicity: Suggests acute tubular necrosis or early kidney disease
- Enlarged kidneys: Suggests acute tubular necrosis, infiltration, or obstruction
- Small kidneys: Suggests chronic disease or dysplasia
- Dilated ureters: Suggests obstruction or reflux

Common Conditions: Recognition and Management

1. ACUTE KIDNEY INJURY (AKI)

What's Happening: Sudden loss of renal function. In neonates, this is usually reversible if the underlying cause is addressed.

Causes:

- Prerenal: Dehydration, shock, sepsis, poor cardiac output,

PDA

- Intrinsic: Acute tubular necrosis (from hypoxia, nephrotoxins), glomerulonephritis, hemolytic uremic syndrome
- Postrenal: Obstruction

Recognition:

- Oliguria or anuria
- Rising creatinine and BUN
- Hyperkalemia
- Metabolic acidosis
- Pulmonary edema (if fluid overloaded)
- Seizures or altered mental status (from electrolyte derangement)

Staging (Modified RIFLE):

- Risk: Creatinine increase 1.5×, or GFR decrease 25%
- Injury: Creatinine increase 2×, or GFR decrease 50%
- Failure: Creatinine increase 3×, or GFR decrease 75%, or anuria >8 hours

What to Do:

Immediate:

- Assess volume status (hypovolemic vs. hypervolemic)
- If hypovolemic: Fluid resuscitation (10-20 mL/kg normal saline)

- If euvolemic or hypervolemic: Fluid restriction (typically 50-60 mL/kg/day)
- Hold nephrotoxic medications
- Adjust medication dosing for renal function

Address underlying cause:

- Sepsis: Antibiotics
- Shock: Inotropes, fluids
- Obstruction: Catheter or surgery
- Hemolysis: Phototherapy, exchange transfusion

Manage electrolytes:

- Hyperkalemia: Calcium gluconate, insulin + glucose, beta-agonists
- Hyponatremia: Fluid restriction
- Hypocalcemia: Calcium gluconate
- Hyperphosphatemia: Phosphate binders

Monitor closely:

- Urine output (may improve with treatment)
- Electrolytes (daily)
- Creatinine (daily)
- Fluid balance
- Weight

Dialysis indications:

- Refractory hyperkalemia (K >6.5 despite medical management)
- Severe pulmonary edema
- Severe metabolic acidosis
- Uremia with seizures or altered mental status
- Inability to provide adequate nutrition due to fluid restriction

Prognosis:

- Most neonatal AKI is reversible if underlying cause is treated
- Oliguria typically resolves within 1-3 weeks
- Creatinine normalizes as maternal creatinine clears
- Some babies may have residual renal dysfunction

2. URINARY TRACT INFECTION (UTI)

What's Happening: Bacterial infection of the urinary tract. Can be cystitis (bladder), pyelonephritis (kidney), or urosepsis (systemic infection).

Risk Factors:

- Male gender (especially uncircumcised)
- Vesicoureteral reflux
- Obstruction

- Indwelling catheter
- Prematurity

Recognition:

- Fever or hypothermia (hypothermia especially concerning)
- Poor feeding
- Jaundice (especially conjugated)
- Sepsis (lethargy, poor perfusion, shock)
- Vomiting or abdominal distension
- Positive urine culture
- Pyuria (WBCs in urine) or bacteriuria on urinalysis

Diagnosis:

- Gold standard: Urine culture (obtained by catheterization or suprapubic aspiration)
- Urinalysis: Leukocyte esterase, nitrites, WBCs, bacteria
- Blood culture (if sepsis suspected)
- Renal ultrasound and VCUG (after acute infection treated)

What to Do:

Immediate:

- Obtain urine for culture (catheterization or SPA)
- Blood culture
- Start empiric antibiotics (after cultures obtained):

  - Ampicillin + gentamicin (covers most uropathogens)
  - Adjust based on culture results
- IV fluids
- Supportive care

Duration:

- Uncomplicated cystitis: 7-10 days IV antibiotics
- Pyelonephritis/urosepsis: 10-14 days IV antibiotics
- Some sources recommend 3-7 days IV followed by oral antibiotics

Imaging:

- Renal ultrasound: Assess for hydronephrosis, abscess
- VCUG: Screen for reflux (done after acute infection treated, usually at 4-6 weeks)

Follow-up:

- Prophylactic antibiotics if reflux present
- Repeat urine culture to document clearance
- Monitor renal function

The Mistake Many Clinicians Make: Missing UTI because they don't think of it. Sepsis in a neonate is urosepsis until proven otherwise.

3. RENAL ARTERY THROMBOSIS

What's Happening: Blood clot in the renal artery, compromising kidney perfusion. More common in infants of diabetic mothers and those with umbilical artery catheters.

Risk Factors:

- Umbilical artery catheter
- Maternal diabetes
- Intrauterine growth restriction
- Sepsis
- Dehydration
- Polycythemia

Recognition:

- Oliguria or anuria
- Hematuria (gross or microscopic)
- Hypertension (can be significant)
- Abdominal mass (enlarged kidney)
- Elevated LDH, elevated creatinine
- Metabolic acidosis

Diagnosis:

- Renal ultrasound with Doppler: Shows absent or diminished blood flow in renal artery
- CT angiography or MR angiography (if ultrasound inconclusive)

What to Do:

- Remove umbilical artery catheter if present"follow your local guidelines of when and how to remove the central lines"
- Supportive care (fluids, management of electrolytes)
- Anticoagulation (controversial; may help prevent progression)
    - Heparin: 50 units/kg bolus, then 20 units/kg/hour infusion
    - Monitor PTT, platelets
- Manage hypertension if present (antihypertensives)
- Monitor renal function
- Long-term: Monitor for chronic kidney disease

Prognosis:

- Many recover renal function if unilateral
- Bilateral thrombosis: Poor prognosis
- Some residual renal dysfunction common

4. RENAL VEIN THROMBOSIS

What's Happening: Blood clot in the renal vein. Similar risk factors to arterial thrombosis.

Recognition:

- Hematuria

- Thrombocytopenia (clot consumes platelets)
- Flank mass (enlarged kidney)
- Oliguria or anuria
- Metabolic acidosis

Diagnosis:

- Renal ultrasound with Doppler: Shows clot in renal vein

What to Do:

- Supportive care
- Anticoagulation (heparin, controversial)
- Monitor renal function and electrolytes
- Manage thrombocytopenia
- Remove umbilical catheter if present

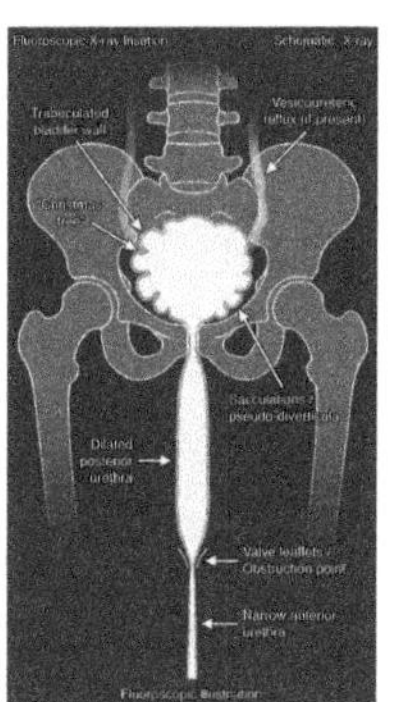

5. URINARY TRACT OBSTRUCTION

Posterior Urethral Valves (PUV):

- Obstructing folds in posterior urethra (males only)
- Presents with oliguria, anuria, or poor urinary stream
- Prenatal history of hydronephrosis
- Diagnosis: VCUG shows dilated posterior urethra

- Management: Catheter drainage initially, then surgical valve ablation

Ureteropelvic Junction Obstruction (UPJ):

- Obstruction at junction of ureter and renal pelvis
- Prenatal history of hydronephrosis
- Usually asymptomatic; detected on imaging
- Management: Monitor renal function; surgery if declining function

Vesicoureteral Reflux (VUR):

- Urine refluxes back up the ureter
- Risk of infection and kidney damage
- Diagnosis: VCUG
- Management: Prophylactic antibiotics; surgery if high-grade reflux or recurrent infections

Recognition of Obstruction:

- Prenatal hydronephrosis (detected on prenatal ultrasound)
- Oliguria or anuria
- Abdominal mass
- Elevated creatinine
- Hypertension
- Imaging findings (hydronephrosis, dilated ureters)

What to Do:

- Renal ultrasound: Assess degree of hydronephrosis and renal function
- VCUG: Assess for reflux and posterior urethral valves
- If significant obstruction: Catheter drainage (suprapubic or urethral)
- Monitor renal function
- Surgical consultation for definitive management
- Prophylactic antibiotics if reflux

6. ELECTROLYTE DISORDERS

Hyperkalemia:

- Serum K >6.0 mEq/L
- Causes: Acute kidney injury, hemolysis, tissue damage, excessive potassium intake
- Signs: Muscle weakness, cardiac arrhythmias, peaked T waves on EKG
- Management:
    - Calcium gluconate: 100-200 mg/kg IV (stabilizes cardiac membrane)
    - Insulin + glucose: 0.1 units/kg insulin + 0.5 g/kg glucose IV (shifts K intracellularly)

    - Beta-agonists: Albuterol nebulized (shifts K intracellularly)
    - Diuretics: Furosemide 1 mg/kg IV (if not oliguric)
    - Sodium polystyrene sulfonate: Oral or rectal (binds K in GI tract)
    - Dialysis: If refractory or severe

Hyponatremia:

- Serum Na <130 mEq/L
- Causes: Excessive free water intake, SIADH, renal disease, sepsis
- Signs: Lethargy, poor feeding, seizures
- Management:
    - If symptomatic: 3% hypertonic saline (0.5-1 mEq/kg IV over 10-20 minutes)
    - If asymptomatic: Fluid restriction
    - Treat underlying cause
    - Avoid rapid correction (risk of pontine myelinolysis)

Hypocalcemia:

- Serum Ca <7.0 mg/dL (ionized Ca <3.5 mg/dL)
- Causes: Hypoparathyroidism, vitamin D deficiency, phosphate retention, sepsis

- Signs: Jitteriness, tremors, seizures, tetany
- Management:
  - Calcium gluconate: 100-200 mg/kg IV over 10-20 minutes (monitor heart rate)
  - Treat underlying cause
  - Vitamin D supplementation if deficiency

Common Pitfalls and Mistakes

Mistake #1: Not Measuring Urine Output Carefully – Estimates are wrong. Measure accurately. Calculate mL/kg/hour. Track trends. This is how you catch problems early.

Mistake #2: Giving Excessive Fluids to an Oliguric Baby – More fluids don't make oliguric kidneys work. Fluid overload causes pulmonary edema and worsens outcomes. Restrict fluids. Wait for the kidneys to recover.

Mistake #3: Missing Hyperkalemia Until It's Critical – Check potassium early and often in babies with renal dysfunction. Don't wait for EKG changes. Treat early.

Mistake #4: Not Considering UTI in a Septic Neonate – UTI is a common source of neonatal sepsis. Get urine culture on every septic workup.

Mistake #5: Delaying Catheter Placement in Anuria – If a baby hasn't urinated in 24 hours and you can't explain it, catheterize to check for obstruction. Don't wait.

Mistake #6: Not Removing Umbilical Artery Catheters Promptly – UACs are a risk factor for thrombosis. Remove when no longer needed. Don't leave them in "just in case."

Mistake #7: Assuming All Hematuria Is Benign – Hematuria can indicate serious pathology (thrombosis, infection, obstruction). Investigate it.

Mistake #8: Not Adjusting Medication Dosing for Renal Function – Many medications are renally cleared. Adjust doses in renal failure to avoid toxicity.

When to Escalate Care

Don't hesitate to escalate if:

- Anuria for >24 hours: Investigate for obstruction. Consider catheterization.
- Severe hyperkalemia (K >7.0): Medical emergency. Get help. Consider dialysis.
- Refractory oliguria: Baby not responding to fluids. Consider transfer for dialysis.
- Suspected thrombosis: Transfer to facility with vascular imaging capability.
- Urosepsis: Aggressive management. Consider transfer if deteriorating.
- Severe electrolyte derangement: Seizures, altered mental status. Get help.
- Signs of urinary obstruction: Get imaging and surgical con-

sultation.

Key Clinical Pearls

1. Urine output is a vital sign. Track it like you track heart rate and blood pressure. It tells you everything.
2. Oliguria is not normal. Investigate it. Don't assume it will resolve.
3. The first urine may be delayed, but by day 3-4, every baby should be making 1-2 mL/kg/hour. If not, something's wrong.
4. Hyperkalemia kills. Check K early, check it often, treat it aggressively.
5. Hematuria needs investigation. It's not benign until you've ruled out serious pathology.
6. Sepsis is urosepsis until proven otherwise. Get urine culture on every septic workup.
7. Fluid overload in a baby with renal failure causes pulmonary edema. Restrict fluids. Don't give more.
8. Ultrasound is your friend. Get renal ultrasound early when you suspect renal pathology.
9. Remove umbilical catheters promptly. They increase thrombosis risk. Don't leave them in unnecessarily.
10. Neonatal renal disease is often reversible. If you catch it early

and manage it well, most babies recover renal function.

Summary

Renal and urologic disorders in neonates range from transient to life-threatening. Your job is recognizing abnormal urine output, investigating systematically, and managing aggressively. The key is understanding normal renal physiology, recognizing when things deviate from normal, and knowing when to hold back (fluids) and when to act (antibiotics, electrolyte management, dialysis).

Remember: the baby with acute kidney injury who recovers is the one whose underlying cause was identified and treated early. The baby who avoids chronic kidney disease is the one whose obstruction was relieved promptly. The baby who survives urosepsis is the one who got antibiotics started before deterioration.

Your clinical judgment, combined with appropriate imaging and laboratory studies, will guide you. When in doubt, measure urine output, get imaging, and escalate. These kidneys are resilient if given the chance to recover.

Chapter Twenty

OPHTHALMOLOGIC DISORDERS IN NEONATES

Introduction: The Eyes as "Windows" into Systemic Disease

If a baby has abnormal eye findings, discharge from the eyes, or you notice something unusual about the appearance or movement of the eyes, you need to pay attention. Ophthalmologic problems in neonates aren't just about vision—they're often signs of systemic disease, infection, or conditions that demand immediate intervention to prevent permanent blindness.

In this chapter, we're focusing on the eye problems you'll actually encounter at the bedside. We're not diving into rare genetic syndromes or subtle refractive errors. We're talking about conjunctivitis, retinopathy of prematurity, cataracts, and other conditions that will test your ability to recognize them early and manage them before they cause irreversible vision loss.

The cardinal rule: Any eye discharge, any abnormal pupil response, any unusual eye appearance or movement requires investigation. Don't assume it's benign. Don't assume it will resolve on its own. Investigate and refer.

Understanding Normal Neonatal Eye Anatomy and Function

What Should Be Happening

At birth, the baby's eyes should be:

- Symmetric and aligned
- Responsive to light (pupils constrict)
- Able to track movement (though tracking may be jerky initially)
- Free of discharge
- Without obvious structural abnormalities

The newborn can see, though vision is blurry. Babies prefer faces and high-contrast patterns. They blink and have a blink reflex. The red reflex (reflection of light from the retina) should be present and symmetric.

When It's Not Normal

You need to recognize red flags:

- Eye discharge: Any purulent, mucopurulent, or bloody discharge
- Conjunctival injection: Red, inflamed conjunctiva
- Eyelid swelling: Suggests infection or obstruction
- Abnormal pupil: Fixed, dilated, or asymmetric
- Absent or abnormal red reflex: Suggests cataract, retinoblastoma, or other pathology
- Nystagmus: Involuntary eye movements (suggests neurologic or ophthalmologic pathology)
- Strabismus: Eyes not aligned (normal in first weeks but should resolve with time)
- Excessive tearing: Suggests nasolacrimal duct obstruction or other pathology
- Photophobia: Light sensitivity (suggests infection or inflammation)
- Corneal opacity: Cloudy cornea (suggests infection, trauma, or metabolic disease)

Recognition: "Reading the Signs"

What You're Looking For

Conjunctivitis (Ophthalmia Neonatorum):

- Eye discharge (clear, mucopurulent, or purulent)
- Conjunctival injection (red eyes)
- Eyelid swelling
- Onset timing: Chemical (within 24 hours), bacterial (24-72 hours), viral (5-14 days)
- Baby may have difficulty opening eyes

Dacryocystitis (Nasolacrimal Duct Infection):

- Swelling and erythema over the nasolacrimal duct (medial canthus)
- Purulent discharge with pressure over the area
- May progress to orbital cellulitis if untreated

Keratitis/Corneal Ulcer:

- Corneal opacity or haziness
- Photophobia
- Tearing
- Pain (baby irritable)

- Suggests HSV infection or other serious pathology

Cataracts:

- Opacity in the lens
- Absent or dull red reflex
- Visible white appearance to the pupil
- May be congenital (TORCH, metabolic) or acquired

Retinopathy of Prematurity (ROP):

- Detected on screening exam (not visible without ophthalmoscopy)
- Risk factors: Prematurity, oxygen exposure, sepsis
- Progression can lead to retinal detachment and blindness

Retinoblastoma:

- Absent or abnormal red reflex (white pupil)
- Strabismus
- Rare but vision-threatening
- Requires urgent referral

Orbital Cellulitis:

- Eyelid swelling and erythema
- Proptosis (eye bulging)
- Fever, systemic signs of infection
- Medical emergency

What to Do Immediately

Your First Actions (Do These at the moment)

1. Perform Red Reflex Screening
    - Use ophthalmoscope or RetCam
    - Look for symmetric, bright red reflexes
    - Absence or asymmetry suggests pathology
    - If abnormal, refer to ophthalmology urgently
2. Examine Eye Discharge
    - Describe: Clear, mucopurulent, purulent, bloody
    - Assess timing of onset
    - Assess unilateral vs. bilateral
3. Assess Conjunctiva and Sclera
    - Inject (redness)
    - Discharge
    - Swelling
    - Corneal clarity
4. Check Pupils
    - Size (should be 2-3 mm)

- Symmetry
- Reactivity to light
- Any fixed or dilated pupils suggest pathology

5. Assess Eye Movement
    - Can baby track?
    - Are eyes aligned?
    - Any nystagmus?
6. Obtain Cultures if Discharge Present
    - Gram stain
    - Culture (bacterial)
    - Consider viral culture or PCR if HSV suspected
    - Chlamydia PCR if indicated
7. Get Labs if Infection Suspected
    - CBC
    - Blood culture
    - Consider systemic workup (sepsis evaluation)
8. Refer to Ophthalmology
    - Abnormal red reflex
    - Significant conjunctivitis
    - Corneal opacity

- Any concern for serious pathology
- Don't wait—refer urgently

9. Start Treatment if Indicated
    - Antibiotic ointment or drops
    - Oral antibiotics if systemic infection
    - Do not delay pending culture results
10. Notify Parents
    - Explain findings
    - Explain management plan
    - Explain importance of follow-up

Diagnostic Approach: Making Sense of the Data

Gram Stain Interpretation

- Gram-Negative cocci: *Neisseria gonorrhoeae*
    - Treat with IV ceftriaxone
    - Prophylaxis with erythromycin ointment should have prevented this
- Gram-Positive Cocci: *Staphylococcus aureus* or *Streptococcus* species

    - Treat with topical and systemic antibiotics

- Gram-Negative Rods: *Pseudomonas* or other gram-negative organism
    - Serious infection; requires systemic antibiotics
- No organisms: Viral or chemical conjunctivitis

Culture Results

- Gonococcus: Treat with IV ceftriaxone + topical antibiotics
- Chlamydia: Treat with oral azithromycin (systemic therapy important to prevent pneumonia)
- HSV: Treat with IV acyclovir
- Pseudomonas: Treat with systemic and topical antipseudomonal antibiotics
- Other bacteria: Treat based on susceptibilities

Ophthalmologic Examination

Dilated Fundus Exam:

- Assesses retina, optic nerve, macula
- Detects ROP, retinoblastoma, other pathology
- Requires ophthalmology expertise

Ultrasound:

- If unable to visualize posterior segment
- Assesses for retinal detachment, masses

Common Conditions: Recognition and Management

1. CONJUNCTIVITIS (OPHTHALMIA NEONATORUM)

What's Happening: Inflammation of the conjunctiva from chemical, bacterial, or viral cause.

Chemical Conjunctivitis:

- From silver nitrate or erythromycin prophylaxis
- Onset: Within 24 hours
- Mild conjunctival injection and watery discharge
- Self-limited; resolves in 24-48 hours
- Treatment: Supportive (warm compresses, gentle cleaning)

Bacterial Conjunctivitis:

Gonococcal: Neisseria gonorrhoeae

- Onset: 2-5 days
- Severe purulent discharge
- Rapid progression to keratitis and blindness if untreated

- Maternal history of untreated gonorrhea
- EMERGENCY: Treat immediately with IV ceftriaxone + topical antibiotics
- Prophylaxis with erythromycin or tetracycline ointment prevents this

Chlamydial: Chlamydia trachomatis

- Onset: 5-14 days
- Mucopurulent discharge
- May progress to chlamydial pneumonia
- Treat with oral azithromycin (systemic therapy important)
- Topical antibiotics less effective; systemic therapy essential

Other bacteria: Staphylococcus aureus, Streptococcus, Pseudomonas, etc.

- Treat with appropriate antibiotics based on culture

Viral Conjunctivitis:

HSV: Herpes simplex virus

- Vesicular rash may be present on eyelid or face
- Conjunctivitis may progress to keratitis or chorioretinitis
- CRITICAL: Treat with IV acyclovir
- Topical antibiotics alone are inadequate
- Risk of disseminated HSV if not treated

Enterovirus: Usually mild, self-limited*Adenovirus:* Conjunctivitis without systemic disease

What to Do:

Chemical conjunctivitis:

- Supportive care
- Warm compresses
- Gentle cleaning with saline
- Resolves spontaneously
- No antibiotics needed

Bacterial conjunctivitis:

- Obtain cultures (gram stain, culture, Chlamydia PCR)
- Start empiric antibiotics while awaiting culture:
    - Gonococcal coverage: IV ceftriaxone 50 mg/kg/day divided BID
    - Chlamydia coverage: Oral azithromycin 10 mg/kg/day
    - Topical: Erythromycin or bacitracin ointment four times daily
- Adjust based on culture results
- Duration: 7-10 days
- Systemic treatment is critical (not just topical)

Viral conjunctivitis (HSV):

- IV acyclovir: 10-15 mg/kg every 8 hours

- Topical trifluridine or vidarabine
- Duration: 10-14 days
- Ophthalmology consultation
- Consider systemic HSV workup (disseminated disease)

When to Escalate:

- Severe purulent discharge (suggests gonococcal)
- Corneal involvement (keratitis)
- Suspected HSV
- No improvement with treatment
- Refer to ophthalmology if any concern

2. DACRYOCYSTITIS (NASOLACRIMAL DUCT INFECTION)

What's Happening: Infection of the nasolacrimal duct, usually from obstruction and stasis.

Recognition:

- Swelling and erythema over nasolacrimal duct (medial canthus)
- Purulent discharge with pressure over the area
- Fever or systemic signs if progressing
- Unilateral typically

- May progress to orbital cellulitis if untreated

What to Do:

Mild (no systemic signs):

- Warm compresses
- Gentle massage over nasolacrimal duct
- Topical antibiotics (erythromycin ointment)
- Most resolve without systemic antibiotics
- Probing may be needed if obstruction persists

Moderate to severe (systemic signs):

- Oral or IV antibiotics (cover Staph and Strep)
- Warm compresses
- Topical antibiotics
- Close monitoring for progression to orbital cellulitis

Orbital cellulitis (emergency):

- IV antibiotics (broad-spectrum)
- Imaging (CT or MRI)
- Possible drainage
- Ophthalmology and ENT consultation

3. NASOLACRIMAL DUCT OBSTRUCTION (Non-Infectious)

What's Happening: Partial or complete obstruction of the nasolacrimal duct, causing tearing and discharge without infection.

Recognition:

- Excessive tearing
- Mucoid discharge (not purulent)
- No fever or systemic signs
- No swelling or erythema over nasolacrimal duct
- Usually unilateral
- Common in first weeks of life

What to Do:

- Reassure parents (usually self-limited)
- Warm compresses
- Gentle massage over nasolacrimal duct
- Topical antibiotics if discharge present (to prevent infection)
- Most resolve by 3-6 months
- Probing indicated if: persistent symptoms at 6-12 months, or signs of infection

4. RETINOPATHY OF PREMATURITY (ROP)

What's Happening: Abnormal retinal vascular development in premature infants, particularly those exposed to high oxygen and other risk factors. Can progress to retinal detachment and blindness.

Risk Factors:

- Prematurity (especially <32 weeks)
- Low birth weight (especially <1500 g)
- Oxygen exposure (both excessive and inadequate)
- Sepsis
- Transfusion
- Respiratory distress syndrome
- PDA

Recognition:

- NOT visible without dilated fundus exam
- Detected on screening ophthalmology exam
- Progression: Vascular abnormalities → fibrovascular proliferation → retinal detachment

Screening Guidelines:

- All infants <30 weeks gestation OR <1500 g birth weight
- First exam: 4 weeks chronologic age or 31 weeks postmenstrual age (whichever is later)
- Frequency: Based on findings (usually every 1-2 weeks initially)

What to Do:

Prevention:

- Avoid excessive oxygen (maintain SpO_2 in target range)
- Avoid excessive hyperoxia
- Manage sepsis aggressively
- Manage PDA
- Maintain adequate nutrition

Screening:

- Ensure all at-risk infants get screened by ophthalmology

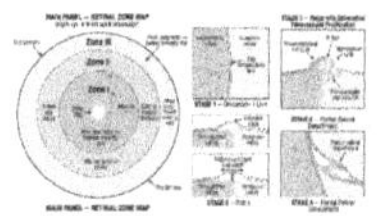

- Don't miss screening windows

Treatment (if indicated):

- Anti-VEGF injections (bevacizumab, aflibercept)
- Laser photocoagulation
- Vitrectomy (for advanced disease)
- Requires ophthalmology expertise

Follow-up:

- Long-term follow-up even if ROP regresses
- Screen for refractive errors, strabismus, amblyopia

5. CONGENITAL CATARACTS

What's Happening: Opacity of the lens present at birth, usually from intrauterine infection, metabolic disease, or genetic factors.

Causes:

- TORCH infections (especially rubella, CMV)
- Metabolic (galactosemia, Lowe syndrome)
- Genetic syndromes
- Idiopathic

Recognition:

- White pupil (leukocoria)
- Absent or dull red reflex
- Visible opacity in lens
- Strabismus (if dense cataract)
- Nystagmus (if bilateral and dense)

What to Do:

Immediate:

- Refer to ophthalmology urgently
- Workup for underlying cause (TORCH titers, metabolic screening, genetic evaluation)
- Don't delay—dense cataracts cause irreversible vision loss if not treated

Treatment:

- Surgical removal (lensectomy) if dense and affecting vision

- Timing critical: Dense unilateral cataracts should be removed by 6 weeks of age to prevent amblyopia
- Bilateral cataracts: Treat the denser one first
- Post-operative: Contact lens, intraocular lens, or glasses for optical rehabilitation

Follow-up:

- Ophthalmology management
- Treat underlying cause
- Screen for complications

6. RETINOBLASTOMA

What's Happening: Malignant tumor of the retina. Rare but vision-threatening and life-threatening if not detected.

Recognition:

- Leukocoria (white pupil): Most common presenting sign
- Absent or abnormal red reflex
- Strabismus
- Eye pain or redness (if advanced)
- Family history (hereditary form)

What to Do:

Immediate:

- Refer to ophthalmology URGENTLY

- Don't delay—this is a medical emergency
- Any abnormal red reflex needs ophthalmology evaluation

Diagnosis:

- Dilated fundus exam
- Imaging (ultrasound, CT, MRI)
- Genetic testing if hereditary form suspected

Treatment:

- Depends on size, location, laterality
- Options: Chemotherapy, laser, cryotherapy, enucleation (eye removal), external beam radiation
- Requires specialized pediatric oncology and ophthalmology expertise

7. HERPES SIMPLEX KERATITIS/CHORIORETINITIS

What's Happening: HSV infection of the cornea or retina, potentially causing scarring and vision loss.

Recognition:

- Conjunctivitis with vesicular rash on eyelid or face
- Corneal opacity or haziness (keratitis)
- Photophobia and tearing
- Chorioretinitis: Whitish infiltrates on fundus exam

- Systemic HSV signs may be present

What to Do:

Immediate:

- IV acyclovir 10-15 mg/kg every 8 hours
- Topical antiviral (trifluridine or vidarabine)
- Ophthalmology consultation
- Systemic HSV workup (CSF, cultures)
- Duration: 10-14 days IV acyclovir

Follow-up:

- Ophthalmology monitoring
- Screen for disseminated HSV
- Long-term follow-up for vision

Common Pitfalls and Mistakes

Mistake #1: Assuming All Eye Discharge Is Benign – Not all conjunctivitis is simple. Gonococcal or HSV conjunctivitis can cause blindness if not treated promptly. Investigate discharge.

Mistake #2: Delaying Ophthalmology Referral – Abnormal red reflex, corneal opacity, or significant conjunctivitis needs ophthalmology evaluation. Don't wait. Don't assume it will resolve.

Mistake #3: Not Doing Red Reflex Screening – Abnormal red reflex can indicate serious pathology (cataract, retinoblastoma, ROP). Screen all babies. Refer abnormal findings.

Mistake #4: Missing ROP Screening – All at-risk infants need ophthalmology screening. Don't miss the screening window. ROP can progress to blindness if not detected.

Mistake #5: Treating Chlamydia Conjunctivitis with Topical Antibiotics Alone – Chlamydia requires systemic (oral) antibiotics. Topical therapy alone is inadequate. Systemic therapy also prevents chlamydial pneumonia.

Mistake #6: Not Starting IV Acyclovir for Suspected HSV Keratitis – Topical antibiotics won't treat HSV. IV acyclovir is essential. Don't delay for culture confirmation.

Mistake #7: Assuming Gonococcal Prophylaxis Prevents All Neonatal Conjunctivitis – Prophylaxis is effective but not 100%. Conjunctivitis still occurs. Investigate all discharge.

Mistake #8: Not Treating Dacryocystitis That's Progressing to Orbital Cellulitis – Dacryocystitis can rapidly progress to orbital cellulitis. Monitor closely. Start systemic antibiotics if signs of progression.

When to Escalate Care

Don't hesitate to escalate if:

- Abnormal red reflex: Refer to ophthalmology urgently
- Severe conjunctivitis with purulent discharge: Suspect gonococcal; treat aggressively
- Corneal involvement: Keratitis is vision-threatening; refer urgently
- Suspected HSV: Start IV acyclovir immediately; refer to ophthalmology

- Suspected orbital cellulitis: IV antibiotics, imaging, refer urgently
- Signs of ROP: Ensure screening is occurring; refer to ophthalmology
- Any concern for retinoblastoma: Refer URGENTLY
- No improvement with treatment: Refer to ophthalmology for further evaluation

Key Clinical Pearls

1. Red reflex screening is essential. Do it on every baby. Refer abnormal findings urgently.
2. Any eye discharge requires investigation. Don't assume it's benign.
3. Gonococcal conjunctivitis is a medical emergency. Treat immediately with IV ceftriaxone.
4. Chlamydia requires systemic antibiotics. Topical therapy alone is inadequate.
5. HSV keratitis requires IV acyclovir. Don't wait for culture confirmation.
6. Prophylaxis prevents but doesn't eliminate conjunctivitis. Stay vigilant.
7. ROP screening is critical. Don't miss at-risk infants or screening windows.

8. Dacryocystitis can progress rapidly. Monitor closely for orbital cellulitis.

9. Nasolacrimal duct obstruction is usually benign. Reassure parents; most resolve spontaneously.

10. When in doubt, refer to ophthalmology. These are your partners in preserving vision.

Summary

Ophthalmologic disorders in neonates range from benign and self-limited to vision-threatening emergencies. Your job is recognizing abnormal findings, distinguishing serious pathology from benign conditions, and knowing when to refer urgently to ophthalmology.

Remember: the baby with gonococcal conjunctivitis who sees is the one who got IV ceftriaxone immediately. The baby with HSV keratitis who retains vision is the one who got IV acyclovir without delay. The baby with ROP who doesn't go blind is the one who got screened and treated appropriately.

Your role is screening, recognizing red flags, initiating treatment, and referring appropriately. Trust your clinical instincts. When something looks wrong with the eyes, it probably is. Refer early. Refer often. Preserve vision.

Chapter Twenty-One

OTOLARYNGOLOGIC DISORDERS IN NEONATES

Introduction: Ears, Nose, and Throat as "Critical Airway Structures"

If a baby has noisy breathing, nasal congestion, ear drainage, or you notice abnormal findings in the ears, nose, or throat, you need to pay attention. Otolaryngologic problems in neonates aren't just about discomfort—they're about airway management, hearing preservation, and recognizing when a baby's breathing is compromised.

In this chapter, we're focusing on the ENT problems you'll actually encounter at the bedside. We're not diving into rare syndromic presentations or subtle hearing loss. We're talking about stridor, nasal obstruction, ear infections, and other conditions that will test your ability to recognize them early and manage them before they compromise the airway or cause permanent hearing loss.

The cardinal rule: Any abnormal breathing sound, any nasal obstruction, any ear drainage requires investigation. Don't assume it's normal. Don't assume it will resolve. Investigate.

Understanding Normal Neonatal ENT Anatomy and Function

What Should Be Happening

At birth, the baby's airways should be:

- Patent and unobstructed
- Producing normal breathing sounds (no stridor, no wheeze, no snoring)
- Symmetric and aligned
- Free of discharge
- Without obvious structural abnormalities

The newborn breathes primarily through the nose. Nasal patency is essential. The ears should be symmetric and positioned appropriately. The throat should allow normal swallowing and feeding.

When It's Not Normal

You need to recognize red flags:

- Stridor: High-pitched breathing sound (inspiratory, expiratory, or biphasic)
- Nasal obstruction: Baby struggling to breathe through nose, mouth breathing
- Ear drainage: Any discharge from the ear canal
- Ear swelling or erythema: Suggests infection or inflammation
- Hearing concerns: No response to sound, abnormal startle response
- Difficulty feeding: Suggests oropharyngeal pathology
- Excessive drooling: Suggests swallowing difficulty or oral pathology
- Asymmetric ears: May indicate syndromic condition
- Cleft palate or lip: Obvious structural abnormality

Recognition: "Reading the Signs"

What You're Looking For

Stridor:

- Inspiratory stridor: High-pitched sound during inspiration (suggests upper airway obstruction at or above glottis)
- Expiratory stridor: High-pitched sound during expiration (suggests intrathoracic obstruction)

- Biphasic stridor: Both inspiration and expiration (suggests fixed obstruction)
- Timing of onset: Congenital (present at birth or early weeks) vs. acquired
- Triggers: Position-dependent, worse with agitation, worse with crying
- Associated symptoms: Feeding difficulty, failure to thrive, cyanosis

Nasal Obstruction:

- Noisy breathing (snoring)
- Mouth breathing
- Difficulty feeding (can't coordinate suck-swallow-breathe through obstructed nose)
- Nasal flaring with breathing
- Visible nasal discharge or crusting
- Asymmetric nares

Otitis Media (Ear Infection):

- Fever
- Irritability
- Pulling at ears
- Ear drainage (if tympanum perforated)

- Fullness or bulging of tympanum on otoscopy
- Reduced tympanogram

Otitis Externa (Ear Canal Infection):

- Ear drainage (purulent or serous)
- Ear pain or irritability with ear manipulation
- Erythema and edema of ear canal
- Itching or discomfort

Cleft Palate:

- Visible cleft in hard or soft palate
- Feeding difficulty
- Nasal regurgitation
- Speech/cry abnormality (if older)
- Associated with syndromes (Pierre Robin, Treacher Collins, etc.)

What to Do Immediately

Your First Actions (Do These NOW)

1. Assess Airway Patency
    - Listen to breathing: Normal, stridor, wheeze?

- Assess work of breathing: Retractions, nasal flaring?
- Assess color: Cyanosis?
- Assess responsiveness: Is baby in distress?

2. Assess Nasal Patency
    - Can you pass a 6-8 Fr catheter through each naris?
    - Is there obvious obstruction?
    - Is the baby mouth-breathing?
    - Can a baby feed from breast or bottle?
3. Examine Ears
    - Otoscopy: Assess tympanum, ear canal
    - Palpate: Tenderness, swelling, warmth
    - Assess for drainage
    - Check hearing: Startle response to sound?
4. Examine Oral Cavity and Throat
    - Cleft palate or lip?
    - Tongue position and size (macroglossia?)
    - Oropharyngeal mass or abnormality?
    - Exudate or inflammation?
    - Ability to swallow?
5. Get Labs if Infection Suspected

- CBC (infection)
- Culture of drainage (if present)
- Blood culture (if systemic signs)

6. Get Imaging if Indicated
   - X-ray (neck/airway): Assess for obstruction, foreign body
   - Ultrasound: Assess for masses, fluid
   - CT or MRI: If complex anatomy or mass suspected (usually after stabilization)
7. Refer to ENT surgeon
   - Significant stridor
   - Nasal obstruction not explained by secretions
   - Cleft palate (especially bilateral or associated with other anomalies)
   - Persistent ear drainage
   - Hearing concerns
   - Any airway compromise
8. Hearing Screening
   - Universal newborn hearing screening (UNHS) should occur before discharge
   - Auditory brainstem response (ABR) or otoacoustic emissions (OAE)

- Refer any baby who doesn't pass screening

9. Manage Airway if Compromised
    - Position for optimal airway: Prone or lateral, neck in neutral position
    - Supplemental oxygen if needed
    - Prepare for possible intubation if severe obstruction
    - Don't agitate baby (agitation worsens stridor)
10. Call for Help
    - Significant stridor or respiratory distress: Get ENT and respiratory support ready
    - Airway emergency: Call for intubation capability
    - Don't manage alone

Diagnostic Approach: Making Sense of the Data

Stridor Classification and Workup

Inspiratory Stridor:

- Suggests obstruction at or above glottis
- Causes: Laryngomalacia (most common), subglottic stenosis, vocal cord paralysis, hemangioma, foreign body
- Workup: Flexible laryngoscopy (gold standard)

Expiratory Stridor:

- Suggests intrathoracic obstruction
- Causes: Tracheomalacia, vascular ring, mediastinal mass
- Workup: Chest X-ray, CT or MRI, bronchoscopy if indicated

Biphasic Stridor:

- Suggests fixed obstruction
- Causes: Subglottic stenosis, hemangioma, web, stenosis
- Workup: Laryngoscopy and bronchoscopy

Flexible Laryngoscopy

What it shows:

- Vocal cord position and movement
- Laryngeal abnormalities (arytenoid prolapse in laryngomalacia, stenosis, etc.)
- Subglottic anatomy
- Tracheal anatomy

Interpretation:

- Laryngomalacia: Arytenoid prolapse, omega-shaped epiglottis, foreshortened aryepiglottic folds
- Vocal cord paralysis: Cords fixed in paramedian or lateral position

- Subglottic stenosis: Narrowing below vocal cords
- Hemangioma: Vascular mass

Hearing Assessment

Auditory Brainstem Response (ABR):

- Objective measure of hearing
- Detects auditory nerve and brainstem response
- Doesn't require behavioral response
- Gold standard for newborn screening

Otoacoustic Emissions (OAE):

- Detects cochlear function
- Faster screening tool
- May miss some hearing loss

Follow-up:

- Any baby who doesn't pass initial screening needs repeat testing
- Confirm hearing loss with diagnostic testing
- Early intervention for hearing loss critical for language development

Common Conditions: Recognition and Management

1. LARYNGOMALACIA

What's Happening: Abnormal supraglottic tissue (arytenoid prolapse, abnormal aryepiglottic folds) causes intermittent airway obstruction. Most common cause of stridor in infants.

Recognition:

- Inspiratory stridor (worse with agitation, better when calm)
- Onset: First weeks to months of life
- Feeding difficulty (especially if severe)
- Failure to thrive
- Position-dependent (worse supine, better prone)
- Normal cry (unlike vocal cord paralysis)
- Self-limited in most cases (resolves by 18-24 months)

Diagnosis:

- Flexible laryngoscopy: Shows arytenoid prolapse, omega-shaped epiglottis

What to Do:

Mild to moderate (no feeding difficulty, no failure to thrive):

- Reassurance (will resolve spontaneously)
- Positioning (prone when possible)
- Monitor growth and feeding
- Follow-up ENT visits

- Avoid agitation

Severe (significant feeding difficulty, failure to thrive, significant work of breathing):

- Surgical intervention: Supraglottoplasty
- Divides aryepiglottic folds, removes excess tissue
- Usually definitive treatment
- ENT surgical consultation

When to Escalate:

- Severe stridor with respiratory distress
- Significant feeding difficulty or failure to thrive
- Cyanosis or apnea

2. CHOANAL ATRESIA

What's Happening: Congenital failure of the nasal cavity to open into the nasopharynx. Bilateral atresia is a neonatal emergency.

Recognition:

Unilateral:

- Unilateral nasal obstruction, rhinorrhea, snoring

Bilateral:

- Severe respiratory distress at birth (baby is obligate nasal breather)
- Cyanosis that improves with crying (mouth open)

- Respiratory distress worsening when baby quiets
- Feeding very difficult
- Associated with CHARGE syndrome (50% of cases)

Diagnosis:

- Inability to pass catheter through naris
- CT or MRI: Shows bony or membranous obstruction
- Nasal endoscopy: Visualizes obstruction

What to Do:

Bilateral (emergency):

- Keep airway open: Oral airway, prone positioning
- Avoid nasal obstruction: Remove any secretions
- May need intubation if severe distress
- Surgical repair: Transnasal or transpalatal approach
- ENT emergency consultation

Unilateral:

- Can usually manage without emergency intervention
- Elective surgical repair
- ENT consultation

3. NASAL OBSTRUCTION FROM SECRETIONS

What's Happening: Normal nasal secretions or blood from delivery causing nasal obstruction.

Recognition:

- Snoring or noisy breathing
- Mouth breathing
- Feeding difficulty
- Visible nasal discharge or crusting
- Usually unilateral
- No systemic signs

What to Do:

- Saline nasal drops (2-3 drops per naris)
- Gentle suctioning if needed
- Humidified air
- Reassurance (usually self-limited)
- Avoid aggressive suctioning (can cause epistaxis)

4. VOCAL CORD PARALYSIS

What's Happening: Paralysis of one or both vocal cords, usually from birth trauma, CNS abnormality, or cardiac surgery.

Risk Factors:

- Birth trauma (forceps delivery, shoulder dystocia)

- Hydrocephalus or other CNS pathology
- Cardiac surgery (left recurrent laryngeal nerve injury)
- Arnold-Chiari malformation
- Idiopathic

Recognition:

Unilateral:

- Weak cry, stridor (may be minimal), feeding difficulty

Bilateral:

- Severe stridor, respiratory distress, weak cry
- Laryngoscopy: Cords fixed in paramedian or lateral position

What to Do:

Unilateral:

- Usually managed conservatively
- May improve spontaneously (especially if birth trauma)
- Monitor for aspiration
- Speech/swallowing therapy
- Surgical intervention (arytenoid adduction, vocal cord injection) if no improvement

Bilateral:

- Airway emergency
- May require tracheostomy

- Surgical intervention: Arytenoidectomy or cordotomy to enlarge airway
- ENT emergency consultation

5. OTITIS MEDIA

What's Happening: Inflammation or infection of the middle ear. Common in neonates, especially those with cleft palate or eustachian tube dysfunction.

Risk Factors:

- Cleft palate (eustachian tube dysfunction)
- Prematurity
- Supine feeding position
- Passive smoke exposure
- Recent upper respiratory infection

Recognition:

- Fever
- Irritability
- Ear pulling or ear pain
- Ear drainage (if perforation)
- Hearing loss
- Otoscopy: Bulging, dull, or retracted tympanum; fluid level

or air-fluid interface

- Tympanometry: Flat or type B pattern

What to Do:

With perforation and drainage:

- Culture drainage (bacterial, viral)
- Topical antibiotic drops (quinolone drops, NOT aminoglycosides if perforation)
- Oral antibiotics (amoxicillin-clavulanate or cephalosporin)
- Pain management
- Keep ear dry
- Follow-up audiology

Without perforation:

- Observation initially (many resolve spontaneously)
- Oral antibiotics if significant symptoms
- Decongestants (limited evidence)
- Pain management
- Follow-up to ensure resolution

With conductive hearing loss:

- Audiologic follow-up
- Repeat audiometry after resolution
- If hearing loss persists, consider tympanostomy tubes

6. CLEFT PALATE AND CLEFT LIP

What's Happening: Failure of palatal shelves to fuse (cleft palate) or failure of lip to fuse (cleft lip). Can be isolated or syndromic.

Recognition:

- Visible cleft in hard or soft palate
- Cleft lip (unilateral or bilateral)
- Feeding difficulty (especially with cleft palate)
- Nasal regurgitation
- Speech abnormality (if older)
- Associated with syndromes: CHARGE, Pierre Robin, Treacher Collins, etc.

What to Do:

Immediate:

- Assess for associated anomalies (cardiac, renal, skeletal)
- Assess for syndromic features
- Feeding: Modified bottles, special nipples, or cup feeding
- Prevent aspiration
- Refer to cleft team (multidisciplinary: Surgery, speech, audiology, genetics)

Feeding strategies:

- Upright position

- Specialized bottles (Pigeon, Mead Johnson, etc.)
- Slow feeding, frequent burping
- May need NG tube if unable to feed adequately

Surgical repair:

- Cleft lip: Usually repaired at 3-6 months ("rule of 10s": 10 lbs, 10 weeks, 10 g/dL hemoglobin)
- Cleft palate: Usually repaired at 12-18 months
- Timing depends on severity and associated conditions

Speech and hearing:

- Audiology screening (cleft palate increases otitis media risk)
- Speech therapy post-repair
- Long-term follow-up

7. SUBGLOTTIC STENOSIS

What's Happening: Narrowing of the subglottic airway, usually from prolonged intubation or congenital anomaly.

Recognition:

- Stridor (inspiratory, expiratory, or biphasic depending on severity)
- History of prolonged intubation
- Croup-like symptoms

- Respiratory distress
- Feeding difficulty

Diagnosis:

- Laryngoscopy and bronchoscopy: Shows narrowing below vocal cords
- Imaging: CT or MRI may show stenosis

What to Do:

- Avoid further airway trauma
- Manage airway: Oxygen, positioning
- May need tracheostomy if severe
- Surgical intervention: Laryngeal reconstruction, dilation
- ENT surgical consultation

8. HEMANGIOMA OF THE AIRWAY

What's Happening: Benign vascular tumor of the airway, can cause obstruction.

Recognition:

- Stridor (usually inspiratory)
- May have visible hemangioma on skin
- Respiratory distress
- Feeding difficulty

- Laryngoscopy: Vascular mass

What to Do:

- Avoid airway trauma
- Propranolol: First-line medical therapy
  - Dosing: 1-3 mg/kg/day divided three times daily
  - Monitor heart rate and blood pressure
  - Taper slowly
- Corticosteroids: Alternative if propranolol contraindicated
- Surgical intervention: If medical therapy fails
- ENT consultation

Common Pitfalls and Mistakes

Mistake #1: Assuming All Stridor Is Laryngomalacia – Laryngomalacia is most common, but other serious causes exist. Workup with flexible laryngoscopy if stridor persists or worsens.

Mistake #2: Not Recognizing Bilateral Choanal Atresia as an Emergency – Bilateral atresia is a neonatal emergency. Baby is an obligate nasal breather. Recognize respiratory distress that improves with crying.

Mistake #3: Aggressive Nasal Suctioning – Can cause epistaxis and further obstruction. Use gentle technique, saline drops first.

Mistake #4: Missing Cleft Palate – Easily missed if you don't look. Always examine the hard and soft palate. Refer to the cleft team early.

Mistake #5: Not Screening for Hearing Loss – Universal newborn hearing screening is critical. Don't miss babies with hearing loss—early intervention is essential.

Mistake #6: Attributing All Ear Drainage to Infection – Can be from perforation, eustachian tube dysfunction, or other causes. Culture drainage and treat appropriately.

Mistake #7: Not Recognizing Vocal Cord Paralysis – Weak cry, stridor, feeding difficulty—think paralysis. Get a laryngoscopy.

Mistake #8: Delaying ENT Referral for Significant Stridor – Significant stridor needs workup. Don't wait. Get a laryngoscopy.

When to Escalate Care

Don't hesitate to escalate if:

- Significant stridor with respiratory distress: Airway emergency. Prepare for intubation.
- Bilateral choanal atresia: Neonatal emergency. Airway management critical.
- Significant nasal obstruction: Feeding difficulty, failure to thrive. ENT referral.
- Ear drainage persisting: Culture and treat. Audiologic follow-up.
- Hearing loss on screening: Confirm with diagnostic testing. Early intervention.
- Cleft palate: Refer to cleft team. Multidisciplinary management.

- Significant airway compromise: Don't manage alone. Get help.

Key Clinical Pearls

1. Stridor is not normal. Investigate it. Get laryngoscopy if persistent or worsening.
2. Laryngomalacia is most common, but don't assume. Workup with flexible laryngoscopy.
3. Babies are obligate nasal breathers. Nasal obstruction is a big problem. Investigate.
4. Bilateral choanal atresia is an emergency. Baby will be in distress at birth. Recognize it.
5. Cleft palate is easy to miss if you don't look. Always examine the palate.
6. Hearing screening is critical. Don't miss hearing loss. Early intervention changes outcomes.
7. Ear drainage needs culture. Don't assume it's benign.
8. Vocal cord paralysis can be serious. Bilateral paralysis is an airway emergency.
9. Otitis media is common in cleft palate. Screen hearing. Manage ear disease.
10. When in doubt, refer to ENT. These are your partners in managing airway and hearing.

Summary

Otolaryngologic disorders in neonates range from benign and self-limited to airway-threatening emergencies. Your job is recognizing abnormal findings, distinguishing serious pathology from benign conditions, and knowing when to refer urgently to ENT or manage as an airway emergency.

Remember: the baby with laryngomalacia who thrives is the one whose condition was recognized and managed expectantly. The baby with bilateral choanal atresia who survives is the one whose airway was recognized as compromised and managed immediately. The baby with hearing loss who develops normal language is the one who got early intervention.

Your role is screening, recognizing red flags, initiating management, and referring appropriately. Trust your clinical instincts. When something sounds or looks wrong with the ears, nose, or throat, it probably is. Refer early. Refer often. Preserve airway and hearing.

Chapter Twenty-Two

GENETIC AND CHROMOSOMAL DISORDERS IN NEONATES: PART 1

Introduction: When the Blueprint Goes Wrong

If a baby has multiple anomalies, unusual facial features, developmental delay, or you can't quite explain a constellation of findings with a single diagnosis, you need to think about genetics. Chromosomal and genetic disorders are common—they affect approximately 3-5% of live births. Some are obvious at birth. Others are subtle and easy to miss if you're not looking carefully.

In this part of Chapter 20, we're focusing on chromosomal and genetic disorders you'll encounter at the bedside. We're talking about

Down syndrome, Trisomy 18, Trisomy 13, Turner syndrome, and other conditions that will test your ability to recognize patterns, understand implications, and counsel families appropriately.

The cardinal rule: If a baby has multiple anomalies or unusual features, think chromosomal disorder. Get genetic testing. Don't assume findings are isolated or coincidental.

Understanding Genetic Principles in Neonates

Chromosomal vs. Genetic Disorders

Chromosomal Disorders:

- Involve entire chromosomes or large segments
- Result from nondisjunction (chromosomes fail to separate during meiosis)
- Examples: Trisomy 21 (Down syndrome), Trisomy 18, Trisomy 13, Monosomy X (Turner syndrome)
- Usually sporadic (not inherited)
- Risk increases with maternal age
- Can often be detected prenatally (screening, ultrasound, cell-free DNA)

Single-Gene Disorders:

- Involve mutation in one gene
- Can be autosomal dominant, autosomal recessive, or

X-linked

- May be inherited or de novo (new mutation)
- Examples: Cystic fibrosis, sickle cell disease, hemophilia
- Often detected through newborn screening

Multifactorial Disorders:

- Result from combination of genetic and environmental factors
- Examples: Cleft palate, congenital heart disease, neural tube defects
- Recurrence risk depends on number of affected relatives

Key Concepts

- Penetrance: The proportion of individuals with a genotype who express the phenotype. Not everyone with a mutation shows the disease.
- Expressivity: The degree to which a genetic disorder is expressed. Two people with the same mutation may have different severity.
- Pleiotropy: One gene affecting multiple traits. This is why chromosomal disorders cause multiple anomalies.
- Mosaicism: Some cells have the abnormality, others don't. Can result in milder phenotype.

Recognition: Reading the Signs

What You're Looking For

Facial Dysmorphism:

- Unusual facial features (hypertelorism, hypotelorism, epicanthal folds, low-set ears)
- Midface hypoplasia
- Micrognathia (small jaw)
- Macroglossia (large tongue)
- Cleft palate or lip
- Unusual nose shape or position

Structural Anomalies:

- Congenital heart disease (ASD, VSD, tetralogy of Fallot, endocardial cushion defects)
- Renal anomalies (hypoplasia, dysplasia, cystic kidneys)
- Limb anomalies (polydactyly, syndactyly, clubfoot)
- Gastrointestinal anomalies (duodenal atresia, esophageal atresia)
- CNS anomalies (hydrocephalus, holoprosencephaly)

Growth and Development:

- Intrauterine growth restriction (IUGR)
- Failure to thrive
- Developmental delay
- Hypotonia (low muscle tone)
- Hypertonia (increased muscle tone)

Skin Findings:

- Unusual pigmentation or patterns
- Skin tags
- Simian crease (single palmar crease)
- Sandal gap (wide space between first and second toes)

Other Signs:

- Unusual cry (high-pitched in some conditions)
- Feeding difficulty
- Hearing loss
- Vision problems
- Seizures
- Metabolic derangement

What to Do Immediately

Your First Actions (Do These at the moment)

1. Perform Detailed Physical Examination
    - Measure and plot all growth parameters
    - Document all dysmorphic features
    - Assess muscle tone (hypotonia vs. hypertonia)
    - Perform complete neurologic exam
    - Assess for structural anomalies (cardiac exam, abdominal exam, extremity exam)
    - Take photographs (with family permission) for documentation
2. Obtain Detailed History
    - Maternal age at delivery
    - Prenatal screening results (triple screen, quad screen, cell-free DNA, ultrasound)
    - Prenatal imaging findings
    - Family history of genetic disorders
    - Consanguinity (parents related)
    - Recurrent pregnancy losses
    - Other affected family members
3. Get Genetic Testing

- Karyotype: Gold standard for chromosomal disorders (results in 1-2 weeks)
- FISH (Fluorescence In Situ Hybridization): Rapid detection of common aneuploidies (results in 24 hours)
- Microarray (CMA): Detects submicroscopic deletions/duplications (results in 1-2 weeks)
- Cell-free DNA testing: If not done prenatally
- Send blood for testing—don't wait

4. Get Imaging as Indicated
    - Echocardiography: Screen for congenital heart disease
    - Abdominal ultrasound: Screen for renal anomalies
    - Head ultrasound or MRI: If CNS anomalies suspected
    - Skeletal survey: If skeletal dysplasia suspected
5. Get Labs
    - CBC (anemia common in some chromosomal disorders)
    - Metabolic panel (hypoglycemia, electrolyte abnormalities)
    - Thyroid function (hypothyroidism common in Down syndrome)
    - Hearing screen (universal newborn hearing screening)
    - Vision screen (ophthalmology referral if needed)
6. Refer to Genetics team

- Genetic counseling essential
- Helps family understand diagnosis, prognosis, recurrence risk
- Discusses prenatal diagnosis options for future pregnancies
- Coordinates multidisciplinary care

7. Coordinate Multidisciplinary Care
    - Cardiology (if cardiac disease present)
    - Neurology (if seizures or developmental concerns)
    - ENT (if hearing loss or airway issues)
    - Orthopedics (if skeletal anomalies)
    - Ophthalmology (if vision concerns)
    - Developmental pediatrics (for developmental support)
8. Discuss with Family
    - Explain diagnosis and what it means
    - Discuss expected complications and surveillance
    - Discuss prognosis and life expectancy
    - Discuss support resources
    - Be honest but compassionate

Diagnostic Approach: Making Sense of the Data

Karyotype Interpretation

Normal Result:

- 46,XX (female with 46 chromosomes, two X chromosomes)
- 46,XY (male with 46 chromosomes, one X and one Y chromosome)

Abnormal Results:

- 47,XX,+21 or 47,XY,+21: Trisomy 21 (Down syndrome)—three copies of chromosome 21
- 47,XX,+18 or 47,XY,+18: Trisomy 18 (Edwards syndrome)—three copies of chromosome 18
- 47,XX,+13 or 47,XY,+13: Trisomy 13 (Patau syndrome)—three copies of chromosome 13
- 45,X: Monosomy X (Turner syndrome)—only one X chromosome
- 47,XXY: Klinefelter syndrome—extra X chromosome in males
- Balanced translocations: Part of one chromosome attached to another (usually no phenotype)
- Unbalanced translocations: Gain or loss of genetic material (causes disease)

FISH Results

- Results available in 24 hours
- Detects trisomy 21, 18, 13 and sex chromosome aneuploidies
- Doesn't detect all chromosomal abnormalities
- Useful for urgent diagnosis while awaiting full karyotype

Microarray Results

Detects:

- Deletions and duplications >50-100 kb
- More sensitive than karyotype for submicroscopic abnormalities
- Can detect pathogenic copy number variations (CNVs)

Interpretation:

- Pathogenic: Clearly associated with disease
- Likely pathogenic: Probably associated with disease
- Uncertain significance: Unknown clinical significance
- Likely benign: Probably not associated with disease
- Benign: Not associated with disease

Common Conditions: Recognition and Management

1. DOWN SYNDROME (TRISOMY 21)

What's Happening: Three copies of chromosome 21 instead of two. Most common chromosomal disorder (1 in 700 births). Risk increases with maternal age (1 in 1,500 at age 20; 1 in 30 at age 45).

Recognition:

Facial features:

- Upslanting palpebral fissures (eyes slant upward)
- Epicanthal folds (skin fold at inner corner of eye)
- Flat facial profile
- Micrognathia (small jaw)
- Open mouth (due to hypotonia and macroglossia)
- Protruding tongue
- Low-set ears
- Brachycephaly (short head)

Extremities:

- Simian crease (single palmar crease)
- Sandal gap (wide space between first and second toes)
- Short stature
- Hypotonia (decreased muscle tone)
- Ligamentous laxity (loose joints)

Cardiac:

- Endocardial cushion defects (40-50% have cardiac disease)
- ASD, VSD, tetralogy of Fallot
- Patent ductus arteriosus

Other:

- Duodenal atresia (10-15%)
- Hirschsprung disease (1%)
- Hearing loss (50-70%)
- Vision problems (refractive errors, strabismus, cataracts)
- Hypothyroidism (15-20%)
- Leukemia risk increased (10-15 times higher)

Diagnosis:

- Karyotype: 47,XX,+21 or 47,XY,+21
- FISH: Rapid confirmation
- Prenatal screening: Triple screen, quad screen, cell-free DNA
- Prenatal ultrasound: Nuchal translucency, other markers

What to Do:

Immediate:

- Confirm diagnosis with karyotype
- Cardiac ultrasound (screen for congenital heart disease)
- Abdominal ultrasound (screen for duodenal atresia, other GI anomalies)

- Hearing screen (audiology referral)
- Vision screen (ophthalmology referral)
- Thyroid function tests (TSH, free T4)
- Feeding assessment (hypotonia affects feeding)

Ongoing surveillance:

- Thyroid function annually (hypothyroidism common)
- Hearing assessment annually (hearing loss progressive)
- Vision assessment annually
- Cardiac follow-up as indicated
- Developmental assessment and early intervention
- Screen for sleep apnea (common)
- Dental care (delayed tooth eruption, malocclusion)
- Orthopedic follow-up (atlantoaxial instability in some)

Family support:

- Genetic counseling
- Information about Down syndrome
- Connection to support groups
- Discuss recurrence risk (1% risk of recurrence plus maternal age risk)
- Discuss prenatal diagnosis options for future pregnancies

Prognosis:

- Most children with Down syndrome survive to adulthood
- Life expectancy: 50+ years (has increased significantly)
- Intellectual disability: Mild to moderate (varies widely)
- Many achieve independence with support
- Quality of life generally good with appropriate support

2. TRISOMY 18 (EDWARDS SYNDROME)

What's Happening: Three copies of chromosome 18. Rare (1 in 6,000 births). Most have poor prognosis; many die in utero or in the first weeks of life. Those who survive have severe disabilities.

Recognition:

Facial features:

- Micrognathia (severe)
- Microstomia (small mouth)
- Low-set ears (often malformed)
- Cleft palate or lip
- Hypertelorism or hypotelorism
- Holoprosencephaly (in some)

Extremities:

- Clenched fists (characteristic)

- Overlapping fingers (especially index over middle, fifth over fourth)
- Clubfoot or rocker-bottom feet
- Polydactyly (extra fingers/toes)
- Syndactyly (fused digits)
- Short stature, IUGR

Cardiac:

- Congenital heart disease (90%)
- VSD, PDA, ASD
- Complex lesions
- Polyvalvular disease

Other:

- Severe developmental delay
- Seizures
- Severe hypotonia
- Renal anomalies
- GI anomalies (esophageal atresia, omphalocele)
- Hearing loss
- Vision problems

Diagnosis:

- Karyotype: 47,XX,+18 or 47,XY,+18
- FISH: Rapid confirmation
- Prenatal screening: Often detected
- Prenatal ultrasound: Multiple markers

What to Do:

Immediate:

- Confirm diagnosis with karyotype
- Cardiac ultrasound (assess for cardiac disease)
- Discuss prognosis with family (most die in first year)
- Assess for comfort and pain management
- Discuss goals of care (full resuscitation vs. comfort care)

Ongoing:

- Supportive care focused on comfort
- Feeding support (may have difficulty swallowing)
- Pain management
- Family support
- Palliative care consultation if appropriate

Prognosis:

- Median survival: 5-10 days
- 90% die by 1 year

- Rare survivors have severe disability
- Most families choose comfort-focused care

3. TRISOMY 13 (PATAU SYNDROME)

What's Happening: Three copies of chromosome 13. Rare (1 in 10,000 births). Severe disorder with high mortality and morbidity.

Recognition:

Facial features:

- Holoprosencephaly (failure of forebrain to divide—most characteristic)
- Cyclopia (single eye, rare)
- Proboscis (trunk-like nose above eye)
- Cleft lip and palate
- Microphthalmia (small eyes)
- Microcephaly
- Low-set malformed ears

Extremities:

- Polydactyly (postaxial—extra digit on ulnar or fibular side)
- Syndactyly
- Clubfoot
- Rocker-bottom feet

- Clenched fists

Cardiac:

- Congenital heart disease (80%)
- VSD, PDA, ASD
- Complex lesions

Other:

- Severe developmental delay
- Seizures (often intractable)
- Severe hypotonia
- Renal anomalies (cystic kidneys common)
- GI anomalies (omphalocele, gastroschisis)
- CNS anomalies (holoprosencephaly, hydrocephalus)
- Hearing loss
- Vision problems

Diagnosis:

- Karyotype: 47,XX,+13 or 47,XY,+13
- FISH: Rapid confirmation
- Prenatal screening: Often detected
- Prenatal ultrasound: Multiple markers

What to Do:

Immediate:

- Confirm diagnosis with karyotype
- Cardiac ultrasound
- Renal ultrasound
- Head ultrasound or MRI (assess for holoprosencephaly)
- Discuss prognosis (most die in first year)
- Assess for comfort and pain management
- Discuss goals of care

Ongoing:

- Supportive care focused on comfort
- Seizure management if needed
- Pain management
- Family support
- Palliative care consultation if appropriate

Prognosis:

- Median survival: 7-10 days
- 90% die by 1 year
- Rare survivors have severe disability
- Most families choose comfort-focused care

4. TURNER SYNDROME (MONOSOMY X)

What's Happening: Complete or partial absence of one X chromosome. Occurs in females only (1 in 2,500 live female births). Can be 45,X (complete monosomy) or mosaic (some cells with 45,X, others with 46,XX).

Recognition:

Neonatal period:

- Lymphedema (especially hands and feet)
- Broad chest with widely spaced nipples
- Short stature (often apparent early)
- Webbed neck
- Cardiac anomalies (bicuspid aortic valve, coarctation of aorta)
- Renal anomalies (horseshoe kidney, hypoplasia)
- Hearing loss
- Micrognathia
- Low posterior hairline

Later childhood:

- Short stature (most obvious feature)
- Ovarian dysgenesis (infertility, lack of secondary sexual characteristics)
- Gonadal dysgenesis

- Infertility (even with hormone replacement)
- Learning difficulties (especially with spatial reasoning)
- Social immaturity

Diagnosis:

- Karyotype: 45,X or mosaic pattern
- FISH: Rapid confirmation
- Prenatal screening: May be detected
- Prenatal ultrasound: Increased nuchal translucency, cardiac anomalies, renal anomalies

What to Do:

Immediate:

- Confirm diagnosis with karyotype
- Cardiac ultrasound (assess for bicuspid aortic valve, coarctation)
- Renal ultrasound (assess for anomalies)
- Hearing screen
- Blood pressure screening (coarctation risk)
- Thyroid function tests (autoimmune thyroiditis common)

Ongoing surveillance:

- Growth monitoring (growth hormone therapy may be indicated)

- Cardiac follow-up (monitor for aortic dissection risk)
- Renal follow-up
- Hearing assessment
- Thyroid function annually
- Bone density screening (osteoporosis risk)
- Educational support
- Endocrinology consultation (hormone replacement therapy at puberty)
- Genetic counseling (discuss fertility options)

Family support:

- Information about Turner syndrome
- Support groups
- Discuss prognosis (normal life expectancy with appropriate management)
- Discuss fertility options (egg donation, adoption)

Prognosis:

- Normal life expectancy with appropriate medical management
- Short stature (average adult height 4'8" without growth hormone)
- Infertility (but pregnancy possible with assisted reproduc-

tion)

- Generally normal intelligence (some specific learning difficulties)
- Quality of life generally good with support

5. KLINEFELTER SYNDROME (47,XXY)

What's Happening: Extra X chromosome in males. Most common sex chromosome disorder in males (1 in 500-1,000 male births). Often undiagnosed until adolescence or adulthood.

Recognition in Neonatal Period:"rarely discovered"

- Often no obvious features at birth
- May have tall stature (relative to family)
- Developmental delay (variable)
- Hypotonia (low muscle tone)

Later manifestations:

- Tall stature with long legs
- Reduced facial and body hair
- Small testes
- Infertility (azoospermia—no sperm production)
- Reduced testosterone
- Learning difficulties

- Social immaturity
- Increased risk of metabolic syndrome
- Learning difficulties (language delay common)
- Behavioral issues (ADHD, autism spectrum)
- Gynecomastia (breast development) may appear in adolescence

Diagnosis:

- Karyotype: 47,XXY
- FISH: Rapid confirmation
- Often detected on prenatal screening
- Often not diagnosed until adolescence or adulthood

What to Do:

Immediate:

- Confirm diagnosis with karyotype
- Developmental assessment (early intervention if needed)
- Hearing screen
- Vision screen

Ongoing surveillance:

- Developmental monitoring
- Educational support
- Behavioral assessment (ADHD, autism screening)

- Endocrinology consultation at puberty
- Testosterone replacement therapy (if indicated in adolescence/adulthood)
- Infertility counseling (sperm retrieval possible for reproduction)
- Genetic counseling

Prognosis:

- Normal or near-normal life expectancy
- Generally normal intelligence (learning difficulties common)
- Infertility (but reproduction possible with assisted techniques)
- Quality of life generally good with appropriate support

6. OTHER CHROMOSOMAL ABNORMALITIES

Balanced Translocations:

- Part of one chromosome attached to another
- Usually no phenotype (person is phenotypically normal)
- Reproductive risk: May produce unbalanced offspring
- Genetic counseling important for family planning

Unbalanced Translocations:

- Gain or loss of genetic material
- Causes disease (phenotype depends on amount of material gained/lost)
- May be inherited from parent with balanced translocation
- Genetic counseling important

Deletions:

- Loss of genetic material
- Examples: DiGeorge syndrome (22q11 deletion), Wolf-Hirschhorn syndrome (4p deletion)
- Severity depends on size of deletion
- Can be detected by microarray

Duplications:

- Gain of genetic material
- Can be detected by microarray
- Severity depends on size and location of duplication

When to Escalate Care

Don't hesitate to escalate if:

- Suspected chromosomal disorder: Get genetic testing immediately. Don't wait.
- Multiple congenital anomalies: Refer to genetics. Don't as-

sume findings are isolated.

- Significant cardiac disease: Cardiology consultation. Some chromosomal disorders have specific cardiac patterns.
- Severe developmental delay or seizures: Neurology consultation. Genetic workup.
- Failure to thrive: Investigate for underlying genetic disorder.
- Prenatal screening abnormalities: Confirm postnatally. Genetic counseling.
- Family history of genetic disorder: Genetic counseling. Discuss recurrence risk.

Key Clinical Pearls - Part 1

1. Multiple anomalies = think chromosomal. Don't assume findings are coincidental.
2. Get genetic testing early. Karyotype or FISH for rapid diagnosis. Don't delay.
3. Cardiac disease is common. Screen all babies with suspected chromosomal disorders with echocardiography.
4. Renal anomalies are common. Screen with renal ultrasound.
5. Hearing loss is common. Universal newborn hearing screening is essential.
6. Down syndrome is the most common chromosomal disor-

der. Know the features.

7. Trisomy 18 and 13 have poor prognosis. Discuss goals of care with families early.
8. Turner syndrome presents with lymphedema and cardiac disease. Screen for coarctation.
9. Klinefelter syndrome is often undiagnosed at birth. May present with developmental delay.
10. Genetic counseling is essential. Helps families understand diagnosis and recurrence risk.
11. Prenatal diagnosis options exist. Discuss with families for future pregnancies.
12. Multidisciplinary care is key. Coordinate with cardiology, neurology, ENT, ophthalmology, endocrinology as needed.

Summary - Part 1

Chromosomal and genetic disorders are common in neonates. Your job is recognizing patterns of multiple anomalies, getting appropriate genetic testing, and understanding the implications for each condition. Down syndrome requires ongoing surveillance for cardiac disease, thyroid dysfunction, and developmental delay. Trisomy 18 and 13 have poor prognoses; goals of care discussions are essential. Turner syndrome requires cardiac screening and growth monitoring. Klinefelter syndrome often goes undiagnosed but requires developmental support.

Remember: the baby with Down syndrome who thrives is the one whose cardiac disease was detected and managed, whose thyroid dysfunction was treated, and who received early developmental intervention. The family that makes informed decisions about Trisomy 18 or 13 is the one that received clear prognostic information and genetic counseling early. The girl with Turner syndrome who reaches her potential is the one whose cardiac disease was managed, whose growth was optimized, and who received appropriate endocrinologic care.

Your role is recognizing red flags, getting appropriate testing, coordinating multidisciplinary care, and supporting families through diagnosis and management. Trust your clinical instincts. When something looks unusual, investigate. When you see multiple anomalies, think chromosomal. Get genetic testing. Refer appropriately.

Chapter Twenty-Three

GENETIC AND CHROMOSOMAL DISORDERS : PART 2

SINGLE GENE DISORDERS

Autosomal Dominant Disorders

Marfan Syndrome

Pathophysiology:

- Mutation in *FBN1* gene encoding fibrillin-1

- Affects connective tissue throughout body
- Autosomal dominant inheritance; 25% new mutations
- Pleiotropy: single gene affects multiple organ systems

Clinical Recognition:

- Tall stature with disproportionate arm span
- Arachnodactyly (long, slender fingers)
- Lens dislocation (ectopia lentis): upward displacement
- Myopia and astigmatism
- Skeletal: pectus deformities, scoliosis, high-arched palate
- Cardiovascular: aortic root dilatation (most serious), mitral valve prolapse, aortic dissection
- Pulmonary: spontaneous pneumothorax
- Skin: striae atrophicae

Diagnostic Approach:

- Clinical diagnosis using Ghent nosology
- Ophthalmology evaluation: slit lamp examination for lens dislocation
- Echocardiography: assess aortic root diameter
- Genetic testing: *FBN1* mutation analysis
- Family screening: examine first-degree relatives

Management:

- Cardiovascular surveillance: Echocardiography at diagnosis and annually; more frequently if aortic root >40 mm
- Beta-blocker therapy: Propranolol or atenolol to reduce aortic wall stress; target heart rate reduction
- ARB therapy: Losartan shown to slow aortic root dilatation; often used alongside beta-blockers
- Activity restriction: Avoid strenuous exercise, contact sports; swimming and walking encouraged
- Ophthalmology care: Annual eye exams; corrective lenses for myopia
- Orthopedic management: Scoliosis screening; bracing if needed; surgical correction if >50 degrees
- Surgical intervention: Aortic root replacement if diameter >5.0 cm or >4.7 cm with risk factors (family history of dissection, desire for pregnancy, need for aortic valve replacement)
- Genetic counseling: 50% recurrence risk in offspring

Achondroplasia

Pathophysiology:

- Mutation in *FGFR3* gene (fibroblast growth factor receptor 3)

- Most common skeletal dysplasia (1:25,000 births)
- 80% new mutations; paternal age effect
- Autosomal dominant; homozygous form lethal

Clinical Recognition:

- Disproportionate short stature (limbs shorter than trunk)
- Rhizomelic shortening (proximal limb shortening)
- Genu varum (bowlegs)
- Limited elbow extension
- Trident hand (fingers spread apart)
- Frontal bossing and midface hypoplasia
- Lumbar lordosis
- Spinal stenosis (progressive with age)
- Normal intelligence
- Hypermobility of joints (except elbows, hips, knees)

Complications:

- Foramen magnum stenosis: hydrocephalus, apnea, sudden death
- Spinal stenosis: leg pain, claudication, neurological deficit
- Otitis media with effusion: hearing loss
- Sleep apnea

- Obesity (predisposition)

Diagnostic Approach:

- Clinical diagnosis based on skeletal features
- X-rays: confirm skeletal dysplasia pattern
- Genetic testing: *FGFR3* mutation analysis
- MRI: assess foramen magnum, spinal canal if symptoms present
- Sleep study: if apnea suspected

Management:

- Neurosurgical evaluation: Assess for foramen magnum stenosis; MRI at diagnosis if symptoms (hypotonia, apnea, developmental delay)
- Growth monitoring: Plot on achondroplasia-specific growth charts
- Orthopedic care: Monitor for genu varum; surgical correction if severe (>20 degrees)
- Spinal surveillance: MRI at diagnosis and periodically; assess for stenosis
- Hearing assessment: Audiometry given high rate of otitis media
- Sleep study: If snoring, witnessed apneas, or daytime somnolence

- Psychosocial support: Address body image, social integration, educational needs
- Limb lengthening: Controversial; consider in motivated families; distraction osteogenesis procedures
- Genetic counseling: 50% recurrence risk if affected parent

Autosomal Recessive Disorders

Cystic Fibrosis (CF)

Pathophysiology:

- Mutation in *CFTR* gene (cystic fibrosis transmembrane conductance regulator)
- Defective chloride channel leads to thick, viscous secretions
- Incidence: 1:2,500-3,500 (varies by ethnicity)
- Autosomal recessive; carrier frequency 1:25-30 in Caucasians
- Progressive multisystem disease

Clinical Recognition:

Respiratory Manifestations:

- Chronic productive cough
- Recurrent/chronic sinusitis and nasal polyps
- Bronchiectasis

- Hemoptysis
- Pneumothorax
- Respiratory failure (late stage)

Gastrointestinal Manifestations:

- Pancreatic insufficiency (85%): steatorrhea, fat-soluble vitamin deficiencies
- Meconium ileus (10-15% of newborns with CF)
- Distal intestinal obstruction syndrome (DIOS): abdominal pain, constipation
- Cystic fibrosis-related diabetes (CFRD): 25-30% by age 30
- Hepatic cirrhosis (5-10%)
- Pancreatic insufficiency-related bone disease

Other Manifestations:

- Infertility: obstructive azoospermia in males; reduced fertility in females
- Failure to thrive
- Fat-soluble vitamin deficiencies (A, D, E, K)
- Salty sweat

Diagnostic Approach:

- Newborn screening: Immunoreactive trypsinogen (IRT) elevated; follow-up testing required

- Sweat chloride test: Gold standard; >60 mEq/L diagnostic; 40-59 mEq/L intermediate
- Genetic testing: *CFTR* mutation analysis (2+ mutations confirm diagnosis)
- Pancreatic function: 72-hour fecal fat, fecal chymotrypsin
- Pulmonary function: Spirometry, chest X-ray
- Glucose tolerance: Annual screening after age 10
- Liver function: Annual LFTs, ultrasound if abnormal

Management:
Multidisciplinary CF Center Care: Essential for optimal outcomes
Pulmonary Management:

- Airway clearance: Chest physiotherapy, high-frequency chest wall oscillation, or positive expiratory pressure (PEP) devices 2-4 times daily
- Bronchodilators: Albuterol before airway clearance to improve clearance
- DNase: Dornase alfa (recombinant human DNase) 2.5 mg inhaled daily; reduces sputum viscosity
- Hypertonic saline: 7% saline nebulized 2 times daily; enhances mucus clearance
- Antibiotics:
    - Prophylactic: Not recommended routinely

  - Acute exacerbations: Oral (ciprofloxacin), IV (tobramycin, ceftazidime), or inhaled (tobramycin, colistin) based on culture
  - Chronic suppression: Inhaled tobramycin or azithromycin for *Pseudomonas aeruginosa*
- CFTR modulators (breakthrough therapy):
  - Ivacaftor (Kalydeco): For G551D and other gating mutations; improves FEV1 by 10-15%
  - Lumacaftor/ivacaftor (Orkambi): For F508del homozygotes; modest FEV1 improvement (~3-4%)
  - Tezacaftor/ivacaftor (Symdeko): Improved potency over Orkambi
  - Elexacaftor/tezacaftor/ivacaftor (Trikafta): For F508del and other mutations; significant FEV1 improvement (13-15%)
- Immunizations: Annual influenza vaccine; pneumococcal vaccine
- Smoking cessation: Counsel family members

Gastrointestinal Management:

- Pancreatic enzyme replacement: Pancrelipase dosed with meals and snacks (typically 500-2,500 lipase units/kg/meal)
- Fat-soluble vitamins:
  - Vitamin A: 400,000-500,000 IU daily (monitor levels)

  - Vitamin D: 400-1,000 IU daily (target 25-OH vitamin D >30 ng/mL)
  - Vitamin E: 200-400 IU daily
  - Vitamin K: 5 mg 2-3 times weekly
- High-calorie diet: 120-150% of recommended daily intake; high fat content
- Nutritional monitoring: Monitor growth, weight, BMI; consider enteral supplementation if inadequate intake
- Acid suppression: Proton pump inhibitor if pancreatic insufficiency present (improves enzyme effectiveness)
- DIOS management: Increased fluid intake, osmotic laxatives (polyethylene glycol), N-acetylcysteine; severe cases may require GI intervention
- CFRD screening and management: Annual oral glucose tolerance test; insulin therapy if CFRD develops
- Hepatic monitoring: Annual LFTs and ultrasound; ursodeoxycholic acid if liver disease develops

Psychosocial Support:

- Counseling for depression and anxiety (common in CF)
- Transition planning to adult CF care
- Genetic counseling for family members
- Support groups and resources

Sickle Cell Disease

Pathophysiology:

- Point mutation in beta-globin gene (glutamic acid → valine at codon 6)
- Results in hemoglobin S (HbS) polymerization under deoxygenation
- Autosomal recessive; carrier frequency varies by ancestry (8-10% African Americans)
- Hemolytic anemia with vaso-occlusive complications

Clinical Recognition:

Infancy:

- Dactylitis (hand-foot syndrome): swelling and pain of hands/feet (first manifestation, often age 6 months-2 years)
- Acute chest syndrome: chest pain, fever, infiltrate on CXR
- Splenic sequestration crisis: acute splenomegaly, anemia, shock
- Overwhelming sepsis (especially with encapsulated organisms)

Childhood:

- Recurrent vaso-occlusive crises: severe bone and joint pain
- Acute chest syndrome
- Stroke: 5-10% by age 18 (transcranial Doppler screening

identifies high-risk patients)

- Avascular necrosis (femoral head, humeral head)
- Priapism: painful penile erection
- Splenic infarction leading to asplenia
- Renal papillary necrosis
- Gallstones (pigmented)
- Leg ulcers
- Retinopathy

Chronic Manifestations:

- Hemolytic anemia (Hb 7-10 g/dL)
- Growth delay
- Delayed puberty
- Pulmonary hypertension
- Chronic kidney disease
- Cognitive impairment (related to stroke history)

Diagnostic Approach:

- Newborn screening: Hemoglobin electrophoresis or HPLC
- Confirmation: Hemoglobin electrophoresis showing HbS
- Complete blood count: Hemoglobin, reticulocyte count, WBC, platelets

- Reticulocyte count: Usually elevated (5-25%)
- LDH and bilirubin: Elevated (hemolysis markers)
- Transcranial Doppler ultrasound: Screen for stroke risk (velocity >200 cm/sec = high risk)
- Chest X-ray: Baseline; acute imaging with chest pain
- Abdominal ultrasound: Assess spleen, gallstones, kidney function
- Ophthalmology: Screen for retinopathy

Management:

Preventive Care:

- Immunizations:
    - Pneumococcal: PCV13 followed by PPSV23; revaccination based on age
    - Meningococcal: MenACWY and MenB
    - *H. influenzae* type b
    - Influenza (annual)
    - COVID-19
- Penicillin prophylaxis: Penicillin V 125 mg BID <5 years; 250 mg BID ≥5 years; continue until age 5 minimum (some continue indefinitely)
- Folic acid: 1 mg daily (increased demand from hemolysis)

- Hydroxyurea therapy:
  - Mechanism: Increases fetal hemoglobin (HbF) production, reducing HbS polymerization
  - Indications: ≥3 vaso-occlusive crises per year, recurrent acute chest syndrome, severe anemia, chronic organ damage
  - Dosing: Start 15 mg/kg/day; titrate to maximum tolerated dose (MTD) over 8-12 weeks
  - Monitoring: CBC every 2 weeks during titration, then monthly; LFTs, renal function
  - Benefits: Reduces vaso-occlusive crises by 50%, reduces mortality by 40%
- Transcranial Doppler screening: Annual from age 2-16 years
- Stroke prevention:
  - High-risk patients (TCD velocity >200 cm/sec): Chronic transfusion program targeting HbS <30%
  - Iron chelation therapy if transfusion-dependent

Acute Crisis Management:

Vaso-occlusive Crisis:

- IV hydration: 1.5 times maintenance
- Analgesia: Opioids (morphine, hydromorphone) for severe pain

- Oxygen: Only if SpO_2 <90% or acute chest syndrome
- Antibiotics: If fever present
- Exchange transfusion: If severe symptoms or complications

Acute Chest Syndrome:

- Hospitalization
- Oxygen to maintain SpO_2 >90%
- IV hydration
- Antibiotics: Broad-spectrum coverage (covers atypical organisms)
- Analgesia
- Blood transfusion or exchange transfusion if severe
- Incentive spirometry to prevent atelectasis

Splenic Sequestration Crisis:

- IV hydration
- Blood transfusion
- Possible emergency splenectomy if life-threatening

Chronic Management:

- Regular hematology follow-up every 3-6 months
- Psychosocial support and pain management
- Transition planning to adult sickle cell care

- Genetic counseling for family members

X-Linked Disorders

Hemophilia A

Pathophysiology:

- Deficiency of clotting factor VIII
- X-linked recessive inheritance
- Incidence: 1:5,000 male births
- Severity correlates with factor VIII level: <1% severe, 1-5% moderate, >5% mild

Clinical Recognition:

- Spontaneous bleeding (severe form)
- Easy bruising
- Hemarthroses (joint bleeding): knees, elbows, ankles
- Muscle hematomas
- Prolonged bleeding after trauma or surgery
- Intracranial hemorrhage (life-threatening)
- Gastrointestinal bleeding
- Hematuria

Diagnostic Approach:

- Prolonged activated partial thromboplastin time (aPTT)
- Normal PT and bleeding time
- Low factor VIII activity level
- Normal von Willebrand factor level
- Genetic testing: *F8* gene mutation

Management:

Factor VIII Replacement:

- Prophylaxis (preferred): Regular infusions to maintain factor VIII level >1%
    - Dosing: 25-40 IU/kg 3 times weekly or every other day
    - Initiated in early childhood; improves joint outcomes
- On-demand therapy: Factor VIII given only with bleeding episodes
    - Dosing: 10-50 IU/kg IV depending on severity and location of bleeding
    - Target levels: 20-40% for minor bleeding, 50-100% for major bleeding/surgery

Factor VIII Products:

- Plasma-derived (less commonly used now due to infection risk history)
- Recombinant factor VIII (preferred)

- Extended half-life recombinant products (allow less frequent dosing)

Complications Management:

- Inhibitor development (10-15% of patients): Immune tolerance induction, bypassing agents (activated prothrombin complex concentrate, recombinant factor VIIa)
- Viral infections: Screen for HIV and hepatitis C; vaccinate for hepatitis A and B
- Joint damage: Physical therapy, pain management, orthopedic intervention if severe

Psychosocial Support:

- Counseling regarding activity restrictions and lifestyle
- Transition planning to adult care
- Genetic counseling for female carriers

MULTIFACTORIAL GENETIC DISORDERS

Congenital Heart Defects (CHD)

Epidemiology:

- Most common birth defect (8-10 per 1,000 live births)
- Result from abnormal cardiac development
- Multifactorial: genetic predisposition + environmental fac-

tors

- Recurrence risk: 2-4% if one parent affected, 3-5% if one sibling affected

Common Types:

- Ventricular septal defect (VSD): 30% of CHD
- Atrial septal defect (ASD): 10% of CHD
- Patent ductus arteriosus (PDA): 10% of CHD
- Tetralogy of Fallot: 8% of CHD
- Transposition of great arteries: 5% of CHD
- Coarctation of aorta: 5% of CHD

Clinical Recognition:

- Cyanosis (blue baby syndrome)
- Murmur on auscultation
- Feeding difficulties
- Failure to thrive
- Dyspnea
- Clubbing (chronic hypoxia)

Diagnostic Approach:

- Prenatal ultrasound
- Postnatal chest X-ray

- Echocardiography (gold standard)
- ECG
- Cardiac catheterization (if intervention planned)
- Genetic testing if syndromic features present (22q11 deletion, trisomy 21, etc.)

Management:

- Medical management: Prostaglandin E1 to keep PDA open if needed for pulmonary or systemic circulation
- Surgical repair: Timing depends on type and severity of defect
- Interventional catheterization: Device closure for certain defects
- Long-term cardiology follow-up
- Genetic counseling regarding recurrence risk

GENOMIC DISORDERS

22q11 Deletion Syndrome (DiGeorge Syndrome)

Pathophysiology:

- Microdeletion of chromosome 22q11.2
- Incidence: 1:4,000 live births

- Autosomal dominant; 90% de novo mutations, 10% inherited
- Results from abnormal neural crest cell migration

Clinical Features (Highly Variable):

- Cardiac: Congenital heart defects (74%): tetralogy of Fallot, VSD, conotruncal defects, aortic arch anomalies
- Palatal: Cleft palate or velopharyngeal insufficiency (speech hypernasality)
- Thymic: Thymic hypoplasia or aplasia; immunodeficiency (T-cell deficiency)
- Hypocalcemia: Due to parathyroid hypoplasia; seizures if severe
- Facial: Micrognathia, short philtrum, hypertelorism, ear abnormalities
- Renal: Renal anomalies (30-40%): hypoplasia, dysplasia
- Skeletal: Vertebral anomalies, limb abnormalities
- Developmental: Developmental delay (70%), intellectual disability (variable)
- Psychiatric: ADHD, anxiety, depression, psychosis (increased risk in adulthood)
- Hearing: Conductive hearing loss (common)

Diagnostic Approach:

- FISH or microarray: 22q11.2 deletion
- Cardiac evaluation: Echocardiography
- Immunological assessment: T-cell counts, immunoglobulin levels
- Calcium and phosphate levels
- Renal ultrasound
- Hearing assessment
- Developmental screening

Management:

- Cardiac: Surgical repair as indicated
- Immunological:
    - Monitor for infections
    - Thymic transplantation if severe immunodeficiency (rarely needed)
    - Avoid live vaccines if immunodeficiency present
- Calcium management: Calcium and calcitriol supplementation if hypocalcemic
- Palatal: Speech therapy; surgical intervention if indicated
- Hearing: Hearing aids if conductive loss
- Developmental: Early intervention, special education

- Psychiatric: Counseling, medication management
- Genetic counseling: 50% recurrence risk if parent affected

MITOCHONDRIAL DISORDERS

General Principles:

- Maternal inheritance pattern
- Heteroplasmy: mixture of normal and mutant mtDNA
- Variable expressivity and age of onset
- Progressive neurological and multisystem involvement common

Common Presentations:

- MELAS (Mitochondrial Encephalomyopathy, Lactic Acidosis, Stroke-like episodes)
- MERRF (Myoclonic Epilepsy with Ragged-Red Fibers)
- Leigh syndrome (subacute necrotizing encephalopathy)
- LHON (Leber Hereditary Optic Neuropathy)

Management:

- Supportive care
- Seizure management
- Stroke prevention
- Metabolic support: L-arginine during acute strokes, CoQ10, carnitine supplementation
- Genetic counseling: Maternal inheritance; all children of affected mothers at risk

GENETIC SCREENING AND COUNSELING

Newborn Screening Programs

Purpose and Scope:

- Early detection of genetic, metabolic, and functional disorders
- Allows intervention before symptoms develop
- Varies by state/country; typically screens 30-60+ conditions
- Performed on dried blood spot from heel stick at 24-48 hours of life

Common Screened Conditions:

- Phenylketonuria (PKU)
- Congenital hypothyroidism

- Sickle cell disease
- Maple syrup urine disease
- Homocystinuria
- Cystic fibrosis
- Biotinidase deficiency
- Medium-chain acyl-CoA dehydrogenase (MCAD) deficiency
- G6PD deficiency "offered in countries with high disease incidence"

Management of Abnormal Newborn Screen:

1. Confirm with repeat testing
2. Initiate diagnostic workup
3. Begin treatment if diagnosis confirmed
4. Provide family counseling and support

Prenatal Genetic Screening

First Trimester Screening (11-14 weeks):

- Maternal serum markers: PAPP-A (pregnancy-associated plasma protein A), hCG
- Ultrasound: Nuchal translucency (NT) measurement
- Detects: Trisomy 21, Trisomy 18, Trisomy 13

- Detection rate: 85-90% with 5% false positive rate

Second Trimester Screening (15-22 weeks):

- Quad screen: AFP, hCG, uE3, inhibin A
- Detection rate: 80% for Down syndrome
- Can be combined with first trimester (sequential or integrated screening)

Cell-Free Fetal DNA Testing (cfDNA/NIPT):

- Non-invasive prenatal testing
- Analyzes fetal DNA fragments in maternal blood
- Can be performed from 10 weeks gestation
- Detection rate: >99% for trisomy 21, 98% for trisomy 18
- False positive rate: <1%
- Advantages: Highly accurate, non-invasive, early timing
- Limitations: Cannot detect balanced rearrangements, requires adequate fetal fraction (typically >4%)
- Expanded panels: Can detect microdeletions (22q11, 5p, etc.)

Diagnostic Testing:

- Chorionic villus sampling (CVS): 11-14 weeks; 0.2-0.5% miscarriage risk
- Amniocentesis: 15-20 weeks; 0.1-0.3% miscarriage risk

- Karyotype analysis
- Microarray
- Targeted genetic testing

Genetic Counseling

Definition and Goals:

- Process of helping individuals and families understand genetic information
- Assess inheritance patterns and recurrence risks
- Support informed decision-making
- Provide emotional support and resources

Key Components:

1. Risk assessment: Obtain detailed family history (pedigree)
2. Education: Explain inheritance patterns, test options, results implications
3. Discussion of options: Prenatal testing, carrier screening, management strategies
4. Support: Address emotional concerns, provide resources
5. Follow-up: Ongoing support after diagnosis or test results

Indications for Genetic Counseling:

- Family history of genetic disorder

- Abnormal prenatal screening
- Diagnosis of genetic disorder in child
- Carrier screening before pregnancy
- Advanced maternal age (≥35 years)
- Recurrent pregnancy loss
- Consanguinity
- Ethnic background with increased risk for specific disorders

CARRIER SCREENING

Purpose:

- Identify couples at risk of having children with genetic disorders
- Allow for informed reproductive decision-making
- Enable prenatal diagnosis if desired

Ethnicity-Specific Screening:

Ashkenazi Jewish:

- Tay-Sachs disease
- Cystic fibrosis

- Canavan disease
- Familial dysautonomia
- Gaucher disease
- Niemann-Pick disease

Mediterranean (Greek, Italian, Turkish):

- Thalassemia
- G6PD deficiency

African:

- Sickle cell disease
- Thalassemia
- G6PD deficiency

Southeast Asian:

- Thalassemia
- G6PD deficiency

Expanded Carrier Panels:

- Screen for 100+ recessive conditions
- Recommended for all couples
- Identifies carriers regardless of ethnicity

Timing:

- Ideally before conception
- Can be offered at first prenatal visit

Results Interpretation:

- Negative: Low risk of affected child (unless test not comprehensive)
- Positive: Carrier of one mutated gene; risk depends on partner's carrier status
- Partner testing: Essential if one partner is carrier

MANAGEMENT OF GENETIC DISORDERS IN CHILDHOOD

Family-Centered Care

Key Principles:

- Involve family in all decisions
- Respect family values and preferences
- Provide clear, compassionate communication
- Offer psychosocial support
- Connect with resources and support groups

Transition Planning (Adolescence to Adulthood)"Neonatal ..Paediatrics..Adult service"

- Prepare for transfer to adult specialists

- Develop self-advocacy skills
- Discuss reproductive health and genetic implications
- Address educational and vocational planning
- Establish adult healthcare providers

Psychosocial Support

Common Issues:

- Grief and adjustment to diagnosis
- Anxiety regarding prognosis and future
- Depression (especially in adolescents)
- Body image concerns
- Social isolation
- Educational challenges
- Sibling adjustment

Interventions:

- Individual and family counseling
- Support groups
- School advocacy and IEP development
- Mental health referrals
- Peer mentorship programs

ETHICAL CONSIDERATIONS IN GENETIC MEDICINE

Informed Consent

- Individuals must understand purpose, benefits, risks, and limitations of genetic testing
- Must be voluntary without coercion
- Right to decline testing
- Right to receive or not receive results

Privacy and Confidentiality

- Genetic information is highly sensitive
- Protect from unauthorized access
- HIPAA compliance
- State laws regarding genetic privacy vary

Genetic Discrimination

- Protect from employment discrimination
- Protect from insurance discrimination

- Genetic Information Nondiscrimination Act (GINA) provides federal protection
- Limitations: Does not cover life insurance, disability insurance, long-term care insurance

Incidental Findings

- Secondary findings discovered during genetic testing
- Examples: *BRCA1/2* mutations, familial hypercholesterolemia
- Ethical obligation to disclose if actionable
- Must discuss possibility before testing

Duty to Relatives

- Genetic information affects family members
- Tension between individual privacy and family benefit
- Encourage communication with at-risk relatives
- Provide support for disclosure

CLINICAL PEARLS AND KEY TAKEAWAYS

Genetic heterogeneity: Similar phenotypes can result from different genetic causes; molecular diagnosis increasingly important

Variable expressivity: Same mutation can cause different severity in different individuals

Penetrance: Not all individuals with disease-causing mutations manifest the phenotype

Anticipation: Trinucleotide repeat disorders show worsening severity and earlier age of onset in successive generations

Imprinting: Some genetic disorders show parent-of-origin effects (e.g., Prader-Willi vs. Angelman syndrome)

Microarray is superior to karyotype: Detects submicroscopic deletions and duplications; recommended as first-line chromosomal testing

Early intervention improves outcomes: Developmental delay, therapy, and support services significantly improve prognosis in many genetic disorders

Multidisciplinary care essential: Genetic disorders often require coordination among multiple specialists

Genetic counseling improves outcomes: Helps families understand diagnosis, make informed decisions, and access support

Rapidly evolving field: New genetic discoveries, therapies, and screening technologies emerging constantly; stay current with literature

Chapter Twenty-Four

CONGENITAL ANOMALIES

INTRODUCTION: WHEN NORMAL DEVELOPMENT GOES AWAY

Congenital anomalies are one of those realities that hits you hard as a neonatal clinician. You're expecting a healthy newborn, and instead you're facing a baby with a visible defect, an unexpected diagnosis, or a condition that will require immediate intervention. The pressure is real—parents are frightened, you need to act decisively, and you often don't have all the answers immediately.

Here's what matters: congenital anomalies occur in 2-3% of live births, and many are compatible with life and good outcomes. Your job isn't to panic or to become an expert surgeon overnight. Your job is to recognize what you're seeing, stabilize the baby, avoid making things worse, and get the right specialists involved quickly.

This chapter focuses on the anomalies you'll actually encounter in the delivery room or first hours of life—the ones where your initial actions matter tremendously. We're talking about conditions that need immediate recognition and intervention: abdominal wall defects, diaphragmatic hernia, esophageal atresia, and other structural problems that can't wait.

The key principle here: Structural anomalies demand respect. They're often part of a bigger picture. Don't get tunnel vision on one defect—think about what else might be wrong. And always, always prioritize stabilization over definitive repair.

ABDOMINAL WALL DEFECTS: GASTROSCHISIS AND OMPHALOCELE

RECOGNITION: THE MOMENT YOU SEE IT

You'll know it immediately. The baby is born with exposed abdominal contents. But here's where most clinicians get confused: gastroschisis and omphalocele look similar at first glance, but they're fundamentally different problems requiring different immediate management.

Gastroschisis: The defect is mostly a small opening (usually 2-4 cm) typically to the right of the umbilical cord. The bowel herniates through and hangs outside the abdomen, often matted together and inflamed-looking. There's no covering membrane. The bowel looks angry—edematous, discolored, sometimes darkened from amniotic fluid exposure.

Omphalocele: This is a larger defect covered by a shiny membrane (the sac). The umbilical cord inserts into the sac itself. The contents include bowel but also often liver or other organs. The sac looks intact, glistening, sometimes quite large.

The critical difference? Gastroschisis is a surgical emergency requiring closure within hours. Omphalocele is urgent but often manageable with staged closure or even non-operative management depending on size.

Red flags you need to recognize immediately:

- Bowel that's dark, necrotic-looking, or obviously damaged (suggests intrauterine volvulus or compromise)
- Signs of sepsis or peritonitis (fever, lethargy, metabolic acidosis)
- Respiratory distress out of proportion to the defect (suggests associated anomalies or tension from visceral packing)
- Bilious drainage from the defect (indicates bowel perforation)

WHAT TO DO IMMEDIATELY

First things first: DO NOT touch that exposed bowel with your bare hands. I know it's tempting to try to push it back in. Don't. Here's your action sequence:

In the delivery room:

1. Keep the baby warm. Exposed viscera lose heat rapidly. Use plastic wrap or sterile drapes to cover the defect—this reduces evaporative losses and contamination.
2. Do NOT attempt closure or reduction. The temptation is strong, but forcing the bowel back into an ab-

domen that's too small causes abdominal "compartment syndrome", compromises perfusion, and kills babies.

3. Establish IV access and begin fluid resuscitation. These babies need aggressive hydration—they're losing fluid through the exposed bowel.

4. Place an orogastric tube and set it to low intermittent suction. Gastroschisis babies often have ileus; gastric decompression prevents aspiration.

5. Start broad-spectrum antibiotics immediately. The exposed bowel is colonized within hours.

6. Call your surgical team NOW. Don't wait for a transfer. Don't wait for imaging. These babies need the OR.

Transport considerations:

- If you're not at a surgical center, this baby needs transport NOW.

- Keep the defect covered with sterile gauze moistened with warm normal saline wrapped in plastic.

- Maintain NPO status.

- Continue IV fluids and antibiotics during transport.

- Have your surgical team aware of ETA.

DIAGNOSTIC APPROACH: WHAT YOU ACTUALLY NEED TO KNOW

Honestly? If you can see the defect clinically, you don't need imaging to confirm it. But here's what matters:

Ultrasound or CT (if available and not delaying transfer):

- Differentiates gastroschisis from omphalocele if unclear
- Assesses for associated anomalies (cardiac, renal, GI malrotation)
- Evaluates bowel viability if concerned about compromise

Associated anomalies to screen for:

- Cardiac defects (echo if time permits)
- Renal anomalies (ultrasound)
- Intestinal malrotation (common with gastroschisis)
- Trisomy 13 or 18 (especially with omphalocele)

Labs:

- CBC, metabolic panel, lactate (baseline for acidosis)
- Blood type and cross-match
- Blood culture (before antibiotics if possible)

But here's the reality: don't let imaging studies delay surgical evaluation. The surgeon needs to see this baby in person.

MANAGEMENT: WHAT HAPPENS NEXT

Gastroschisis: This is a surgical emergency. Most will go to the OR for primary closure within 6-12 hours. If the defect is small and reduction causes significant tension, surgeons may use a staged approach with a "silo" (a temporary plastic pouch) that's gradually reduced over days.

Your role: Keep the baby stable, maintain fluids, prevent infection, and don't interfere with surgical planning.

Omphalocele: This depends on size. Small defects (<5 cm) often close primarily. Larger defects may need staged closure, and some surgeons will manage them non-operatively with topical agents (silver sulfadiazine, iodine-based solutions) allowing the defect to epithelialize over weeks to months.

The key is that omphalocele isn't always an immediate OR case like gastroschisis is.

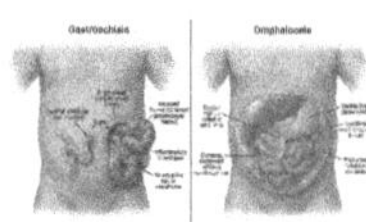

COMPLICATIONS AND RED FLAGS

Abdominal compartment syndrome is the nightmare complication of attempted primary closure. Signs include:

- Severe respiratory distress after closure
- Oliguria despite adequate fluid resuscitation
- Elevated peak airway pressures
- Metabolic acidosis
- Decreased perfusion

If you see this, notify your surgical team immediately. The closure may need to be partially undone or converted to a silo.

Infection is a constant threat. These babies are on antibiotics for weeks. Watch for:

- Fever (not always present with neonatal sepsis)

- Leukopenia or left shift
- Increasing lactate
- Feeding intolerance
- Bowel perforation (free air on imaging)

Bowel dysfunction is expected. Gastroschisis babies often have prolonged ileus, dysmotility, and feeding difficulties. Some develop short bowel syndrome if significant bowel is necrotic.

COMMON PITFALLS AND MISTAKES

Mistake #1: Trying to close the defect yourself. I've seen this. A clinician thinks they're helping by reducing the bowel. Result? The baby goes into respiratory distress, develops compartment syndrome, and needs emergency decompression. Let the surgeons make that call.

Mistake #2: Underestimating fluid needs. These babies need aggressive resuscitation—often 100-150 mL/kg/day initially. They're losing fluids through exposed viscera, and they're often growth-restricted. Don't be stingy with fluids.

Mistake #3: Delaying antibiotics. Exposed bowel is colonized rapidly. Start broad-spectrum coverage immediately. Don't wait for culture results.

Mistake #4: Missing associated anomalies. Especially with omphalocele—this is associated with Beckwith-Wiedemann syndrome, trisomy 13, and cardiac defects. Screen carefully.

Mistake #5: Assuming omphalocele needs emergency surgery. It doesn't. Many omphaloceles are managed conservatively. Don't create urgency where it doesn't exist.

WHEN TO ESCALATE CARE

- Any abdominal wall defect = immediate surgical consultation. Full stop.
- Signs of bowel compromise (dark, perforated, necrotic appearance) = emergency OR.
- Respiratory distress after closure = possible compartment syndrome; notify surgeon immediately.
- Sepsis = escalate antibiotics, consider ICU-level care.
- Feeding intolerance or abdominal distension = imaging and surgical evaluation.

DIAPHRAGMATIC HERNIA: THE DEFECT THAT "STEALS LUNG SPACE"

RECOGNITION: THE SUBTLE PRESENTATION THAT CATCHES YOU OFF GUARD

Unlike abdominal wall defects, diaphragmatic hernia doesn't announce itself. The baby looks relatively normal at birth—maybe a little grunty, maybe needing some oxygen. Then over the first hours, respiratory distress worsens. You're bagging the baby, thinking "this is RDS," but something feels off. The baby's not responding the way you'd expect.

Here's what's happening: there's a hole in the diaphragm (usually left-sided, sometimes right). Abdominal contents herniate into the chest cavity during fetal development, compressing the lungs. The baby is born with hypoplastic lungs—lungs that never developed normally because they were squeezed by liver, bowel, or spleen.

Clinical presentation:

- Respiratory distress within first hours (can be subtle or dramatic)
- Barrel-shaped chest (from hyperinflation)
- Scaphoid (sunken) abdomen (because organs are in the chest)
- Bowel sounds heard in the chest
- Asymmetrical breath sounds (usually decreased on affected side)
- Heart sounds displaced (often to the right if left-sided hernia)
- Cyanosis that doesn't respond well to oxygen

The critical insight: This baby's problem isn't primarily respiratory failure—it's that there's not enough lung tissue. You can bag and mask all day, but you're trying to ventilate lungs that are only 40-50% of normal size.

WHAT TO DO IMMEDIATELY

Here's where most clinicians go wrong: they aggressively bag the baby, trying to get oxygen in and CO_2 out. This makes things worse. Why?

Because aggressive bagging inflates the bowel in the chest cavity, compressing the lungs further and shifting the mediastinum. You're making it worse.

Your action sequence:

1. Place an orogastric tube immediately and set it to low intermittent suction. This is critical. Bowel in the chest will distend with air during bagging, worsening compression. Decompressing the GI tract is your first priority.

2. Gentle ventilation only. Use low pressures (14-16 cm H_2O initially). Watch chest rise—you want gentle movement, not aggressive inflation. You're not trying to achieve "normal" blood gases; you're trying to avoid making things worse.

3. Consider high-frequency oscillatory ventilation (HFOV). Many centers use HFOV from the start with diaphragmatic hernia because it uses lower tidal volumes and lower mean airway pressures—less likely to cause barotrauma and mediastinal shift.

4. Avoid CPAP. Continuous positive airway pressure will inflate the bowel in the chest. Don't use it.

5. Get IV access and start fluids. These babies often need pressors because of mediastinal shift and compromised cardiac output.

6. Call your surgical team and your ECMO center. Diaphragmatic hernia is a surgical emergency, and many babies will need ECMO. Don't wait.

7. Prepare for possible ECMO cannulation. Many babies with

diaphragmatic hernia need ECMO support before, during, or after surgery. Have your ECMO team aware.

DIAGNOSTIC APPROACH: CONFIRMING WHAT YOU SUSPECT

Chest X-ray: This is your confirmation. You'll see:

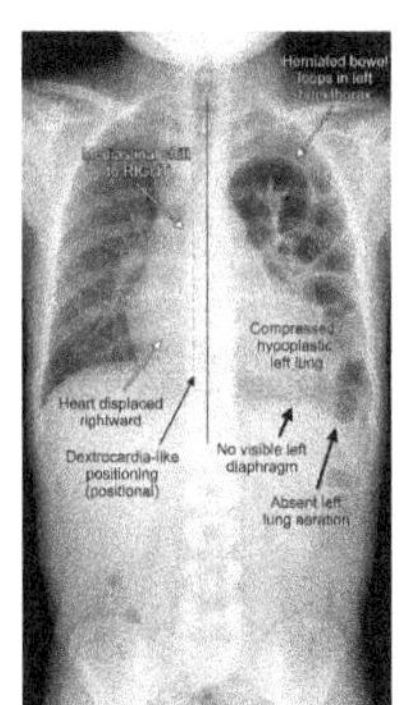

- Bowel loops in the chest cavity
- Mediastinal shift (heart displaced)
- Hyperinflation of remaining lung tissue
- Possibly stomach or liver in the chest

The X-ray might show the defect more clearly than your clinical exam.

Ultrasound or CT: Helps define the defect, assess liver position (if liver is in chest, prognosis is worse), and estimate lung volumes.

Associated anomalies:

- Cardiac defects (10-15%)
- Vertebral anomalies
- Esophageal atresia
- Cardiac echo if time permits

MANAGEMENT: THE LONG GAME

Preoperative stabilization: Your goal is not to "fix" the baby's oxygenation before surgery. Your goal is to keep the baby stable enough to reach the OR or ECMO cannulation site.

- Gentle ventilation with low pressures
- Keep orogastric tube to suction
- Maintain blood pressure with fluids and pressors (dopamine, dobutamine)
- Permissive hypercapnia: accept CO_2 levels of 50-60 mmHg if needed. You're not curing the lungs; you're keeping the baby alive until surgery.
- Avoid agitation (use sedation if needed)

ECMO consideration: Many babies with diaphragmatic hernia need ECMO support. Some go on ECMO preoperatively to stabilize, then have surgery. Others go on ECMO intraoperatively if they can't tolerate repair. This is a surgical/ECMO team decision.

Surgical repair: This happens when the baby is stable enough. The surgeon closes the diaphragmatic defect, allowing the abdominal contents back into the abdomen. The challenge is that the lungs are hypoplastic—even with the defect closed, the baby still has limited lung capacity.

Postoperative management: Often more challenging than surgery itself. These babies have:

- Persistent pulmonary hypoplasia
- Pulmonary hypertension
- Potential for barotrauma and volutrauma

- Prolonged ventilator dependence

Management focuses on gentle ventilation, managing pulmonary hypertension (inhaled nitric oxide, sildenafil), and gradual weaning.

COMPLICATIONS AND RED FLAGS

Pulmonary hypertension is the major post-repair complication. Signs include:

- Acute desaturation
- Right-to-left shunting
- Hypotension
- Decreased urine output

Management includes inhaled nitric oxide, milrinone, and sometimes ECMO support.

Mediastinal shift during ventilation can compromise cardiac output. If you see sudden hypotension or decreased perfusion during bagging, you've shifted the mediastinum. Stop aggressive ventilation.

Liver in chest (right-sided hernia with liver herniation) carries worse prognosis. Lung hypoplasia is more severe.

Recurrent hernia occurs in 5-10% of cases. Watch for recurrent respiratory distress weeks to months after repair.

COMMON PITFALLS AND MISTAKES

Mistake #1: Aggressive bagging. This is the big one. Clinicians see a baby in distress and instinctively bag hard. Result? Bowel inflates, mediastinum shifts, baby crashes. Gentle ventilation only.

Mistake #2: Forgetting the orogastric tube. This is your secret weapon. Decompressing the GI tract often dramatically improves ventilation and oxygenation before surgery.

Mistake #3: Trying to "normalize" blood gases. You can't. The baby has limited lung tissue. Accept higher CO_2 and lower pH. Your goal is perfusion and oxygenation adequate for survival, not normal values.

Mistake #4: Missing the diagnosis. If a baby has scaphoid abdomen + respiratory distress + bowel sounds in chest, think diaphragmatic hernia. Don't assume it's RDS.

Mistake #5: Using CPAP. This will inflate the bowel in the chest. Don't do it.

WHEN TO ESCALATE CARE

- Any suspicion of diaphragmatic hernia = immediate surgical consultation and ECMO center notification.
- Worsening respiratory status despite gentle ventilation = ECMO evaluation.
- Signs of pulmonary hypertension = increase inhaled nitric oxide, consider milrinone.
- Hemodynamic instability = pressors, consider ECMO.
- Persistent hypoxemia despite all interventions = ECMO.

ESOPHAGEAL ATRESIA AND TRACHEOESOPHAGEAL FISTULA

RECOGNITION: THE BABY WHO CAN'T HANDLE SECRETIONS

This one has a classic presentation if you know what to look for. The baby is born and immediately starts drooling excessively. You try to feed, and the baby chokes or gags. There's respiratory distress, sometimes cyanosis. The baby sounds congested.

What's happening: the esophagus ends in a blind pouch (atresia), and there's usually a fistula connecting the trachea to the distal esophagus. Saliva and gastric contents reflux into the trachea, causing aspiration and respiratory symptoms.

Clinical red flags:

- Excessive drooling within first hours of life
- Choking or gagging with feeding attempts
- Respiratory distress
- Cyanotic episodes (from aspiration)
- Abdominal distension (if there's a distal fistula, air enters the stomach)
- Inability to pass an orogastric tube into the stomach

Associated anomalies (VACTERL association):

- Vertebral defects
- Anorectal malformations
- Cardiac defects

- Tracheoesophageal fistula
- Renal anomalies
- Limb anomalies

If you see EA/TEF, screen for the other VACTERL components.

WHAT TO DO IMMEDIATELY

1. NPO—nothing by mouth. Stop feeding immediately. Any oral intake will aspirate.
2. Place a large-bore orogastric tube (10-12 Fr) and leave it to continuous low suction. This decompresses the blind esophageal pouch, reducing aspiration risk. Don't try to pass the tube into the stomach; if there's a blind pouch, the tube will just sit there draining secretions.
3. Position the baby prone or semi-prone with head elevated. This reduces aspiration risk.
4. Prepare for intubation. Many of these babies need airway protection because of aspiration risk. Have your equipment ready.
5. Start broad-spectrum antibiotics. These babies have aspirated; cover for respiratory infection.
6. Call your surgical team immediately. This is a surgical emergency requiring repair, usually within 24-48 hours.
7. Obtain a chest X-ray with the orogastric tube in place. If the

tube coils in the upper esophageal pouch, you've confirmed the diagnosis. If you see air in the stomach and bowel, there's a distal fistula.

DIAGNOSTIC APPROACH

Clinical suspicion + imaging = diagnosis:

Chest X-ray:

- Shows the orogastric tube coiling in the blind pouch
- May show aspiration pneumonia
- If air is in the stomach/bowel, confirms distal fistula

Contrast study:

- Sometimes done to confirm anatomy, but imaging delays surgery. If you're confident clinically, don't delay.

Associated anomaly screening:

- Cardiac echo (look for cardiac defects)
- Renal ultrasound
- Spine imaging if vertebral anomalies suspected
- Anorectal exam

MANAGEMENT

Preoperative:

- NPO

- Continuous suction on orogastric tube
- IV fluids
- Antibiotics
- Minimal handling; avoid agitation
- Intubate if aspiration risk high or respiratory distress significant

Surgical repair: Usually primary repair of the fistula and anastomosis of the esophageal segments. Timing depends on the baby's stability and associated anomalies.

Postoperative:

- Chest tube often placed
- NPO for several days
- Parenteral nutrition
- Gradual advancement to feeding once anastomosis healed
- Watch for stricture formation (common complication)

COMPLICATIONS AND RED FLAGS

- Aspiration pneumonia is common. Signs include fever, infiltrates on X-ray, respiratory deterioration.
- Esophageal stricture develops in 10-40% of cases, usually weeks after repair. Baby has feeding difficulties, regurgitation, or respiratory symptoms.

- Anastomotic leak is a surgical emergency. Signs include fever, subcutaneous emphysema, pneumothorax, sepsis.
- Recurrent fistula can occur if the fistula wasn't completely divided.

COMMON PITFALLS

Mistake #1: Feeding the baby before diagnosis. If you feed a baby with EA/TEF, you're aspirating formula. Don't do it.

Mistake #2: Trying to pass the orogastric tube into the stomach. It won't go. Leave it in the blind pouch for suction.

Mistake #3: Using CPAP. If there's a distal fistula, CPAP will inflate the stomach and bowel, worsening abdominal distension and splinting the diaphragm.

Mistake #4: Missing associated anomalies. Screen for VACTERL components.

WHEN TO ESCALATE

- Any suspicion of EA/TEF = immediate surgical consultation.
- Aspiration pneumonia = increase antibiotics, consider ICU-level care.
- Respiratory distress = intubate and protect airway.
- Anastomotic leak = emergency surgical evaluation.

KEY CLINICAL PEARLS

Abdominal wall defects need immediate surgical evaluation, but not all need emergency surgery. Gastroschisis is urgent; omphalocele can often be managed more deliberately.

Gentle ventilation is your friend with diaphragmatic hernia. Aggressive bagging makes things worse. Decompress the GI tract first.

The orogastric tube is your most powerful tool. Whether it's abdominal wall defect, diaphragmatic hernia, or EA/TEF, decompressing the GI tract improves outcomes.

Structural anomalies often come in packages. Look for associated defects. VACTERL association is real.

Your job is stabilization, not definitive repair. Get these babies to surgery safely. Let the surgeons make the technical calls.

Permissive hypercapnia is acceptable. You're not trying to achieve normal blood gases; you're keeping the baby alive until surgical intervention.

Infection is a constant threat. Start antibiotics early and keep coverage broad until you know what you're dealing with.

These babies need aggressive fluid resuscitation. Exposed viscera, ongoing losses, and third-spacing mean higher fluid requirements than you'd expect.

Don't let imaging studies delay surgical evaluation. If you're confident clinically, get the baby to the surgeon. Imaging can happen there.

Parental support matters. These diagnoses are frightening. Be honest about what you know and don't know. Connect families with surgical teams and support resources early.

Chapter Twenty-Five

PERINATAL ASPHYXIA AND HYPOXIC-ISCHEMIC ENCEPHALOPATHY

INTRODUCTION: WHEN THE OXYGEN AND ITS CARRIER RUN OUT

Perinatal asphyxia is one of those moments that defines your career as a neonatal clinician. Everything was going fine, and then suddenly it wasn't. The baby's heart rate plummets. The meconium is thick. The baby comes out limp, not breathing, with an Apgar score that makes your stomach drop.

Here's the reality: perinatal asphyxia is terrifying, but panic is your enemy. What matters is what you do in the next few minutes. Your decisions—about resuscitation, about when to push harder, about when to step back—will shape this baby's entire life.

Let me be direct: not every baby with a low Apgar score has asphyxia. Not every baby with asphyxia will develop hypoxic-ischemic encephalopathy (HIE). And not every baby with HIE will have permanent injury. But the babies who do—they need you to recognize it early, treat it aggressively, and avoid making things worse.

This chapter is about recognizing the signs, understanding what's actually happening at the cellular level, and knowing when therapeutic hypothermia can change the trajectory of a baby's life.

UNDERSTANDING PERINATAL ASPHYXIA: WHAT'S REALLY HAPPENING

THE PATHOPHYSIOLOGY YOU NEED TO UNDERSTAND

When oxygen delivery fails—whether from placental abruption, cord prolapse, maternal hypotension, or fetal distress—the baby's cells start dying. But it's not immediate. There are phases, and understanding them matters because it changes how you respond.

Phase 1: Primary Asphyxia (Minutes 0-5)

The oxygen runs out. The baby's cells shift to anaerobic metabolism. Lactate accumulates. The pH drops. The baby's heart rate drops (from vagal stimulation and hypoxia). Breathing stops. This is the "gasping" phase—the baby makes some respiratory efforts but they're ineffective.

Here's the critical part: during this phase, the baby is still salvageable. If you restore oxygen now, the baby recovers. The damage is minimal.

Phase 2: Secondary Asphyxia (Minutes 5-20)

If oxygen isn't restored, things get worse. The baby's heart rate drops further. Blood pressure falls. Perfusion to vital organs (brain, heart, kidneys) becomes compromised. The baby enters a state of "apparent recovery"—heart rate comes back up a bit, there might be some gasping. Clinicians sometimes mistake this for improvement. It's not. It's the baby's dying gasp.

During this phase, if you restore oxygen, there's still hope—but the damage is accumulating.

Phase 3: Terminal Asphyxia (Minutes 20+)

The baby's heart rate drops to nothing. Breathing stops completely. Without intervention, this is death. But here's where resuscitation saves lives: you're providing oxygen artificially, buying time for the baby's own systems to recover.

The cellular damage during phases 2 and 3 is what causes HIE—the hypoxic-ischemic encephalopathy that can lead to cerebral palsy, developmental delay, and death.

THE WINDOW THAT MATTERS

Here's what you need to know: there's a "window" after asphyxia where the damage is still reversible. It's called the latent phase—usually 6 hours after the insult. During this window, therapeutic hypothermia works. After this window closes, hypothermia doesn't help.

This is why timing matters so much. If you identify asphyxia early and get the baby cooled within 6 hours, you can reduce the risk of death or severe disability by about 50%. Miss this window, and you've lost a critical intervention.

RECOGNITION: IDENTIFYING THE BABY WITH ASPHYXIA

THE IMMEDIATE SIGNS YOU NEED TO SPOT

At birth:

- Apgar score of 0-3 at 1 minute and below 5 at 10 minutes(severely depressed)
- No respiratory effort or only gasping
- No heart rate or heart rate <100
- Limp, no muscle tone
- Pale or cyanotic appearance
- Meconium-stained amniotic fluid (not diagnostic alone, but concerning)

The baby who doesn't respond to resuscitation: You're bagging the baby, providing chest compressions, giving epinephrine—and the baby's not responding. Heart rate stays low or absent. Perfusion doesn't improve. This is profound asphyxia.

The baby with metabolic acidosis: Arterial or umbilical cord blood gas shows:

- pH <7.0
- Base deficit >12 mEq/L
- Lactate >18 mg/dL

This isn't just low oxygen—this is profound metabolic derangement from anaerobic metabolism.

The baby with seizures in the first hours: If a baby has seizures within the first 24 hours of life and there's no other obvious cause (infection, metabolic disorder), think of asphyxia. HIE causes seizures.

CRITERIA FOR ASPHYXIA-RELATED ENCEPHALOPATHY

Not every baby with a low Apgar score has asphyxia-related HIE. Here are the criteria that actually matter:

Essential criteria (must have all three):

1. Profound metabolic acidosis (pH <7.0 or base deficit ≥12 mEq/L in umbilical artery blood)
2. Apgar score of 0-3 for longer than 5 minutes
3. Neonatal encephalopathy (see below)

Neonatal encephalopathy signs (must have at least one):

- Altered consciousness (lethargy, stupor, coma)
- Seizures
- Abnormal muscle tone (hypotonia or hypertonia)
- Abnormal reflexes

- Difficulty feeding
- Respiratory depression

Supportive criteria:

- Fetal heart rate abnormalities before delivery
- Placental abruption or cord prolapse
- Maternal hypotension or trauma
- Meconium-stained fluid

Here's the key: you need the metabolic acidosis AND the low Apgar AND the encephalopathy signs. If you only have one or two, it's not asphyxia-related HIE—it's something else.

GRADING ENCEPHALOPATHY SEVERITY

Understanding severity matters because it guides your treatment decisions.

Mild encephalopathy (Sarnat Grade 1):

- Hyperalertness or irritability
- Normal or slightly increased muscle tone
- Normal reflexes
- No seizures
- Normal feeding
- Usually resolves within 24-48 hours

- Prognosis: generally good

Moderate encephalopathy (Sarnat Grade 2):

- Lethargy
- Hypotonia (decreased muscle tone)
- Weak suck, difficulty feeding
- Seizures (usually present)
- Abnormal reflexes
- May have bradycardia, hypotension
- Usually lasts 5-7 days
- Prognosis: variable; depends on severity and response to treatment

Severe encephalopathy (Sarnat Grade 3):

- Stupor or coma
- Severe hypotonia initially, then hypertonia
- No suck or feeding ability
- Frequent seizures, often difficult to control
- Absent or severely abnormal reflexes
- Severe cardiovascular instability
- May have respiratory depression
- Prognosis: poor; high risk of death or severe disability

Clinical reality: mild encephalopathy often doesn't need hypothermia. Moderate to severe encephalopathy is where hypothermia makes a difference.

WHAT TO DO IMMEDIATEL

RESUSCITATION: THE FIRST MINUTES

You know the NRP algorithm. But let me emphasize the parts that matter most for asphyxiated babies:

At delivery:

1. Dry the baby and stimulate. Even if the baby looks terrible, dry and stimulate for 10 seconds. You're buying time for the baby's respiratory center to respond.

2. Assess: Is the baby breathing? Is the heart rate >100? If yes to both, observe and warm. If not, move to the next step.

3. If not breathing or heart rate <100: Start positive pressure ventilation. Use a rate of 40-60 breaths per minute. Watch for chest rise. If you see it, you're ventilating adequately.

4. Reassess at 15 seconds. Is the heart rate >100 now? Is the baby starting to breathe? If yes, continue PPV. If not, check your technique—are you getting a good seal? Is the airway open?

5. If heart rate is still <100 after 30 seconds of adequate PPV: Start chest compressions. Use the two-thumb technique. Compress at a rate of 90 compressions per minute with 30 breaths per minute (3:1 ratio). Yes, this is different from adult CPR. This is what works for newborns.

6. Get IV access and give epinephrine. IV is preferred (umbilical vein), but if you can't get it quickly, intraosseous access works. Dose: 0.01-0.03 mg/kg (10-30 mcg/kg) IV. Repeat every 3-5 minutes if asystole or severe bradycardia persists.

7. Intubate if you're going to be doing this for more than a minute or two. Bag-mask ventilation works, but if you need sustained resuscitation, get the airway secured.

The critical decision point: How long do you continue resuscitation? Here's what matters: if the baby has a heartbeat at any point, keep going. If the baby is asystolic for 20 minutes without response to resuscitation, you might consider stopping. But honestly? Many asphyxiated babies respond to prolonged resuscitation. I've seen babies who required more than 20 minutes of resuscitation make recoveries with hypothermia therapy."The decision to stop CPR is kept for the most senior neonatologist at handy"

Don't give up too early. These babies can surprise you.

INITIAL STABILIZATION

Once the baby is resuscitated (or resuscitation is ongoing):

1. Get a blood gas immediately. Umbilical artery blood gas is ideal. You need to know the pH and base deficit.

2. Get blood glucose. Asphyxiated babies often have hypoglycemia. Check it and treat if low.

3. Get a lactate level. This is another marker of the severity of asphyxia.

4. Establish IV access if not already done. You'll need it for

medications and fluids.

5. Maintain normothermia (or mild hypothermia if you're considering cooling). Don't overheat the baby. Active cooling should start as soon as possible if criteria are met."Rem ember that warming every newborn soon after delivery is the standard care for all babies even if you believe that this baby may be a candidate of cooling therapy "

6. Avoid hypoxia and hyperoxia. Target SpO_2 90-95% (not 100%). Supplemental oxygen is fine, but don't overdo it—hyperoxia causes oxidative stress.

7. Avoid hypocapnia. Target PCO_2 of 45-55 mmHg. Hypocapnia (low CO_2) causes cerebral vasoconstriction and worsens ischemic injury.

8. Treat seizures aggressively. If the baby seizes, load with phenobarbital (20 mg/kg IV) or levetiracetam (20-40 mg/kg IV). Don't wait for a second seizure.

THERAPEUTIC HYPOTHERMIA: THE INTERVENTION THAT WORKS

"It is the only worldwide-approved ,evidence-based treatment for HIE at the moment"

WHEN TO USE IT

Not every baby with asphyxia needs hypothermia. You need to meet the criteria:

Inclusion criteria:

- Gestational age ≥36 weeks
- Postnatal age <6 hours (ideally <3 hours)
- Metabolic acidosis (pH <7.0 or base deficit ≥12 mEq/L in umbilical artery or arterial blood)
- AND at least ONE of the following:
    - Apgar score ≤5 at 10 minutes
    - Continued need for resuscitation at 10 minutes
    - Neonatal encephalopathy (moderate to severe)

Exclusion criteria:

- Gestational age <36 weeks
- Severe congenital anomalies incompatible with life
- Severe growth restriction (estimated fetal weight <1800 g)
- Severe infection/sepsis"septic shock"
- Severe metabolic disorder unrelated to asphyxia

Here's the reality: if you're unsure whether to cool, the data suggests cooling is safe even if the baby doesn't meet strict criteria. The risk-benefit favors cooling in borderline cases.

HOW TO DO IT

Whole-body cooling (preferred method): The baby's core temperature is lowered to 33-34°C and maintained for 72 hours.

Equipment:

- Cooling blanket or cooling cap (many devices available)
- Continuous temperature monitoring (esophageal, rectal, or bladder probe)
- Servo-controlled system to maintain target temperature

Protocol:

1. Initiate cooling as soon as possible (within 6 hours of birth, ideally within 3 hours).
2. Cool to 33-34°C over 4-6 hours. Don't cool too rapidly; this can cause arrhythmias.
3. Maintain at 33-34°C for 72 hours total.
4. Rewarm slowly (0.5°C per hour) over 6-12 hours. Rapid rewarming worsens outcomes.

What to monitor during cooling:

- Core temperature (every 15-30 minutes until target reached, then hourly, however mostly the cooling machine would monitor body temperature throughout the cooling period through a rectal sensor)
- Heart rate and rhythm (cooling can cause bradycardia; this is expected)
- Blood pressure (may drop; usually doesn't need intervention unless significant)

- Glucose (cooling impairs glucose metabolism; check frequently)
- Coagulation studies (cooling affects clotting; check baseline and periodically)
- Platelet count (may drop; usually recovers after rewarming)
- Seizures (cooling reduces seizure frequency but doesn't eliminate them)

Medications during cooling:

- Anticonvulsants: Phenobarbital or levetiracetam for seizure prevention/treatment
- Sedation: Morphine or midazolam to prevent shivering and agitation
- Paralysis: Sometimes used to prevent shivering (vecuronium or cisatracurium)

Honestly? Sedation and paralysis make cooling easier to manage, but they make it harder to assess the baby's neurological status. Use them judiciously.

WHAT HYPOTHERMIA ACTUALLY DOES

Let me be clear about what hypothermia does and doesn't do:

What it does:

- Reduces cerebral metabolic rate (the brain uses less oxygen)
- Reduces inflammation and excitotoxicity

- Reduces seizure frequency
- Reduces cell death “apoptosis”in the first 72 hours
- Improves outcomes: reduces death or severe disability by about 50%

What it doesn't do:

- It doesn't reverse damage that's already happened
- It doesn't prevent all brain injury
- It doesn't guarantee a normal outcome
- It doesn't work if started after 6 hours

The babies who benefit most from hypothermia are those with moderate encephalopathy. Mild encephalopathy has good outcomes anyway. Severe encephalopathy often has poor outcomes even with hypothermia.

COMPLICATIONS AND RED FLAGS DURING COOLING

EXPECTED EFFECTS OF HYPOTHERMIA

These are normal and expected:

- Bradycardia: Heart rate often drops to 80-100 bpm. This is fine as long as perfusion is adequate.
- Hypotension: Blood pressure may drop slightly. Usually it doesn't need intervention.

- Increased glucose: Cooling impairs glucose metabolism and insulin secretion. Hyperglycemia is common.
- Coagulopathy: Platelet count may drop, PT/PTT may lengthen. Usually reversed with rewarming.
- Reduced urine output: Cooling decreases renal perfusion. Oliguria is expected.
- Reduced seizure frequency: This is the goal.

RED FLAGS REQUIRING INTERVENTION

- Severe bradycardia (<60 bpm): Notably ,if blood pressure drops significantly, consider epinephrine infusion."if persistently kept below 60 bpm then commence CPR measures"
- Severe hypotension: If systolic pressure <40 mmHg or baby looks poorly perfused, give fluid bolus (10 mL/kg normal saline) or start dopamine.
- Arrhythmias: Cooling can cause atrial fibrillation or other arrhythmias. Usually self-limited. If hemodynamically significant, consider amiodarone or treating the underlying cause (hyperkalemia, hypocalcemia).
- Hyperkalemia: Asphyxia causes cellular breakdown and potassium release. Cooling worsens this. Check K^+ frequently. If >6.5 mEq/L, treat with calcium gluconate, insulin/glucose, and possibly sodium bicarbonate.
- Infection: Don't miss sepsis in a cooled baby. Fever is absent

(baby is hypothermic), so you have to rely on other signs. Check CBC, blood culture, and start antibiotics if concerned.

- Renal failure: Asphyxia damages kidneys. Hypothermia worsens this. Monitor urine output, creatinine, and BUN. If oliguria persists, be cautious with fluid administration.

- Bleeding: Coagulopathy from hypothermia can cause bleeding. Check coagulation studies. Most resolve with rewarming, but be ready to give FFP or platelets if needed.

DIAGNOSTIC APPROACH: WHAT IMAGING TELLS YOU

WHEN TO IMAGE AND WHY

Imaging doesn't change acute management, but it helps with prognosis and planning.

Head ultrasound:

- Can be done at bedside
- Detects gross abnormalities: intraventricular hemorrhage, severe edema, stroke
- Limited resolution compared to MRI
- Useful for screening; doesn't replace MRI

MRI (preferred for prognostic information):

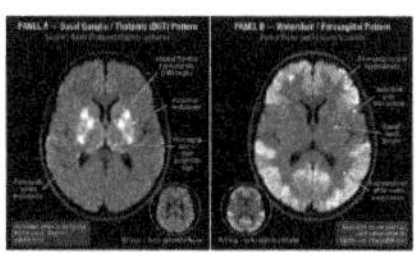

- Best imaging modality for HIE
- Shows pattern of injury: basal ganglia/thalamic pattern (typical for HIE) vs. watershed pattern (suggests timing differences)
- Should be done at 4-7 days of life (earlier MRI may look normal even with significant injury)
- Helps predict neurodevelopmental outcomes
- Doesn't change acute management but guides family counseling

EEG:

- Helps assess seizure activity
- Prognostic value: severely abnormal background predicts poor outcome
- Should be done early and repeated
- Helps guide anticonvulsant therapy

Amplitude-integrated EEG (aEEG):

- Continuous EEG monitoring
- Useful for seizure detection during cooling
- Good prognostic tool

WHAT TO TELL FAMILIES ABOUT PROGNOSIS

This is hard. Parents want to know: *will my baby be okay?* And honestly, you don't know yet. Here's what you can say:

Mild encephalopathy: "Most babies with mild encephalopathy do well. We expect your baby to recover over the next few days. We'll watch carefully for seizures and any other problems."

Moderate encephalopathy with cooling: "Your baby has significant injury from the lack of oxygen. We're using cooling therapy, which has been shown to reduce the risk of severe disability by about 50%. We won't know the full extent of any long-term effects for months or years. We'll do imaging and careful monitoring to help guide us."

Severe encephalopathy: "Your baby has very severe injury. Even with all our treatments, the risk of death or severe disability is high. We're going to do everything we can to support your baby and help you through this. We'll talk about comfort care if things don't improve."

Be honest. Be compassionate. Don't promise outcomes you can't guarantee.

COMMON PITFALLS AND MISTAKES

Mistake #1: Giving up on resuscitation too early. Asphyxiated babies can take a long time to respond. I've seen babies who required more than 20 minutes of resuscitation make promising recoveries with hypothermia. Don't stop for 20 minutes.

Mistake #2: Overheating the baby. Hyperthermia worsens outcomes in asphyxia. Keep the baby normothermic until you decide about cooling. Don't use warming blankets or heat lamps aggressively.

Mistake #3: Hyperventilating. High CO_2 is harmful in asphyxia. Target PCO_2 of 45-55 mmHg. Don't hyperventilate trying to correct acidosis.

Mistake #4: Missing the 6-hour window. Cooling only works if started within 6 hours. If you identify asphyxia at 7 hours, cooling mostly won't help. Make sure your transport and referral systems move quickly.

Mistake #5: Using 100% oxygen. Hyperoxia causes oxidative stress and worsens outcomes. Target SpO_2 90-95%.

Mistake #6: Cooling without sedation. Shivering during cooling is counterproductive. Sedate the baby appropriately.

Mistake #7: Rapid rewarming. Slow rewarming (0.5°C per hour) is critical. Rapid rewarming worsens outcomes.

Mistake #8: Not treating seizures aggressively. Seizures in HIE are harmful. Load with phenobarbital or levetiracetam at the first seizure, not after three seizures.

Mistake #9: Assuming all low Apgar scores are asphyxia. Some babies have low Apgar scores from prematurity, infection, or congenital anomalies. You need the metabolic acidosis AND encephalopathy to call it asphyxia-related HIE.

Mistake #10: Abandoning supportive care. Even with severe HIE, these babies need meticulous care. Infection, metabolic derangement, and secondary injuries can be prevented. Don't give up.

WHEN TO ESCALATE CARE

- Any baby with profound asphyxia requiring resuscitation = Tertiary NICU-level care, in rare cases you might consider referral to ECMO center.

- Metabolic acidosis with encephalopathy = immediate consideration for cooling (may need transfer).
- Seizures not controlled with phenobarbital = add levetiracetam, consider other agents, aEEG monitoring.
- Hemodynamic instability despite fluids = pressors.
- Renal failure = nephrology consultation, prepare for possible dialysis.
- Severe coagulopathy = “consider rewarming from cooling if initiated” , transfusion of FFP and injection of vitamin K is warranted .
- Severe respiratory depression = intubate and ventilate.

KEY CLINICAL PEARLS

Not every low Apgar is asphyxia. You need metabolic acidosis AND encephalopathy to make the diagnosis.

The first 6 hours are critical. Therapeutic hypothermia only works if started within this window.

Gentle ventilation is better than aggressive bagging. Avoid hypocapnia and hyperoxia.

Seizures are common and harmful. Treat them aggressively with phenobarbital or levetiracetam at the first seizure.

Cooling is safe even in borderline cases. If you're unsure, the data supports cooling.

Rewarming is as important as cooling. Slow rewarming (0.5°C per hour) over 6-12 hours is critical.

These babies need meticulous supportive care. Prevent secondary injuries: maintain normoglycemia, avoid infection, manage fluid and electrolytes carefully.

Prognostic information comes over time. Early imaging and aEEG help, but long-term outcomes aren't clear for months. Be honest about uncertainty.

Family support is critical. These families are traumatized. Connect them with resources, support groups, and long-term follow-up care.

Don't give up too early. Asphyxiated babies can surprise you. With aggressive resuscitation, cooling, and supportive care, outcomes can be better than expected.

Chapter Twenty-Six

MULTIPLE BIRTHS AND COMPLICATIONS

INTRODUCTION: WHEN ONE BABY BECOMES TWO (OR MORE)

Multiple births are a different beast entirely. You're not just managing one baby—you're managing two, three, or more newborns who share a placenta, share intrauterine space, and often share complications that single babies never see. The complexity multiplies exponentially.

Here's what matters: multiple births account for about 3% of all deliveries, but they account for a disproportionate amount of neonatal morbidity and mortality. Twins are more premature, smaller, and sicker than singletons. And if they're monochorionic (sharing a placenta), they face unique complications that can be devastating if you don't recognize them early.

This chapter is about understanding the different types of multiple births, recognizing the complications that are specific to multiples, and knowing when one baby's problem becomes both babies' problem. It's also about practical management—because managing multiples in the NICU is logistically different from managing singletons.

Let me be direct: if you don't understand chorionicity and amnionicity, you're flying blind with multiple births. This is foundational knowledge that changes everything about how you approach these babies.

CHORIONICITY AND AMNIONICITY: THE FOUNDATION YOU NEED

WHAT IT MEANS AND WHY IT MATTERS

When we talk about twins, we're really talking about three different scenarios, and each one has completely different risks:

Dichorionic-Diamniotic (DCDA) Twins:

- Two placentas (may appear fused)
- Two amniotic sacs
- Most common type of dizygotic (fraternal) twins
- Also occurs in about 30% of monozygotic (identical) twins
- Lowest risk for complications

- Each baby has independent placental circulation
- Complications are usually independent (one baby's problem doesn't automatically affect the other)

Monochorionic-Diamniotic (MCDA) Twins:

- One placenta
- Two amniotic sacs
- Results from monozygotic twinning (identical twins) that split after day 3-8 of conception
- Moderate risk for complications
- Placental vascular anastomoses are common (connections between the two babies' circulations)
- Twin-to-twin transfusion syndrome (TTTS) is the major risk
- Selective intrauterine growth restriction (sIUGR) can occur

Monochorionic-Monoamniotic (MCMA) Twins:

- One placenta
- One amniotic sac
- Results from monozygotic twinning that splits after day 8 of conception
- Highest risk for complications
- Cord entanglement is common and dangerous

- TTTS risk is high
- Congenital anomalies more common
- Often delivered by cesarean section before term to avoid cord entanglement

HOW TO DETERMINE CHORIONICITY

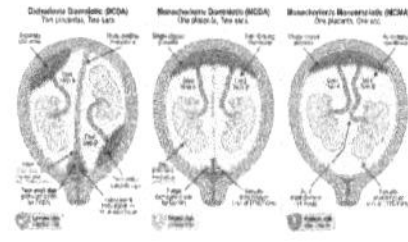

Prenatal ultrasound (most accurate):

- First trimester: Look for number of gestational sacs and yolk sacs
- Second/third trimester: Look for number of placentas, thickness of intertwin membrane, presence of "twin peak" sign (indicates dichorionic), presence of "T sign" (indicates monochorionic)
- Ultrasound determination of chorionicity is 95%+ accurate if done in first/second trimester

Placental examination after delivery:

- Number of placentas
- Number of amniotic membranes
- Presence of vascular anastomoses on placental surface
- Same-sex vs. opposite-sex (opposite-sex = definitely dichori-

onic)

Cord blood testing:

- DNA testing can determine if twins are monozygotic or dizygotic
- Useful if prenatal chorionicity unknown

Why this matters clinically: If you don't know the chorionicity, you don't know what complications to watch for. A mother arriving in labor with twins and no prenatal care? You need to know if they're DCDA (relatively straightforward) or MCMA (potentially catastrophic). This changes your entire approach.

TWIN-TO-TWIN TRANSFUSION SYNDROME (TTTS): THE EMERGENCY WITHIN THE EMERGENCY

WHAT'S HAPPENING

TTTS occurs only in monochorionic twins (shared placenta). Here's the pathophysiology: the placenta has vascular connections between the two babies' circulations. In TTTS, there's net blood flow from one twin (the donor) to the other (the recipient).

The donor twin loses blood volume and becomes anemic, growth-restricted, and oligohydramnios develops (not enough urine = not enough amniotic fluid). The recipient twin receives extra blood volume, becomes polycythemic, and polyhydramnios develops (too much urine = too much amniotic fluid).

If this goes unchecked prenatally, the donor twin can become severely compromised, and the recipient can develop heart failure from volume overload.

RECOGNITION: PRENATAL AND POSTNATAL

Prenatal diagnosis (Quintero criteria): For TTTS to be diagnosed prenatally, all four of these must be present:

1. Monochorionic-diamniotic pregnancy
2. Polyhydramnios in recipient twin (deepest vertical pocket >8 cm in second trimester, >10 cm in third trimester)
3. Oligohydramnios in donor twin (deepest vertical pocket <2 cm)
4. Discordant growth (though this is less specific)

Stages of severity:

- Stage 1: Polyhydramnios and oligohydramnios present; recipient's bladder still visible
- Stage 2: Recipient's bladder not visible on ultrasound
- Stage 3: Abnormal Doppler studies (umbilical artery, ductus venosus)
- Stage 4: Hydrops in one or both twins
- Stage 5: Death of one or both twins

Postnatal recognition: When twins deliver with TTTS, the physical findings are often striking:

Donor twin:

- Pale, anemic-looking
- Small (growth-restricted)
- Lethargic
- Oligohydramnios meant less fetal movement; may have contractures
- Low hemoglobin (often <12 g/dL)
- Respiratory distress (from anemia and prematurity)
- Potential for acute blood loss if placental transfusion occurs after delivery

Recipient twin:

- Plethoric (red, congested-looking)
- Larger
- More active, sometimes irritable
- Polyhydramnios meant more fetal movement and potential for more meconium
- High hemoglobin (often >18 g/dL)
- Potential for polycythemia-related complications: seizures, hypoglycemia, hypocalcemia
- Heart murmur possible (from volume overload and tricuspid regurgitation)

- Potential for congestive heart failure

WHAT TO DO IMMEDIATELY

For the donor twin:

- Anticipate prematurity and growth restriction. Have a resuscitation team ready; these babies are often small and sick.
- Avoid aggressive fluid administration early. The donor is volume-depleted, but aggressive hydration can precipitate pulmonary edema in the recipient.
- Monitor for anemia-related complications. Severe anemia can cause high-output heart failure. Have transfusion capability ready.
- Get a CBC immediately. You need to know the hemoglobin.
- Watch for hypoglycemia. Growth-restricted babies are at high risk.
- Assess for contractures or other anomalies. Oligohydramnios babies can have joint contractures from limited movement.

For the recipient twin:

- Monitor for polycythemia complications. High hemoglobin causes hyperviscosity, which can lead to seizures, NEC, renal failure, and CNS injury.
- Get a CBC immediately. Hematocrit >65% or hemoglobin >20 g/dL suggests polycythemia.

- Check glucose frequently. Polycythemic babies have high metabolic demands and are prone to hypoglycemia.
- Monitor for signs of heart failure. Tachycardia, tachypnea, hepatomegaly, murmur.
- Assess for hydrops. If the recipient had hydrops prenatally, look for ascites, pleural effusion, pericardial effusion.
- Consider partial exchange transfusion if severely polycythemic and symptomatic.

MANAGEMENT OF POLYCYTHEMIA IN THE RECIPIENT TWIN

This is where it gets tricky. Not all polycythemia needs treatment, but severe symptomatic polycythemia can cause serious complications.

When to treat:

- Hematocrit >65% AND symptoms (seizures, hypoglycemia, lethargy, poor feeding)
- Hematocrit >70% even without symptoms (risk of thrombosis)
- Signs of hyperviscosity (poor perfusion, oliguria)

How to treat: Partial exchange transfusion:

- Goal: Reduce hematocrit to 50-55%
- Formula: Volume to exchange = (Observed Hct – Desired Hct) / Observed Hct × Blood volume

- Blood volume in newborn ≈ 85-90 mL/kg
- Use normal saline or 5% albumin as replacement fluid
- Remove blood from umbilical vein (or peripheral artery if umbilical vein not available)
- Infuse replacement fluid into umbilical vein
- Do this slowly over 30 minutes to avoid sudden hemodynamic changes

Alternative: Isovolemic hemodilution

- Infuse normal saline or albumin without removing blood
- Less commonly used but effective

Supportive care:

- Frequent glucose monitoring and treatment of hypoglycemia
- Adequate hydration (but not excessive)
- Monitor for seizures; treat if occur
- Monitor urine output; oliguria suggests hyperviscosity

MANAGEMENT OF ANEMIA IN THE DONOR TWIN

The donor twin's anemia is usually mild to moderate at birth. The key is not to make it worse.

What NOT to do:

- Don't do an immediate partial exchange transfusion. The donor is volume-depleted; removing blood and replacing it with fluid can precipitate circulatory collapse.
- Don't over-hydrate. This can precipitate pulmonary edema.

What to do:

- Support with gentle fluid management and oxygen as needed
- Monitor hemoglobin; transfuse if <12 g/dL or if symptomatic with respiratory distress
- Allow physiologic increase in hemoglobin over first week as RBC production increases
- Most donor twins don't need transfusion if hemoglobin >10 g/dL and they're tolerating feeding

SELECTIVE INTRAUTERINE GROWTH RESTRICTION (sIUGR)

WHAT'S DIFFERENT FROM TTTS

sIUGR occurs in monochorionic twins when there's discordant growth (one twin significantly smaller) without meeting full TTTS criteria. The smaller twin isn't necessarily the "donor" in a TTTS pattern.

There are different types:

- Type 1 (sIUGR with normal Doppler): Growth-discordant but normal umbilical artery Doppler in smaller twin. Generally better prognosis.

- Type 2 (sIUGR with abnormal Doppler): Growth-discordant with abnormal umbilical artery Doppler (elevated resistance). Worse prognosis; higher risk of fetal loss.

- Type 3 (sIUGR with reverse flow): Umbilical artery reverse diastolic flow in smaller twin. Very high risk; often results in fetal loss or severe morbidity.

POSTNATAL RECOGNITION AND MANAGEMENT

The smaller twin in sIUGR presents like any growth-restricted baby:

- Small for gestational age
- Thin, wasted appearance
- Potential for hypoglycemia
- Potential for polycythemia (from chronic intrauterine hypoxia)
- Respiratory distress (from prematurity and growth restriction)
- Potential for feeding difficulties

Management:

- Aggressive glucose monitoring and treatment
- Careful feeding advancement (high risk for NEC)

- Monitor for polycythemia
- Anticipate need for longer NICU stay
- Close follow-up for growth and development

ACUTE TWIN ANEMIA-POLYCYTHEMIA SEQUENCE (ATAPS)

WHEN ONE TWIN'S PROBLEM BECOMES BOTH TWINS' PROBLEM

This is a scenario that can happen at delivery or in the immediate postnatal period. One twin becomes severely anemic while the other becomes severely polycythemic. This can occur with:

- Monochorionic twins with acute placental transfusion at delivery
- Delayed cord clamping in one twin but not the other
- Velamentous cord insertion with rupture

RECOGNITION

Clinical picture:

- One twin is pale, lethargic, potentially in shock
- Other twin is plethoric, potentially hypertensive

- Hemoglobin difference is extreme (>5 g/dL)
- Symptoms develop acutely at or shortly after delivery

MANAGEMENT

For the anemic twin:

- Aggressive resuscitation
- IV access and fluid support
- Transfusion (packed RBCs) to raise hemoglobin
- Support for shock if present

For the polycythemic twin:

- Partial exchange transfusion if symptomatic
- Fluid support
- Close monitoring for complications

CORD COMPLICATIONS IN MONOCHORIONIC-MONOAMNIOTIC TWINS

THE UNIQUE RISK: ENTANGLEMENT

Monoamniotic twins share not just a placenta but an amniotic sac. This means their umbilical cords are in the same space. The risk: the cords can become entangled, and if one twin moves, it can cut off the other twin's blood flow.

Prenatal management:

- Close ultrasound surveillance (often weekly after viability)
- Many centers deliver monoamniotic twins at 32-34 weeks to avoid cord entanglement catastrophe
- Some centers manage expectantly with daily monitoring

Postnatal implications: If one twin in a monoamniotic pair dies in utero or is severely compromised at delivery, think cord entanglement. The surviving twin may have been deprived of blood flow.

MANAGEMENT OF CORD ENTANGLEMENT COMPLICATIONS

- Aggressive resuscitation if twin is depressed
- Anticipate severe asphyxia; consider therapeutic hypothermia if criteria met
- Prepare for possible long-term neurologic sequelae
- Support for the surviving twin and family

VANISHING TWIN SYNDROME

WHAT HAPPENS

One twin dies in utero (usually early in pregnancy), and the other survives. The dead twin's tissue is resorbed or mummified.

Prenatal presentation:

- Ultrasound shows two gestational sacs initially, then only one fetus survives
- Occurs in 10-15% of multiple pregnancies
- More common with monochorionic twins

Postnatal implications:

- Surviving twin is usually unaffected
- Risk of preterm delivery (may be increased)
- Risk of growth restriction (if monochorionic)
- Rare risk of coagulopathy in survivor (from fetal-fetal transfusion of thromboplastin from dead twin)

MANAGEMENT

- Anticipate prematurity
- Screen for coagulopathy if concerned
- Otherwise, manage as singleton
- Provide family support; they're often grieving the loss of one twin while adjusting to the birth of another

PRACTICAL NICU MANAGEMENT OF MULTIPLES

LOGISTICS AND ORGANIZATION

Identification:

- Use consistent identifiers (wristbands with "Twin A" and "Twin B" or names)
- Some centers use different colored tape or markers
- Be obsessive about this; mistakes happen, and twin mix-ups are catastrophic

Separate charts:

- Keep separate medical records for each twin
- Even if they share complications, each has their own course
- Document which twin is which in every note

Separate care plans:

- Each twin has their own care plan, even if similar
- Orders are written for each baby individually
- Medications are labeled for each baby

Rooming in:

- Many parents want twins roomed together
- This is fine, but make sure identification is crystal clear

- Some units separate twins if one is much sicker than the other

FEEDING MULTIPLES

Breastfeeding:

- Some mothers want to breastfeed both; this is possible but challenging
- Tandem nursing (both at once) is possible
- Sequential nursing (one at a time) is more common
- Pumping and bottle-feeding is an option if breastfeeding isn't working
- Lactation support is crucial; twins are harder than singletons

Formula feeding:

- Standard approach; each baby gets their own bottle
- Make sure you're feeding the right baby
- Some units use color-coding (formula bottles with different colored tape)

Advancement:

- If twins are different sizes or have different complications, advancement may be different
- The smaller or sicker baby may advance slower
- Don't rush to get them on the same schedule if they're not

ready

DISCHARGE PLANNING FOR MULTIPLES

Timing:

- Ideally, both babies go home together
- If one is significantly more premature or sick, one may go home first
- This creates logistical challenges for families (two locations, divided attention)
- Coordinate closely with parents about what's realistic

Preparation:

- Parents need to be confident managing two babies
- More support at home may be needed
- Consider home nursing if available
- Make sure they have resources for both babies

Follow-up:

- Both babies need follow-up
- Schedule appointments at different times if possible (so parents don't have to manage both at once in clinic)
- Corrected age for development is based on gestational age, not on being born as a twin

COMMON PITFALLS AND MISTAKES

Mistake #1: Not knowing chorionicity. This is foundational. If you don't know whether these are DCDA, MCDA, or MCMA twins, you're missing critical complications.

Mistake #2: Treating both twins identically when they're not the same. One may be larger, one may be sicker. Individualize their care.

Mistake #3: Underestimating polycythemia in the recipient twin. Polycythemia can cause seizures, hypoglycemia, and NEC. Take it seriously.

Mistake #4: Over-transfusing the donor twin. The donor is volume-depleted. Aggressive fluids can precipitate pulmonary edema. Support gently.

Mistake #5: Twin mix-ups. This is rare but catastrophic. Be obsessive about identification.

Mistake #6: Missing TTTS because you didn't know the chorionicity prenatally. Ask the mother: "Did you have an ultrasound? Do you know if your twins share a placenta?" If you don't know, treat it as high-risk.

Mistake #7: Not screening for associated anomalies. Monozygotic twins have higher rates of congenital anomalies. Don't assume both babies are healthy just because one is.

Mistake #8: Giving up on one twin too early. If one twin is severely compromised at delivery, aggressive resuscitation may still result in good outcomes with therapeutic hypothermia and supportive care.

Mistake #9: Not involving both parents in decision-making. Multiples are complex; families need clear communication about what's happening with each baby.

Mistake #10: Discharging one twin significantly before the other without addressing family logistics. This is stressful for parents. Coordinate timing if possible.

WHEN TO ESCALATE CARE

- Any monochorionic twin with signs of TTTS = immediate specialist consultation (fetal medicine prenatally, neonatology at delivery)
- Severe polycythemia in recipient twin = consider partial exchange transfusion
- Severe anemia in donor twin with respiratory distress = transfusion
- One twin with severe asphyxia = consider therapeutic hypothermia; ECMO center notification
- Signs of entanglement or acute transfusion in monoamniotic twins = aggressive resuscitation
- Coagulopathy in surviving twin after vanishing twin = transfusion medicine consultation
- One twin significantly sicker than the other = consider separate care areas; individualize management

KEY CLINICAL PEARLS

Chorionicity determines risk. DCDA twins are relatively low-risk. MCDA twins have TTTS risk. MCMA twins have entanglement risk.

TTTS can be devastating if not recognized. The donor twin is anemic and growth-restricted. The recipient is polycythemic and at risk for heart failure.

Polycythemia in the recipient needs treatment if symptomatic. Partial exchange transfusion reduces hematocrit and prevents complications.

The donor twin's anemia is usually manageable without transfusion. Support gently; don't over-hydrate.

sIUGR is different from TTTS. It's growth discordance without full TTTS criteria. Still requires careful management of the smaller twin.

Monoamniotic twins are high-risk. Cord entanglement is a real threat. Many are delivered early to avoid catastrophe.

Identification of multiples is critical. Use consistent markers. Twin mix-ups are rare but catastrophic.

Individualize care for each twin. Don't assume they need the same management just because they're twins.

Screen for associated anomalies in monozygotic twins. Congenital anomalies are more common.

Family support is crucial. Parents of multiples, especially with complications, are stressed and need clear communication, resources, and emotional support.

Chapter Twenty-Seven

NEONATAL EMERGENCIES AND CRITICAL CARE

INTRODUCTION: WHEN EVERYTHING GOES WRONG AT ONCE

Neonatal emergencies are different from other medical emergencies. You're working with a patient who can't tell you what's wrong, whose physiology is fundamentally different from older children and adults, and whose margin for error is razor-thin. A baby can deteriorate from stable to dead in minutes. You need to think fast, act decisively, and know when to call for help.

This chapter isn't about rare conditions or exotic diagnoses. It's about the emergencies you'll actually face: the baby who suddenly crashes, the baby with a tension pneumothorax, the baby with severe sepsis, the baby whose heart stops. These are the moments that define your career as a neonatal clinician.

Here's what matters: most neonatal emergencies follow predictable patterns. If you understand the physiology, recognize the early signs, and have a systematic approach to resuscitation and stabilization, you can save lives. Panic is your enemy. Protocol is your friend.

Let me be direct: if you're not comfortable with emergency procedures—intubation, chest compressions, emergency medications—this is not the time to learn. Practice on mannequins. Know your algorithms. Know where your equipment is. When the emergency comes, muscle memory and preparation will carry you through.

THE CRASHING BABY: SYSTEMATIC APPROACH TO SUDDEN DETERIORATION

RECOGNITION: THE MOMENT YOU KNOW SOMETHING'S WRONG

You're charting, and suddenly an alarm goes off. Or a nurse calls: "The baby's not looking good." Or you walk into the room and immediately sense something is wrong—the baby looks gray, or the monitors show a heart rate that's dropping, or you hear abnormal breath sounds.

Your first instinct might be panic. Don't. Your second instinct should be protocol.

The immediate assessment (takes 10 seconds):

- Look: Is the baby breathing? Is the chest moving? Is the baby pink or cyanotic or pale?

- Listen: Are there breath sounds? Is the baby making any sounds? Are there bilateral differences in equality of sounds in the chest (suggests pneumothorax)?

- Feel: Is the baby warm? Can you feel a pulse? Is the chest moving with your hand?

- Check monitors: What's the heart rate? Is it dropping? Is the SpO_2 falling? Is the blood pressure dropping?

This takes 10 seconds. In those 10 seconds, you've determined whether this is a respiratory emergency, a cardiac emergency, or something else.

THE ABCDE APPROACH TO EMERGENCY STABILIZATION

A = Airway – Is the airway open? Can the baby breathe? If not, you need to open it.

- Positioning: Head in neutral position (not extended, not flexed)

- Suction: Clear secretions, blood, meconium

- Airway adjuncts: Oral airway if indicated (rarely needed in neonates)

- Intubation: If you can't maintain the airway or if the baby needs mechanical ventilation

B = Breathing – Is the baby breathing? Are the lungs inflating?

- If spontaneously breathing: Support with oxygen as needed
- If not breathing: Provide positive pressure ventilation
- If severe respiratory distress: Consider intubation

C = Circulation – Is there a heartbeat? Is perfusion adequate?

- Check pulse (umbilical artery, femoral artery)
- If heart rate <60: Start chest compressions
- If hypotension: IV access, fluids, pressors
- If no pulse: Full resuscitation protocol

D = Disability (Neurologic) – Is the baby conscious? Seizing? Altered?

- Assess responsiveness
- Check pupils
- Look for seizure activity
- Get glucose immediately if altered

E = Exposure – Look at the whole baby. What's the problem?

- Examine for trauma, bleeding, rash
- Check abdomen for distension, tenderness
- Look at skin: is there mottling? Cyanosis? Pallor?

SPECIFIC EMERGENCIES AND HOW TO MANAGE THEM

TENSION PNEUMOTHORAX: THE EMERGENCY THAT DEMANDS IMMEDIATE ACTION

What's happening: Air has entered the pleural space. Normally, this would just collapse the lung. But in tension pneumothorax, the air keeps building up, compressing the lung, shifting the mediastinum, and compromising cardiac output. The baby deteriorates rapidly.

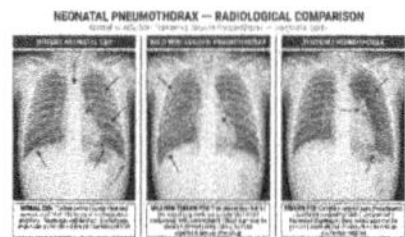

Recognition (classic presentation):

- Sudden respiratory distress
- Cyanosis that doesn't improve with oxygen
- Unequal breath sounds (decreased on affected side)
- Hyperresonance to percussion on affected side (if you have time to percuss)
- Heart sounds displaced to opposite side
- Hypotension
- Bradycardia (from vagal stimulation)
- Shock

What NOT to do: Don't wait for a chest X-ray. Don't call radiology. "Transillumination would help". If you're confident this is tension pneumothorax, treat it now.

What to do immediately:

1. Give 100% oxygen. This helps the air resorb faster.
2. Needle decompression NOW. This is your emergency intervention.
   - Site: 2nd intercostal space, midclavicular line (upper chest)
   - Equipment: 22-gauge needle on a syringe (or needle with catheter)
   - Technique: Insert perpendicular to chest wall, aiming just above the rib below (to avoid neurovascular bundle)
   - You'll hear a rush of air if it's tension pneumothorax
   - Leave the catheter in, remove the needle
3. Get chest X-ray to confirm and assess for other injuries.
4. Place a chest tube. After needle decompression, the baby needs a proper chest tube.
   - Site: 4th-5th intercostal space, anterior axillary line
   - Size: 8-14 Fr tube (depending on baby size)
   - Connect to water seal or Heimlich valve
5. Support ventilation as needed while you're doing this.

The critical point: Tension pneumothorax kills babies. If you wait, the baby will code. Needle decompression takes 30 seconds. Do it.

SEVERE BRADYCARDIA OR ASYSTOLE

When to start chest compressions:

- Heart rate <60 bpm in a baby who's not responding to ventilation
- No pulse palpable
- No cardiac output on ultrasound

Chest compression technique:

- Hand position: Two thumbs encircling the chest, fingers supporting the back (preferred method for neonates)
- Compression rate: 90 compressions per minute
- Ventilation rate: 30 breaths per minute (3:1 ratio)
- Depth: About 1/3 of chest diameter (roughly 1.5 inches for term infant)
- Recoil: Let the chest fully recoil between compressions

Medications:

- Epinephrine: 0.01-0.03 mg/kg IV every 3-5 minutes
    - IV route preferred (umbilical vein)
    - If no IV access: Intraosseous (IO) access in proximal tibia
    - Higher doses (0.1 mg/kg) if IO used

- Sodium bicarbonate: 1 mEq/kg IV for severe metabolic acidosis (pH <7.0)
- Calcium gluconate: 100-200 mg/kg IV if hyperkalemia suspected
- Dextrose: 250-500 mg/kg (2-4 mL/kg of 10% dextrose) if hypoglycemia

Duration of resuscitation:

- Continue for at least 10 minutes if there's any sign of life
- Many babies respond after prolonged resuscitation
- Asphyxiated babies especially can respond after 15-20 minutes
- Don't give up too early

SEVERE SEPSIS AND SEPTIC SHOCK

Recognition: Sepsis in neonates can be subtle. You might not see the classic signs of older children. Instead, look for:

- Temperature instability (fever OR hypothermia)
- Lethargy or poor tone
- Poor feeding
- Vomiting or diarrhea
- Mottled skin

- Tachycardia
- Tachypnea
- Metabolic acidosis
- Thrombocytopenia (dropping platelet count)
- Coagulopathy

Shock signs:

- Hypotension
- Prolonged capillary refill (>3 seconds)
- Cool extremities
- Oliguria
- Altered mental status
- Lactate elevation

Immediate management:

1. Blood culture (before antibiotics if possible, but don't delay antibiotics)
2. Start broad-spectrum antibiotics immediately.
    - Ampicillin + gentamicin (covers Group B Strep, gram-negatives)
    - Add vancomycin if concern for resistant organisms or if baby is very sick
    - Empiric coverage; adjust when cultures return

3. IV access and aggressive fluid resuscitation.
    - 20 mL/kg normal saline bolus over 15-30 minutes
    - Reassess; may need additional boluses
    - Watch for signs of pulmonary edema (respiratory distress, crackles)
4. Vasopressors if hypotensive despite fluids.
    - Dopamine: 5-20 mcg/kg/min
    - Dobutamine: 5-20 mcg/kg/min (for cardiogenic shock)
    - Consider commencing on Hydrocortisone iv "if required 2 pressor medications" :1:2 mg/kg/dose 8-6 houly
    - Epinephrine or/and Norepinephrine : 0.1-1 mcg/kg/min (for severe shock)
    - Vasopressin "in severe hypotension not responding to usual pressors " :0.01-0.1 unit/kg/h
5. Supportive care:
    - Oxygen and ventilation as needed
    - Glucose monitoring and treatment
    - Correction of coagulopathy (FFP, platelets, cryoprecipitate as needed)
    - Renal support if acute kidney injury develops

The critical point: Sepsis kills babies fast. If you suspect it, start antibiotics now. You can narrow the spectrum later when cultures return.

SEVERE HYPOGLYCEMIA

Recognition:

- Seizures (most common presentation)
- Tremor, jitteriness
- Lethargy, poor tone
- Apnea
- Cyanosis
- Bradycardia

Immediate management:

1. Check blood glucose immediately. Point-of-care testing (POC) or lab draw.
2. If symptomatic and glucose <40 mg/dL: Give dextrose immediately.
    - IV dextrose: 250-500 mg/kg (2-4 mL/kg of 10% dextrose) IV push
    - OR 5-10 mL/kg of 10% dextrose if IV not available (but IV is better)
3. Recheck glucose in 15 minutes. You want it >60 mg/dL.

4. Start continuous dextrose infusion to maintain glucose.
    - D10 at 5-8 mg/kg/min initially
    - Adjust based on glucose checks
5. Treat seizures if present (phenobarbital or levetiracetam).

Prevention:

- Early feeding (glucose from breast milk or formula)
- Frequent glucose monitoring in at-risk babies
- Avoid prolonged fasting

SEVERE HEMORRHAGE

Recognition:

- Pale, cool baby
- Tachycardia
- Hypotension
- Weak pulses
- Oliguria
- Metabolic acidosis
- Shock
- Visible bleeding (cord stump, GI bleeding, other source)

Immediate management:

1. Identify the source of bleeding. Where is the blood coming from?
    - Umbilical cord: Apply pressure, clamp the stump
    - GI: NPO, NG tube to suction, prepare for possible transfusion
    - Internal: Imaging (ultrasound, CT) to identify source
2. Two large-bore IVs (or IO access if can't get IV)
3. Type and cross-match blood immediately.
4. Fluid resuscitation:
    - 20 mL/kg normal saline bolus
    - Reassess; may need more
5. Blood transfusion:
    - O-negative blood if type unknown
    - Packed RBCs (10-15 mL/kg) to raise hemoglobin
    - Fresh frozen plasma and platelets if coagulopathy
6. Correct coagulopathy (FFP, platelets, cryoprecipitate)
7. Prepare for surgical intervention if bleeding is internal and not stopping

The critical point: Babies don't have much blood volume. They can lose 10-15% of their blood volume and still look okay. Then they crash suddenly. Don't wait for the crash. If you suspect significant bleeding, act aggressively.

SEVERE HYPOTENSION

Recognition:

- Systolic BP <50 mmHg (term infant) or <40 mmHg (preterm)
- Signs of poor perfusion: mottled skin, cool extremities, weak pulses, altered mental status
- Oliguria
- Metabolic acidosis

Causes:

- Sepsis
- Hypovolemia (bleeding, fluid loss)
- Cardiogenic shock (myocarditis, arrhythmia)
- Medication effect
- Pneumothorax (mediastinal shift)

Management:

1. Identify and treat the cause.
    - If sepsis: antibiotics, fluids, pressors
    - If bleeding: transfusion, surgery

- If cardiogenic: echo, cardiology consultation
- If pneumothorax: needle decompression, chest tube

2. Fluid resuscitation: 20 mL/kg normal saline bolus
3. Vasopressors if hypotensive despite fluids:
   - Dopamine: 5-20 mcg/kg/min
   - Dobutamine: 5-20 mcg/kg/min
   - Epinephrine , and/or Norepinephrine: 0.1-1 mcg/kg/min
4. Monitoring: Continuous BP monitoring, urine output, lactate

SEVERE HYPERKALEMIA

Recognition:

- Peaked T waves on ECG
- Widened QRS
- Bradycardia
- Cardiac arrhythmias
- Cardiac arrest
- K^+ >7 mEq/L

Causes:

- Renal failure
- Massive hemolysis
- Tissue breakdown (asphyxia, rhabdomyolysis)
- Acidosis
- Medications (ACE inhibitors, NSAIDs)

Immediate management:

1. Calcium gluconate: 100-200 mg/kg IV over 2-5 minutes
    - Stabilizes cardiac membrane
    - Doesn't lower K^+, but prevents arrhythmias
    - Can repeat in 10 minutes if ECG changes persist
2. Shift K^+ into cells:
    - Insulin: 0.1 unit/kg IV with dextrose (1 g/unit)
    - Sodium bicarbonate: 1-2 mEq/kg IV
    - Beta-agonist: Albuterol nebulized or IV
3. Remove K^+ from body:
    - Diuretics: Furosemide if urine output intact
    - Ion exchange resin: Sodium polystyrene sulfonate (Kayexalate) oral or rectal
    - Dialysis: If renal failure or if above measures fail

4. Continuous cardiac monitoring

5. Recheck K^+ in 30-60 minutes

The critical point: Hyperkalemia can kill in minutes. If you see peaked T waves on ECG, treat immediately. Don't wait for confirmation.

EMERGENCY PROCEDURES: WHEN YOU NEED TO ACT NOW

EMERGENCY INTUBATION

When to intubate:

- Apnea or severe respiratory distress
- Unable to maintain airway
- Need for mechanical ventilation
- Aspiration risk
- Severe asphyxia

Equipment:

- Laryngoscope (Miller blade, straight blade preferred for neonates)
- Endotracheal tubes: 2.5 mm (preterm), 3.0 mm (term)
- Suction

- Stylet (optional but helpful)
- Tape or tube holder

Technique:

1. Prepare: Have everything ready before you start
2. Position: Neutral head position; slight neck extension
3. Preoxygenate: Give 100% oxygen for 30 seconds if time allows
4. Insert laryngoscope: Blade into mouth, visualize vocal cords
5. Insert tube: Pass through vocal cords; listen for bilateral breath sounds
6. Confirm: Chest X-ray, end-tidal CO_2 detector, condensation in tube
7. Secure: Tape tube in place; note depth at lip

Common mistakes:

- Inserting tube too deep (enters right mainstem bronchus)
- Inserting tube too shallow (tube slips out)
- Not visualizing vocal cords (tube in esophagus)
- Inserting tube with stylet too far (perforates trachea)

EMERGENCY UMBILICAL VENOUS CATHETERIZATION

When to use:

- Need for emergency IV access
- Central access for medications and fluids
- Measurement of central venous pressure

Technique:

1. Identify umbilical vein: Usually single, larger vessel in umbilical cord
2. Prepare: Sterile field, catheter (3.5 or 5 Fr)
3. Insert: Advance catheter into vein until blood returns
4. Confirm position: Chest X-ray (tip should be at junction of IVC and right atrium)
5. Secure: Suture in place

Complications:

- Perforation of vein or liver
- Infection
- Thrombosis
- Pericardial effusion if tip too far

EMERGENCY INTRAOSSEOUS ACCESS

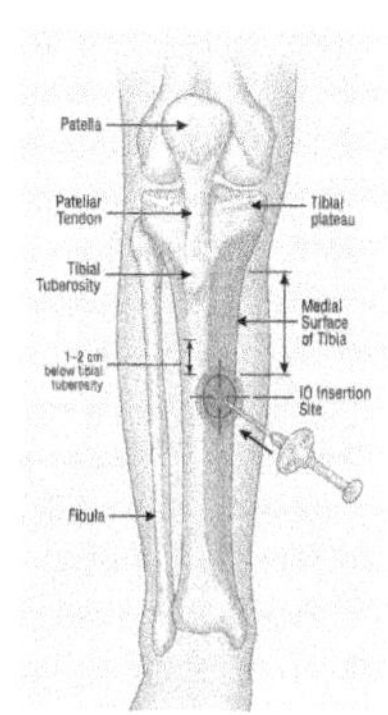

When to use:

- Can't get IV access in resuscitation
- Need for immediate vascular access

Technique:

- Site: Proximal tibia (medial, below tibial tuberosity)
- Equipment: IO needle (15-18 gauge)
- Insert: Perpendicular to bone, twist until "pop" felt
- Confirm: Needle stands without support; fluid infuses easily
- Medications: Can give any medication IV through IO

Advantages:

- Quick access
- High success rate in resuscitation
- Can give all medications

CRITICAL CARE PRINCIPLES FOR SICK NEONATES

MONITORING THE CRITICALLY ILL BABY

Continuous monitoring:

- Heart rate and rhythm
- Respiratory rate
- Blood pressure (invasive or non-invasive)
- SpO_2
- Temperature
- Urine output
- Fluid balance

Frequent labs:

- Blood gas (arterial preferred) every 4-6 hours or after changes
- Glucose every 2-4 hours
- Electrolytes daily or more often if abnormal
- CBC daily
- Lactate if shock or sepsis
- Coagulation studies if bleeding or sepsis

Assessment:

- Physical exam every 4 hours minimum
- More frequently if unstable
- Look for deterioration, improvement, or complications

VENTILATOR MANAGEMENT IN CRITICAL ILLNESS

Modes of ventilation:

- Conventional ventilation: Pressure-controlled or volume-controlled
- High-frequency ventilation: For severe lung disease refractory to conventional
- ECMO: For babies who fail maximal medical therapy

Goals:

- Adequate oxygenation (SpO_2 90-95%)
- Adequate ventilation (pH 7.20-7.35, PCO_2 45-55)
- Minimize barotrauma and volutrauma
- Permissive hypercapnia acceptable

Weaning:

- Gradual reduction in support as baby improves
- Based on blood gases, clinical status, lung compliance
- Extubation when baby can maintain airway and adequate spontaneous breathing

FLUID AND ELECTROLYTE MANAGEMENT IN CRITICAL ILLNESS

Fluid strategy:

- Aggressive hydration in shock (boluses)
- Restrictive fluids in pulmonary edema or renal failure
- Balanced approach: adequate perfusion without overload

Electrolyte monitoring:

- Sodium: target 130-145 mEq/L
- Potassium: target 3.5-5.5 mEq/L (lower in severe illness)
- Calcium: target >7 mg/dL
- Glucose: target 60-150 mg/dL

Correction:

- Gradual correction (avoid sudden shifts)
- Address underlying cause, not just lab value

INFECTION PREVENTION IN CRITICAL CARE

Hand hygiene:

- Most important intervention
- Before and after every baby contact
- Alcohol-based sanitizer or soap and water

Line care:

- Sterile technique for insertion
- Regular assessment for infection signs

- Remove lines as soon as no longer needed
- Dressing changes per protocol

Antibiotic stewardship:

- Start broad-spectrum empirically
- Narrow based on cultures
- Duration appropriate to diagnosis
- Avoid unnecessary prolonged antibiotics

COMMON PITFALLS AND MISTAKES

Mistake #1: Hesitating in a true emergency. If you're confident it's tension pneumothorax, do needle decompression. Don't wait for an X-ray.

Mistake #2: Hyperventilating the baby. This causes hypocapnia, which worsens cerebral perfusion. Target PCO_2 45-55, not 30-35.

Mistake #3: Using 100% oxygen routinely. Hyperoxia causes oxidative stress. Target SpO_2 90-95%.

Mistake #4: Giving up on resuscitation too early. Asphyxiated babies can respond after prolonged resuscitation. Keep going.

Mistake #5: Not treating sepsis aggressively enough. If you suspect it, start antibiotics now. You can narrow the spectrum later.

Mistake #6: Ignoring subtle signs of deterioration. A baby doesn't have to crash suddenly. Watch for gradual changes: increasing oxygen needs, rising lactate, worsening metabolic acidosis.

Mistake #7: Forgetting the basics. When everything is chaotic, remember ABCDE. Airway, breathing, circulation, disability, exposure. Systematic approach saves lives.

Mistake #8: Not communicating with the team. In emergencies, everyone needs to know the plan. Call for help early. Delegate tasks. Communicate clearly.

Mistake #9: Continuing ineffective interventions. If something isn't working after a reasonable trial, try something else. Don't persist with failure.

Mistake #10: Not debriefing after an emergency. After the crisis passes, take time to review what happened, what worked, what didn't. Learn from it.

WHEN TO CALL FOR HELP

Call immediately if:

- Baby is deteriorating despite your interventions
- You're unsure what to do
- You need another set of hands
- You need specialist input (cardiology, surgery, etc.)
- Baby needs ECMO evaluation
- Baby needs transfer to higher level of care

Don't wait for:

- Perfect diagnosis
- Confirmation from imaging

- Specialist to be available
- Baby to crash completely

Calling for help early often prevents the crash from happening.

KEY CLINICAL PEARLS

Systematic approach beats panic. ABCDE every time. It works.

Trust your gut. If something feels wrong, investigate. Babies deteriorate fast.

Tension pneumothorax is an emergency. Needle decompression takes 30 seconds. Do it.

Sepsis kills babies fast. If you suspect it, start antibiotics now.

Hypoglycemia causes seizures. Check glucose immediately in any seizing baby.

Hypotension is a late sign. By the time BP drops, the baby is already in shock. Look for earlier signs: mottled skin, weak pulses, poor perfusion.

Resuscitation works. Babies can respond to prolonged resuscitation. Don't give up too early.

Permissive hypercapnia is acceptable. You don't need to "normalize" blood gases. Adequate perfusion matters more.

Fluid boluses save lives in shock. 20 mL/kg normal saline can turn things around.

Communication is critical. In emergencies, everyone needs to know the plan. Clear communication prevents mistakes and saves lives.

Chapter Twenty-Eight

DISCHARGE PLANNING AND FOLLOW-UP

INTRODUCTION: THE HOME TRANSITION IS WHERE REAL PARENTING BEGINS

You've done it. The baby made it through the NICU. The critical illness has resolved. The feeding is established. The baby is gaining weight. Now comes a moment that many clinicians underestimate: discharge planning. This is where the hospital care ends and real life begins—and it's terrifying for parents.

Here's what matters: discharge planning isn't just paperwork. It's not just making sure the baby has a car seat and follow-up appointments scheduled. Discharge planning is about setting families up for success, preventing readmissions, catching problems early, and giving parents confidence that they can actually do this.

Let me be direct: a well-planned discharge with good follow-up prevents complications, catches problems early, and changes outcomes. A discharge done hastily, without proper preparation and follow-up, results in readmissions, missed diagnoses, and families in crisis.

This chapter is about the practical, systematic approach to getting babies home safely and keeping them healthy after discharge. It's about understanding what families actually need, what follow-up actually matters, and how to catch problems before they become emergencies.

DISCHARGE READINESS: IS THE BABY ACTUALLY READY?

THE CRITERIA THAT MATTER

You can't just discharge a baby because the parents are eager or the bed is needed. There are real criteria that predict safe discharge. If the baby doesn't meet them, problems happen.

Physiologic stability:

- Maintaining body temperature in open crib (not under heat source)
- Respiratory stability: no significant apnea or bradycardia spells, SpO_2 stable on room air or minimal supplemental oxygen
- Cardiovascular stability: heart rate and blood pressure nor-

mal for age, no significant murmur requiring intervention

- Feeding: taking full volume by mouth (breast or bottle), gaining weight consistently, no significant reflux or feeding intolerance
- Elimination: normal urine and stool output
- Jaundice: resolved or managed with outpatient phototherapy if needed
- No active infection or fever

Neurologic stability:

- Alert and responsive
- Normal muscle tone
- No seizures or concerning neurologic signs
- Appropriate feeding behaviors

Metabolic stability:

- Normal glucose
- Normal electrolytes
- No significant acid-base disturbance
- No active metabolic disorder requiring treatment

Infectious disease clearance:

- Negative cultures if sepsis was concern
- Appropriate antibiotic course completed if needed

- Immunizations up to date
- Screening tests (hearing, metabolic, cardiac) completed or scheduled

Parental readiness:

- Parents demonstrate understanding of baby's condition
- Parents can perform necessary care (feeding, medication administration, equipment use)
- Parents have support system in place
- Parents understand warning signs and when to seek help
- Parents have follow-up appointments scheduled
- Parents have resources and contact information

THE BABY WHO'S NOT QUITE READY

Sometimes babies meet most criteria but not all. This is where clinical judgment matters.

Mild apnea/bradycardia: If the baby is having occasional episodes but they're self-resolving and not requiring intervention, discharge may be appropriate with home monitoring. But the family needs to understand the signs, know how to respond, and have a plan if episodes increase.

Mild jaundice: If bilirubin is rising but not at phototherapy threshold, outpatient phototherapy can work. But you need reliable follow-up (next day) and a system to check bilirubin levels.

Feeding challenges: If the baby is feeding but not gaining optimally, you have options: discharge with close follow-up, lactation support at home, or brief additional hospitalization. The key is having a clear plan and follow-up.

Medication requirements: If the baby needs medications (diuretics, antibiotics, anticonvulsants), discharge is appropriate if parents are reliable and follow-up is arranged.

The critical point: don't discharge a baby who's not ready just because you want to free up a bed. Readmissions are worse than keeping a baby an extra day or two.

PREPARING FAMILIES FOR DISCHARGE

EDUCATION: WHAT PARENTS ACTUALLY NEED TO KNOW

Parents are often overwhelmed. They've been through trauma—their baby was sick, they've been in the hospital, and now they're being sent home with this tiny, fragile human. You need to give them information in digestible pieces, written down, and reviewed multiple times.

Basic care:

- Feeding: how much, how often, how to know if baby is getting enough
- Diaper output: what's normal
- Sleep: safe sleep practices (back sleeping, firm surface, no pillows/blankets)
- Bathing: when to bathe, how to keep baby warm

- Cord care: if umbilical cord still present, how to keep it clean and dry
- Circumcision care: if applicable
- Temperature: how to take it, when to call doctor

Special care if applicable:

- Medication administration: exact dosing, timing, how to give it
- Equipment use: monitors, oxygen, feeding tubes, pumps
- Symptom monitoring: what to watch for
- Positioning: if baby has specific needs (reflux, hip dysplasia)
- Activity restrictions: if any

Warning signs: When to call the doctor immediately:

- Fever >100.4°F (38°C)
- Not feeding or refusing feeds
- Vomiting (not just spit-up)
- Diarrhea or constipation
- Lethargy or unusual sleepiness
- Irritability or high-pitched cry
- Difficulty breathing or increased work of breathing
- Cyanosis or pallor

- Seizures or abnormal movements
- Jaundice that's worsening
- Bleeding from any site
- Rash that doesn't blanch with pressure
- Apnea or prolonged pauses in breathing
- Inability to wake the baby

When to go to the emergency room:

- Severe respiratory distress
- Unresponsiveness
- Suspected sepsis (fever, lethargy, poor feeding)
- Seizures
- Severe bleeding
- Signs of shock (pale, cool, weak pulses)
- Suspected abuse or injury

Provide written information for everything. Parents won't remember verbal instructions. Give them a handout they can reference.

EQUIPMENT AND SUPPLIES AT HOME

Essential supplies:

- Diapers (appropriate size)

- Wipes
- Formula (if not breastfeeding) and bottles
- Feeding supplies (sterilizer, bottle brush)
- Clothing (appropriate for season)
- Blankets and bedding (safe sleep setup)
- Thermometer
- Medications (if prescribed)
- Equipment (monitors, oxygen, pumps, etc.)

Equipment training:

- If baby needs home monitoring (apnea monitor, pulse oximeter), parents need to understand how to use it, how to respond to alarms, and troubleshooting
- If baby needs oxygen, parents need to understand flow rates, how to deliver it, and safety precautions
- If baby has feeding tube or pump, parents need to understand operation, troubleshooting, and emergency procedures
- If baby needs medications via specific route (IV, IM), parents need training and demonstration

Equipment safety:

- Ensure equipment is properly functioning before discharge
- Provide instruction manuals

- Provide emergency contact for equipment company
- Arrange for equipment company to follow up at home if needed
- Make sure parents know how to respond if equipment fails

PSYCHOSOCIAL PREPARATION

Parents of NICU babies are traumatized. They've been through a crisis. Discharge is exciting but also scary. They're worried about:

- Whether they're capable of caring for their baby
- Whether something will go wrong at home
- Whether they're missing something
- Separation anxiety from the NICU team
- Sleep deprivation and exhaustion
- Financial stress from time away from work
- Relationship stress from NICU experience

What you can do:

- Acknowledge their experience and their feelings
- Reassure them that their anxiety is normal
- Connect them with resources: parent support groups, mental health services, lactation support
- Provide clear information about follow-up care

- Encourage them to call with questions
- Normalize the transition; most babies do well at home
- Offer to review their discharge instructions one more time before leaving

Special consideration for parents with depression/anxiety: Screen for postpartum depression and anxiety. Refer to mental health services if needed. Don't assume parents are fine just because their baby is.

DISCHARGE MEDICATIONS AND PRESCRIPTIONS

WHAT MEDICATIONS GO HOME

Common discharge medications:

- Vitamins (iron, vitamin D, multivitamin if indicated)
- Antibiotics (if completing course started in hospital)
- Diuretics (if baby has chronic lung disease or cardiac condition)
- Anticonvulsants (if seizure disorder)
- Reflux medications (H2 blockers, proton pump inhibitors)
- Bronchodilators (if chronic lung disease)
- Inhaled corticosteroids (if chronic lung disease)

- Blood pressure medications (if hypertension)
- Other condition-specific medications

Prescription clarity:

- Write prescriptions clearly with:
  - Medication name
  - Dose (in weight-based dosing, provide both dose in mg and volume in mL)
  - Frequency
  - Route
  - Duration
  - Indication
- Make sure parents understand how to measure and administer
- Consider pharmacy consultation if complex dosing
- Provide written information about each medication: what it does, side effects, when to give it

Medication safety:

- Ensure parents understand exact dosing
- Avoid dosing errors (don't just say "one dropper"—specify volume)
- Provide syringes or droppers as appropriate

- Consider pill organizer or calendar if multiple medications
- Warn about interactions with over-the-counter medications
- Clarify what to do if dose is missed

FOLLOW-UP APPOINTMENTS: THE SAFETY NET THAT CATCHES PROBLEMS

SCHEDULING FOLLOW-UP BEFORE DISCHARGE

Don't send families home without follow-up appointments scheduled. This is your safety net.

Primary care visit:

- Timing: Within 3-7 days of discharge (or sooner if any concerns)
- Purpose: Assess baby's adjustment at home, feeding, jaundice, weight, general health
- What to communicate: Baby's diagnosis, any special needs, medications, warning signs
- Ensure: Primary care provider has discharge summary before appointment

Specialty follow-up (as indicated):

- Cardiology: If cardiac defect or murmur
- Nephrology: If renal disease

- Neurology: If seizure disorder or significant neurologic concern
- Ophthalmology: If ROP risk or other eye concerns
- Audiology: If hearing loss or failed hearing screen
- Pulmonology: If chronic lung disease
- Gastroenterology: If feeding disorder or GI disease
- Surgery: If surgical follow-up needed
- Genetics: If genetic disorder
- Developmental pediatrics: If high-risk for developmental delay

Timing of specialty follow-up:

- Urgent issues: within 1-2 weeks
- Important issues: within 2-4 weeks
- Routine follow-up: within 1-3 months

Communication:

- Send discharge summary to all providers
- Highlight key issues and medications
- Provide contact information for coordination
- Make sure providers know who the primary coordinator is

WHAT HAPPENS AT FOLLOW-UP VISITS

Primary care follow-up:

- Weight check: is the baby gaining appropriately?
- Feeding assessment: is the baby taking adequate volume? Signs of reflux or feeding difficulty?
- Jaundice assessment: is jaundice resolved or worsening?
- General health: fever, infection signs, general well-being?
- Medication review: are medications being given correctly? Any side effects?
- Parental concerns: address any questions or worries
- Examination: general health check, listen to heart, check abdomen
- Plan: if all is well, routine follow-up in 2 weeks or at next scheduled visit; if concerns, more frequent follow-up or specialist referral

Specialty follow-up:

- Assessment specific to condition
- Medication adjustment if needed
- Imaging or testing if indicated
- Coordination with primary care
- Plan for ongoing management

EARLY INTERVENTION AND DEVELOPMENTAL FOLLOW-UP

IDENTIFYING BABIES AT RISK FOR DEVELOPMENTAL DELAY

High-risk factors:

- Prematurity (especially <32 weeks)
- Intrauterine growth restriction
- Perinatal asphyxia or HIE
- Seizures
- Severe infection/sepsis
- Chronic lung disease
- Intraventricular hemorrhage
- Necrotizing enterocolitis
- Congenital anomalies
- Genetic or metabolic disorders
- Maternal substance use
- Maternal infection (TORCH, GBS)
- Low birth weight (<1500 g)

Not all high-risk babies develop delays, but they need close monitoring.

EARLY INTERVENTION PROGRAMS "Applied in some developed countries"

It is an Early intervention program that provides free or low-cost services to infants and toddlers (birth to 3 years) with developmental delays or at-risk conditions.

Services provided:

- Speech-language pathology
- Physical therapy
- Occupational therapy
- Developmental specialist services
- Family support services
- Coordination of care

How to access:

- Referral from pediatrician or hospital
- Self-referral by family
- Contact local early intervention program (varies by state)
- Evaluation by multidisciplinary team
- Development of Individualized Family Service Plan (IFSP)
- Services provided in home or community setting

Timing:

- Refer before discharge or at first follow-up visit
- Evaluation typically within 30 days of referral
- Services can start while evaluation is pending

Corrected age:

- For developmental assessment, use corrected age (chronologic age minus weeks of prematurity) until age 3 years
- Important for accurate developmental assessment and intervention planning

DEVELOPMENTAL SCREENING AT FOLLOW-UP VISITS

What to screen for:

- Gross motor: head control, sitting, crawling, walking
- Fine motor: reaching, grasping, pincer grasp
- Language: sounds, words, understanding
- Social: smiling, interaction, play
- Cognitive: problem-solving, play skills

Tools:

- Denver Developmental Screening Test (DDST)
- Ages and Stages Questionnaire (ASQ)

- Bayley Scales of Infant and Toddler Development
- Mullen Scales of Early Learning

When to refer for formal evaluation:

- Scores below expected for corrected age
- Parent concerns about development
- Neurologic findings concerning for cerebral palsy or other disorder
- Regression in skills
- Hearing or vision problems affecting development

MANAGING COMMON POST-DISCHARGE PROBLEMS

FEEDING DIFFICULTIES

Inadequate intake:

- Assess breastfeeding: latch, duration, frequency
- If bottle feeding: volume, frequency, type of formula
- Weight gain: is the baby gaining appropriately?
- Wet diapers and stools: adequate output?
- Signs of dehydration: dry mucous membranes, decreased skin turgor, fontanelle depression

Interventions:

- Lactation consultation for breastfeeding problems
- Feeding therapy if oral motor dysfunction
- Formula adjustment if intolerance
- More frequent feeds if inadequate intake
- Supplementation if needed
- Nasogastric tube feeding if unable to take adequate oral intake

JAUNDICE MANAGEMENT

Persistent or rising jaundice:

- Recheck bilirubin level
- Plot on nomogram for age
- Determine if phototherapy indicated
- Assess feeding and weight gain
- Consider underlying cause (hemolysis, infection, thyroid disorder)

Home phototherapy:

- Can be done with portable phototherapy units
- Requires reliable follow-up for bilirubin checks
- Parents must understand importance of frequent feeds

- Recheck bilirubin in 24 hours
- Continue phototherapy until bilirubin below phototherapy threshold

REFLUX AND FEEDING INTOLERANCE

Signs:

- Frequent spit-up (beyond normal newborn spit-up)
- Vomiting
- Irritability after feeds
- Poor weight gain
- Signs of aspiration (cough, wheeze, respiratory distress)
- Arching or discomfort

Management:

- Positional: keep head elevated 30 degrees after feeds
- Feeding: smaller, more frequent feeds
- Formula: consider thickened formula or specialized formula for reflux
- Medication:Proton pump inhibitor (omeprazole) if significant
- Evaluation: if severe, assess for pyloric stenosis or other obstruction

WEIGHT GAIN PROBLEMS

Inadequate gain (<15-20 g/day):

- Assess caloric intake: volume and caloric density
- Assess feeding frequency and duration
- Assess for malabsorption: stool character, frequency
- Assess for increased energy expenditure: fever, tachypnea, increased work of breathing
- Assess for underlying disease: infection, cardiac disease, metabolic disorder

Interventions:

- Increase caloric density: add fortifier to breast milk, use higher-calorie formula
- Increase feeding frequency
- Assess and treat underlying cause
- Lactation support if breastfeeding
- Consider supplementation if inadequate intake
- Refer to dietitian if complex case

JAUNDICE REBOUND

Definition: Bilirubin rises again after phototherapy stopped or after discharge.

Risk factors:

- Early discharge
- Breastfeeding difficulty
- Hemolytic disease
- Infection
- Hypothyroidism

Management:

- Recheck bilirubin
- Plot on nomogram
- Restart phototherapy if indicated
- Assess feeding
- Investigate for underlying cause
- More frequent follow-up

SPECIAL POPULATIONS: DISCHARGE CONSIDERATIONS

BABIES ON HOME OXYGEN

Requirements before discharge:

- Oxygen saturation stable on prescribed flow rate
- Family trained on oxygen delivery and safety
- Equipment arranged and in home before discharge
- Backup oxygen supply available
- Pulse oximeter at home for monitoring
- Cardiopulmonary monitor if indicated
- Emergency plan if oxygen runs out

Safety:

- No smoking around baby
- No open flames
- Keep oxygen away from heat sources
- Know how to respond if SpO_2 drops
- Regular equipment maintenance

Weaning:

- Gradual reduction in flow rate as tolerated
- Monitor SpO_2 during weaning
- May take weeks to months
- Coordinate with pulmonology

BABIES ON FEEDING TUBES

Nasogastric tube (NG):

- Temporary; usually for transition to full oral feeds
- Parents trained on tube placement, feeding, care
- Tube changed regularly (weekly or as needed)
- Transition plan to full oral feeds
- Follow-up to ensure transition progressing

Gastrostomy tube (G-tube):

- More permanent; for ongoing feeding support
- Surgical placement
- Parents trained on feeding, flushing, care, troubleshooting
- Regular follow-up for tube function
- Plan for eventual transition to oral feeds if possible
- Infection prevention around stoma

BABIES ON MEDICATIONS FOR CHRONIC CONDITIONS

Chronic lung disease:

- Diuretics, bronchodilators, inhaled corticosteroids
- Regular monitoring: respiratory status, growth, electrolytes
- Pulmonology follow-up

- Plan for weaning medications as lungs improve

Seizure disorder:

- Anticonvulsant dosing and monitoring
- Signs of breakthrough seizures
- Medication side effects
- Neurology follow-up
- When to go to ER (prolonged seizure, status epilepticus)

Cardiac disease:

- Heart failure medications (diuretics, ACE inhibitors)
- Regular monitoring: heart rate, blood pressure, respiratory status
- Cardiology follow-up
- Activity restrictions if indicated
- When to seek help (respiratory distress, syncope, chest pain)

BABIES WITH SPECIAL NEEDS OR DISABILITIES

Cerebral palsy or neurologic impairment:

- Early intervention referral
- Physical therapy, occupational therapy
- Monitoring for contractures, positioning needs

- Developmental follow-up
- Adaptive equipment as needed

Hearing loss:

- Audiology follow-up
- Hearing aids if indicated
- Early intervention for speech and language
- Parent education about communication strategies

Vision problems:

- Ophthalmology follow-up
- Glasses or contact lenses if needed
- Early intervention for visual stimulation
- Adaptive strategies for daily care

COMMON PITFALLS AND MISTAKES

Mistake #1: Discharging a baby who's not ready. The pressure to free up beds is real, but discharging too early leads to readmissions. Be honest about readiness.

Mistake #2: Not scheduling follow-up before discharge. Families won't do it on their own. Schedule it for them. This is your safety net.

Mistake #3: Assuming parents understand discharge instructions. They don't. Go over them multiple times. Provide written information. Ask them to teach back.

Mistake #4: Not addressing parental anxiety. Parents are scared. Acknowledge it. Provide resources. Normalize their feelings.

Mistake #5: Inadequate communication with primary care. Send a detailed discharge summary. Make sure the primary care provider knows the baby's history and any special needs.

Mistake #6: Missing postpartum depression in mothers. Screen for it. Refer if needed. Don't assume mothers are fine.

Mistake #7: Not referring high-risk babies to early intervention. Babies with risk factors need developmental monitoring. Don't wait for obvious delays.

Mistake #8: Inadequate medication instructions. Unclear dosing leads to errors. Be specific. Provide syringes or droppers. Verify understanding.

Mistake #9: Not addressing feeding problems before discharge. Babies sent home with feeding difficulties often end up back in the hospital. Optimize feeding before discharge.

Mistake #10: Assuming follow-up will happen. It won't unless you make it happen. Call to confirm appointments. Follow up if families miss visits.

WHEN TO READMIT

Reasons for readmission:

- Inadequate feeding and weight loss
- Persistent or worsening jaundice
- Suspected infection or sepsis
- Respiratory distress

- Seizures
- Severe reflux or vomiting
- Dehydration
- Metabolic abnormality
- Equipment failure (monitor, oxygen)
- Parental inability to cope
- Suspected abuse or neglect

Readmission should not be seen as a failure. Sometimes babies need additional time in the hospital. Better to readmit than to have a baby deteriorate at home.

KEY CLINICAL PEARLS

Discharge readiness is about more than just medical stability. Parental readiness and support system matter equally.

Follow-up within 3-5 days is critical. This is where problems are caught early.

Written information is essential. Parents won't remember verbal instructions. Provide handouts for everything.

Early intervention is powerful. Babies with risk factors benefit from early developmental support.

Feeding problems should be resolved before discharge. Inadequate feeding is the most common reason for readmission.

Jaundice management requires reliable follow-up. If you're not confident about follow-up, don't discharge with borderline jaundice.

Medication errors are common. Be specific about dosing. Verify understanding. Provide appropriate measuring devices.

Parental mental health matters. Screen for postpartum depression and anxiety. Refer for help.

Primary care coordination is critical. Don't assume primary care knows what happened in the NICU. Tell them explicitly.

Readmission isn't failure. Sometimes babies need more time. Better to readmit than to have a baby deteriorate at home.

Chapter Twenty-Nine

PROCEDURES IN NICU: SAFE, PRACTICAL PROTOCOLS

Setting the Scene

It is 2 AM. You are on call. The nurse calls you because a 28-weeker is deteriorating—his oxygen requirements have jumped in the last hour and you can hear decreased breath sounds on the left. You know there is air in the pleural space. You have done this before, but you also know that a needle in the wrong place at the wrong speed can make things dramatically worse. This is the world of NICU procedures:

high stakes, often urgent, almost always nerve-wracking even for experienced hands.

Procedures in neonatology are not optional extras. They are core survival skills. A baby with a tension pneumothorax who does not get chest decompression within minutes will die. A premature infant with deteriorating perfusion who cannot get vascular access will not receive the medications and fluids that might save him. And a baby who gets an umbilical catheter placed incorrectly—or with poor aseptic technique—may develop a devastating complication that would not have happened otherwise.

This chapter is not a substitute for hands-on supervised training. Read it, understand the concepts, know the pitfalls—but then practice under guidance, watch videos, use simulators, and never perform a procedure you have not been taught properly without having a senior colleague available. That is the non-negotiable rule in this unit and it should be yours too.

What follows is organized by procedure. For each one, you will get the clinical context, the equipment you need, the steps to follow, the common mistakes people make, and the red flags that should make you stop and call for help. Safety first. Always.

The Golden Rule of NICU Procedures

★ Every procedure carries risk. The question is always: does the benefit outweigh the risk for THIS baby at THIS moment?

★ If you are not sure, call your senior. Uncertainty is not weakness—it is clinical wisdom.

★ Good aseptic technique is non-negotiable. Every time. No exceptions.

★ Document everything: time, technique, catheter position, complications, and who was in the room.

Section 1: Vascular Access

Umbilical Venous Catheter (UVC)

Why and When

The umbilical vein is your first choice for central access in a sick neonate—particularly in the delivery room or within the first few days of life. It is large, accessible, and allows you to deliver hypertonic fluids, blood products, and vasoactive drugs that peripheral veins simply cannot handle. You will place a UVC in resuscitations, in very preterm infants who need parenteral nutrition from day one, and in any baby where you need reliable central access urgently.

The umbilical vein remains accessible for catheterization up to about 7-10 days of life, though it gets progressively harder as the cord dries and retracts. In most cases, the earlier the better.

Equipment

- Sterile gloves, gown, mask, drape
- Umbilical catheter (3.5 Fr for infants <1500g; 5 Fr for larger infants)
- Three-way stopcock, 10 mL syringes
- Heparinized flush (0.5-1 unit/mL)
- Silk suture (2-0 or 3-0) and needle holder
- Scalpel or blade

- Povidone-iodine or chlorhexidine solution
- Measuring tape
- Tape and/or suture for securing

Determining the Target Length

The UVC tip should sit at the junction of the inferior vena cava and right atrium—ideally just above the diaphragm, at the level of T8-T9 on chest X-ray. Use the Shukla formula as your starting point: (birth weight in kg x 1.5) + 5.5 = length in cm from the skin level of the cord. This is a guide, not a guarantee—always confirm with imaging.

Alternatively, shoulder-umbilicus distance (SUD) charts give you a reliable estimate based on body length. Many units now keep a laminated reference card with these values at the bedside. If yours does not, make one.

Step-by-Step

1. Set up your sterile field. Open all equipment onto the sterile drape without contaminating anything.
2. Clean the umbilical stump and surrounding skin with antiseptic solution. Allow it to dry.
3. Place a loose purse-string suture at the base of the cord stump—this controls bleeding and helps you secure the catheter.
4. Cut the cord cleanly with your scalpel approximately 1-2 cm from the skin surface. You will see two thick-walled arteries (small, round, often constricted) and one thin-walled vein (large, gaping, usually at the 12 o'clock position).
5. Flush the catheter with heparinized saline before insertion.

Make sure there are no air bubbles.

6. Gently dilate the vein opening with the tip of your forceps if needed, then advance the catheter to the pre-calculated length, rotating gently if you meet resistance.

7. Confirm blood return by aspirating gently. Bright red pulsatile return is a warning—you may be in the hepatic arterial system or too far advanced into the heart.

8. Secure the catheter with the purse-string suture and tape it safely to the cord stump.

9. Obtain a chest X-ray immediately to confirm position before using the line.

UVC RED FLAGS — Stop and Reassess

- ! Pulsatile bright red blood return: tip likely in arterial territory or cardiac chamber — pull back and recheck

- ! Resistance to advancement: do NOT force — you may be in the portal venous system

- ! Unable to aspirate blood: catheter may be malpositioned or kinked

- ! X-ray shows tip in liver or in right atrium: reposition before use — infusing TPN into liver causes serious hepatic injury

- ! Sudden cardiac arrhythmia after placement: catheter is too far in — pull back immediately

Common Mistakes

- Advancing too far: the most common error. If in doubt, a

UVC tip at the level of the ductus venosus is safer than one sitting in the right atrium.

- Poor fixation: UVCs are notorious for dislodging. A catheter that was perfectly positioned at 0200 may be halfway out by morning rounds if not secured properly.
- Forgetting to flush before insertion: introducing air into the umbilical vein is dangerous. Always flush first.
- Using chlorhexidine on premature skin: standard chlorhexidine is not recommended for infants under 28 weeks due to skin absorption and chemical burns. Know your unit protocol.

Umbilical Arterial Catheter (UAC)

Why and When

The umbilical arteries give you continuous arterial blood pressure monitoring and easy access for frequent blood gases—invaluable in any ventilated premature infant or any baby where you expect to be following blood gases multiple times per day. A UAC is also your route for delivering certain medications, though this should be done carefully and according to strict protocols about what is safe to infuse arterially.

High-Line vs. Low-Line Position

This is one of the great debates in neonatology, and most units will have a strong preference. A high line sits at T6-T10 (above the celiac and mesenteric arteries). A low line sits at L3-L4 (below the renal arteries). Both are acceptable. High lines are generally associated with fewer complications in very preterm infants, but check your unit's protocol and follow it consistently.

Use the same approach as UVC for length estimation: (birth weight in kg x 3) + 9 for a high line, or (birth weight in kg x 1.5) + 3.5 for a low line. Again, imaging confirms.

Key Technical Differences from UVC

The arteries are smaller, thicker-walled, and in spasm after delivery. You will need forceps to dilate the artery gently—patience is essential here. Advance the catheter in a smooth, steady motion. If you hit resistance, a small amount of steady continuous pressure often gets past a spasm, but do NOT force it through. Forcing a UAC through a vessel wall is the kind of mistake that ends with a neonatal surgical emergency.

UAC COMPLICATIONS TO KNOW

- ! Vasospasm: the affected leg or buttock turns white or blue. Remove the catheter immediately.
- ! Thrombosis: watch for diminished pulses or limb discoloration hours after placement.
- ! Aortic thrombosis: rare but catastrophic — sudden deterioration, limb ischemia, renal failure.
- ! Necrotizing enterocolitis has been associated with malpositioned UACs — confirm position before use.
- ! Accidental dislodgement: a UAC that pulls out can bleed massively — always keep the baby on continuous BP monitoring.

Peripherally Inserted Central Catheter (PICC)

Why and When

When umbilical access is no longer available—typically after day 7-10—and you still need reliable central access for TPN or long-term medications, a PICC line is your answer. PICC lines can also be placed earlier in some units as an alternative to UAC/UVC, particularly in centers with strong nursing PICC programs.

The technique involves threading a fine silastic catheter through a peripheral vein—most commonly the antecubital, saphenous, or axillary vein—advancing it toward the SVC or IVC. This is a skilled procedure requiring specific training and most units have dedicated PICC teams or trained nurses who perform these. Know who does PICCs in your unit and involve them early rather than waiting until you have lost all other access.

Vascular Access Pearls

- ★ Always confirm central line position with X-ray before starting any infusion, especially TPN or vasoactive drugs.
- ★ Document insertion site, catheter length at skin, and tip position on the bedside chart every shift.
- ★ Any line that stops working should be investigated — a kinked or malpositioned catheter is safer out than in.
- ★ Central line-associated bloodstream infections (CLABSIs) are preventable. Aseptic technique and line care bundles save lives.
- ★ In Saudi tertiary units, dedicated PICC teams have dramatically reduced CLABSI rates — use them.

Section 2: Airway Management

Endotracheal Intubation

When You Need to Intubate

There are babies who need to be intubated immediately and there are babies where you have time to think. Apnea that does not respond to stimulation or CPAP, severe respiratory failure despite non-invasive support, airway obstruction, need for surfactant administration, and certain surgical emergencies—these are the main reasons you reach for the laryngoscope. In the delivery room, any baby who is not breathing adequately after initial steps and positive pressure ventilation may need intubation.

The key decision is not just 'does this baby need to be intubated' but 'am I the right person to do it right now?' Know your skill level honestly. If you are not confident, get your senior. Thirty seconds of good bag-mask ventilation while you call for help is far better than a traumatic failed intubation attempt.

Equipment

- Laryngoscope with Miller blade (size 0 for premature, size 1 for term)
- Endotracheal tubes: 2.5 mm for <1000g; 3.0 mm for 1000-2000g; 3.5 mm for >2000g
- Stylet if used in your unit (optional)
- CO_2 detector or waveform capnography

- Suction device and suction catheters
- Tape or tube-securing device
- Bag and mask connected to oxygen
- Pulse oximeter and cardiac monitor running

Step-by-Step

1. Pre-oxygenate the baby with blow-by oxygen or bag-mask ventilation.
2. Position the baby in the sniffing position. A small shoulder roll helps open the airway in preterm infants.
3. Hold the laryngoscope in your left hand. Open the mouth gently with your right hand.
4. Insert the blade along the right side of the mouth, sweeping the tongue to the left. Advance to the base of the tongue.
5. Lift the laryngoscope blade upward and forward (NOT backward — this is a common mistake). You should see the glottis.
6. Pass the ETT through the vocal cords under direct vision. Watch the tip pass between the cords.
7. Advance the tube to the appropriate lip-length mark: weight (kg) + 6 cm is a commonly used guide.
8. Remove the laryngoscope. Confirm position immediately.
9. Confirmation: chest rise with ventilation, CO_2 detection,

equal air entry bilaterally, improving oxygen saturations.

10. Secure the tube immediately before obtaining a chest X-ray to confirm the tip position (ideally T2-T3).

The whole process from blade in mouth to confirmed tube should take no more than 30 seconds. If you are not in by then, stop. Take the laryngoscope out. Ventilate with bag and mask. Let the baby recover. Then try again or call for senior help.

Intubation Red Flags

- ! 30-second rule: if you have not secured the airway in 30 seconds, stop and ventilate with a bag-mask.
- ! Only breath sounds heard over the stomach: tube is in the esophagus — remove immediately and ventilate.
- ! Unilateral chest rise only: right mainstem intubation — pull the tube back 0.5-1 cm and recheck.
- ! No CO_2 detection after intubation: assume esophageal intubation until proven otherwise.
- ! Severe bradycardia or desaturation during attempt: stop, oxygenate first, then reattempt when stabilized.
- ! Bloody secretions from tube: trauma to airway — reassess and escalate.

Medications for Intubation

Except in the delivery room resuscitation where there is no time, elective intubations should use premedication. The evidence clearly shows that intubation without analgesia and sedation is painful, causes adverse physiological responses, and is harder technically because the baby moves and coughs. Most units now use a protocol involving atropine (to prevent bradycardia), an opioid such as morphine or fentanyl, and a muscle relaxant such as succinylcholine or rocuronium. Know your unit's premedication protocol before you need it.

Surfactant Administration

Once the baby is intubated and the tube position is confirmed, surfactant can be administered via the ETT. In most protocols, the dose is 100-200 mg/kg depending on the agent. Instill the surfactant in one aliquot (or divided doses as per protocol), apply positive pressure to distribute it, and watch for the rapid improvement in oxygenation that confirms it has worked. Transient desaturation and bradycardia can occur during instillation—have someone ready at the bag. After INSURE (INtubate, SURfactant, Extubate), the goal is back to CPAP as quickly as tolerated.

Extubation

Extubation is a procedure too, and failed extubation is common and preventable. Before you extubate, make sure the baby is on minimal or no ventilator support, is breathing spontaneously with adequate drive, has a stable temperature and acceptable blood gases, and has CPAP or HFNC ready to go immediately after. Suction the ETT and oropharynx just before extubation. After removing the tube, place the baby immediately on non-invasive support and observe closely for the first hour. Extubating at 3 AM when you have no CPAP ready and no one immediately available is not safe planning—choose your timing wisely.

Section 3: Thoracic Procedures

Needle Aspiration for Pneumothorax

The Emergency Scenario

A baby deteriorates acutely. He goes from stable to gasping in minutes. The oxygen requirement jumps, the blood pressure drops, and when you transilluminate the chest, one side glows. The breath sounds are asymmetric. You have diagnosed a tension pneumothorax. This is one of the few situations in neonatology where you act first and confirm later. Do not wait for an X-ray. Get the needle in.

Equipment for Needle Aspiration

- 23-gauge butterfly needle or 22-gauge angiocath
- 10 mL syringe
- Three-way stopcock
- Antiseptic wipe
- Assistant to hold the baby still

Technique

1. Identify the second intercostal space, midclavicular line on the affected side.
2. Clean the skin quickly with an antiseptic wipe.
3. Insert the needle perpendicular to the skin, just above the third rib (to avoid the intercostal vessels that run below each rib).
4. Advance slowly until you feel the 'pop' of entering the pleural space, then stop.
5. Aspirate air with the syringe. Significant air return with im-

mediate clinical improvement confirms your diagnosis.

6. Remove the needle once the baby stabilizes and proceed to chest tube if needed.

Needle aspiration is a bridge, not a definitive treatment. If the pneumothorax re-accumulates—and in a ventilated baby it usually will—you need a chest tube. Have someone prepare for that while you are performing the needle aspiration.

Chest Tube Insertion

When You Need a Tube, Not Just a Needle

Any baby on positive pressure ventilation with a pneumothorax will almost certainly need a chest drain rather than repeated needle aspirations. The same applies to significant pleural effusions, chylothorax, or empyema. A chest drain provides ongoing drainage rather than a one-time decompression.

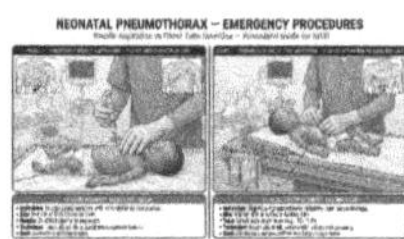

Equipment

- Chest drain (8-10 Fr for most preterm infants; 10-12 Fr for term)
- Underwater seal or Heimlich valve
- Sterile gloves, gown, drape
- Local anesthetic (1% lidocaine)
- Suture material (2-0 silk), scalpel, and artery forceps

- Occlusive dressing

Step-by-Step

1. Position the baby supine with the affected side elevated slightly.

2. Identify the insertion point: 4th or 5th intercostal space, anterior axillary line. This avoids the breast tissue and neurovascular structures.

3. Clean the area with antiseptic and apply a sterile drape.

4. Infiltrate local anesthetic if time permits and the baby is not in extremis.

5. Make a small skin incision (5-10 mm) just above the lower rib.

6. Blunt dissect through the subcutaneous tissue and intercostal muscle with artery forceps.

7. Push the forceps through the pleura with a controlled forward motion. Open the forceps to widen the tract. Do NOT use a trocar in neonates—it is dangerously uncontrolled.

8. Advance the drain through the tract, directing it anteriorly and superiorly for pneumothorax, or posteriorly and inferiorly for effusion.

9. Connect to the underwater seal immediately. Watch for swinging with respiration (confirming position) and air or fluid drainage.

10. Secure with suture and an occlusive dressing. Obtain a chest

X-ray to confirm position.

Chest Tube Complications to Watch For

- ! Lung perforation: the tube went too far — if air return stops and the baby deteriorates, check position urgently.
- ! Subcutaneous emphysema around insertion site: tube may be partially out of the pleural space.
- ! Blocked tube: if output suddenly stops and the baby deteriorates, try flushing gently or consider replacement.
- ! Tube displacement: check external length marking at every nursing assessment.
- ! Infection: any erythema or discharge from the insertion site in a febrile baby needs urgent attention.

Section 4: Lumbar Puncture

Why LPs Are Often Skipped (And Why They Shouldn't Be)

Let us be honest about something. Lumbar punctures are often the most skipped investigation in sick neonates, and it is a problem. Babies are too sick. The LP is deferred. Antibiotics get started. And then nobody ever goes back to do the LP, so we never know if there was meningitis or not. The consequence is a baby who may have been undertreated—or one who gets a full 21-day meningitis course when shorter treatment might have been appropriate.

Do the LP when it is clinically indicated. Do it early. If the baby is too unstable for the procedure at that moment, document why and plan for it as soon as it is safe. Do not just leave it off indefinitely.

Indications

- Any baby with suspected bacterial meningitis
- Positive blood culture (to determine if CNS seeding has occurred)
- Persistent bacteremia despite appropriate antibiotics
- Any clinical picture concerning for encephalitis or meningitis
- Evaluation of HSV CNS disease

Contraindications

- Severe cardiorespiratory instability: defer until more stable
- Coagulopathy or thrombocytopenia (platelets <50,000): consider FFP/platelet transfusion first
- Skin infection over the proposed site
- Signs of raised intracranial pressure (bulging fontanelle, Cushing's triad): imaging first

Equipment

- Spinal needle: 22-gauge, 1.5 inches for most term infants; shorter for very preterm
- Sterile gloves and drape
- Three collection tubes and one for glucose

- Antiseptic solution
- An assistant who knows how to hold a neonate correctly for LP

Positioning Is Everything

You have two choices: lateral decubitus (baby on their side, curled into a C shape) or sitting up (baby held upright, leaning slightly forward). Both work. Whatever position you choose, the key is maximal flexion of the lumbar spine without compromising the airway. In premature infants, a curled-up position that also kinks the airway is dangerous—the monitor should be on and someone should be watching the oxygen saturations throughout.

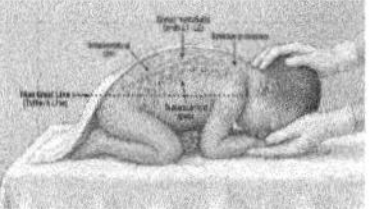

Your target is the L3-L4 or L4-L5 interspace. Find the iliac crest: the line connecting the two iliac crests crosses at approximately L4. Go one space up or one space down from there.

Technique

1. Clean the skin with antiseptic. Allow it to dry.
2. Identify the L3-L4 interspace by palpating the spinous processes.
3. Insert the needle in the midline, aiming slightly toward the umbilicus, bevel up.
4. Advance slowly. You will feel a change in resistance when the needle passes through the ligamentum flavum and then the dura. In premature infants, this 'pop' is subtle.
5. Remove the stylet and look for CSF flow. If you get blood, replace the stylet, wait a moment, and reassess.

6. Collect 1 mL in each tube. Do not aspirate—CSF should drip freely.

7. Replace the stylet before removing the needle. This reduces the risk of post-LP headache (rare in neonates, but good practice).

A traumatic tap—blood in the CSF from the needle passing through a vessel—is common in neonates and does not mean the procedure failed. Compare the first and last tubes: if the blood clears across the tubes, it is likely a traumatic tap. The laboratory can also help you correct white cell counts for a bloody tap. Document clearly.

CSF Interpretation in Neonates

- ★ Normal neonatal CSF can have up to 20 white cells/mm^3 and protein up to 150 mg/dL — very different from adult normals.

- ★ Low CSF glucose (<50% of simultaneous blood glucose) is concerning for bacterial meningitis.

- ★ A Gram stain positive result is highly specific — treat aggressively even if the culture takes days to return.

- ★ Send HSV PCR on the CSF if there is any clinical concern — do not miss neonatal herpes.

Section 5: Abdominal Procedures

Abdominal Paracentesis

When You Need to Tap the Belly

Hydrops fetalis, spontaneous intestinal perforation, NEC with ascites, and certain metabolic disorders can cause significant abdominal fluid accumulation that compromises respiration and circulation. When ascites is causing respiratory embarrassment or hemodynamic compromise, drainage can provide meaningful relief.

This is not a first-line procedure and is not without risk. Before you consider it, make sure you have confirmed the presence of fluid (ultrasound is your friend here—do not blindly needle an abdomen without knowing where the fluid is), that the cause is understood, and that you have discussed it with your senior.

Equipment and Technique

- 22-24 gauge angiocath or paracentesis needle
- 20-60 mL syringe with three-way stopcock
- Sterile gloves and cleaning supplies
- Ultrasound if available to identify the fluid pocket and mark the site

Insert the needle in the right or left lower quadrant, lateral to the rectus muscle (to avoid the inferior epigastric vessels). Use a Z-track technique: displace the skin before advancing, then release after. Aspirate gently. If you get bowel content (brown or feculent material), withdraw immediately—you have perforated bowel—and call surgery urgently.

Gastric Lavage and Decompression

Gastric decompression via nasogastric or orogastric tube is a procedure many treat as routine but it is not without risk in neonates. The tube can enter the airway—particularly in babies who are not alert. Always confirm placement before using the tube: aspirate stomach contents (bile-stained or with gastric pH), listen for air insufflation, or use X-ray in uncertain cases. In a baby with confirmed or suspected oesophageal atresia, stop immediately if you meet resistance advancing the tube—you are likely in a blind-ending pouch, not the stomach.

Section 6: Blood Sampling Techniques

Heel Lance

The heel lance is the most common painful procedure in the NICU—and the one most often performed with inadequate pain management. Every heel lance should be preceded by non-pharmacological analgesia at minimum: sucrose, non-nutritive sucking, or skin-to-skin contact. Warm the heel for 2-3 minutes to increase blood flow. Use a spring-loaded lancet calibrated for neonates (not a standard adult lancet). The lateral aspects of the heel are the safe zones—the central heel has important nerves and vessels. Squeeze gently and intermittently rather than continuously, which causes more pain and hemolysis.

Document that analgesia was given. It takes seconds and makes a real difference to the baby's pain experience and long-term outcomes.

Peripheral Venous Blood Draw

Antecubital, dorsal hand, and saphenous veins are your targets. Scalp veins can be used in infants where limb access is impossible, but they distress families and provide limited volume—reserve them for truly refractory situations. As with heel sticks, provide analgesia before the needle goes in. Stabilize the limb, clean the skin, insert at a low angle (15-20 degrees), and aspirate gently. Hemolysis from aggressive aspiration ruins samples and creates false results—pull the plunger slowly.

Arterial Blood Gas via Radial Artery

When you need an arterial sample and have no arterial line in place, the radial artery is your first choice. Confirm radial patency with the Allen test first (compress both radial and ulnar arteries, release ulnar, and confirm the hand flushes pink). Use a 24-gauge needle, insert at a 30-45 degree angle, advance toward the pulse, and collect into a heparinized syringe. Apply firm pressure for at least 5 minutes after withdrawal. Radial artery puncture in neonates is a genuinely difficult skill—practice and get supervised until you are reliable.

Blood Sampling Pearls

- ★ Every painful procedure requires documented analgesia — this is standard of care, not optional.
- ★ Label samples at the bedside immediately — mislabeled samples in a NICU cause potentially fatal errors.
- ★ Minimum volumes: use neonatal-specific tubes and order only the tests you actually need.
- ★ Hemolyzed samples tell you almost nothing useful — technique matters for result quality.

- ★ In jaundiced babies, bilirubin samples must be protected from light — cover the syringe or tube immediately.

Section 7: Resuscitation-Specific Procedures

Intraosseous Access

When a baby is in cardiac arrest or severe shock and you cannot get intravenous access within 60-90 seconds, the intraosseous (IO) route saves lives. In neonates, the proximal tibia is the standard site. IO access is underused in neonatal emergencies because people hesitate—but in a true resuscitation, it is the right call. The proximal anteromedial tibia, about 1-2 cm below the tibial tuberosity, is your target. A dedicated IO device or a spinal needle can be used in very small infants. Confirm placement by aspirating marrow or flushing easily without subcutaneous extravasation, then flush rapidly to establish flow before giving medications.

IO lines are temporary emergency access only. They should not remain in place for more than 24 hours. As soon as the baby is stable enough, establish proper IV or central access.

Cardiac Compressions and Emergency Drugs

NICU cardiac arrest is managed per current NRP guidelines. Two-thumb encircling technique for chest compressions is recommended over two-finger technique in neonates because it generates better coronary perfusion pressure. The compression-to-ventilation ratio remains 3:1. Epinephrine (0.01-0.03 mg/kg IV/IO) is the drug of choice when heart rate remains below 60 despite 30 seconds of coordinated CPR. The intratracheal route is less effective and should only be used if IV/IO access is genuinely impossible.

Volume resuscitation with normal saline (10 mL/kg IV/IO) can be given if hypovolemic arrest is suspected—particularly after fetal-maternal hemorrhage or cord accidents. Do not give volume blindly in every arrest; know why you are doing it.

Section 8: Infection Control and General Procedural Safety

Aseptic Technique Is Not Negotiable

Central line-associated bloodstream infections are among the most preventable complications in the NICU, and they kill babies. A CLABSI in a 500-gram premature infant is not a minor inconvenience—it is a potential death sentence. Yet they happen because clinicians rush, because 3 AM does not feel like the right time for a full sterile setup, because the nurse was pulling on gloves while also trying to help hold the baby still. None of these are acceptable reasons.

Every invasive procedure gets full sterile technique: sterile gloves, gown, mask, drape, and antiseptic preparation of the site. In Saudi tertiary units, compliance with CLABSI bundles has been transformative in units where it has been implemented rigorously. This is not bureaucracy—it is the difference between a baby going home and a baby getting a fungal sepsis that destroys their brain.

Time-Out Before Every Procedure

Before any significant procedure, do a brief pause. Confirm the correct patient (check the wristband). Confirm the correct procedure and the correct side for lateralized procedures—wrong-side chest tubes have happened in the best units in the world. Confirm that equipment is ready and that you have appropriate support. This takes 30 seconds and prevents catastrophic errors.

Documentation

Document every procedure immediately: time, indication, technique, catheter type and size, insertion length, complications, and the position confirmed on imaging. If a procedure is performed by a trainee under supervision, document who supervised. Good documentation is not just a legal requirement—it is how the team knows what happened at 3 AM when the day shift takes over and the baby's status has changed.

Pain Management Is Part of Every Procedure

This bears repeating because it is too often inadequately addressed. Neonates feel pain. Premature infants feel more pain sensitization, not less, compared to term infants. Every procedure that causes pain requires a documented pain management plan. Non-pharmacological measures (sucrose, non-nutritive sucking, facilitated tucking, skin-to-skin) should be offered for minor procedures. Pharmacological analgesia should be used for intubation, chest tube insertion, and any other significantly painful invasive procedure. There is no excuse for routinely performing painful procedures without analgesia in 2024.

Section 9: When to Ask for Help

There is a culture in medicine that valorizes performing procedures independently and views asking for help as weakness. This culture gets babies hurt. Let us be very clear about when you must involve a senior colleague:

- You have attempted a procedure twice and have not succeeded: get help rather than attempting a third time on an increasingly compromised baby.
- The baby is deteriorating during the procedure: stop what you are doing and stabilize the baby first.
- You encounter unexpected findings: blood where there should be air, resistance where passage should be smooth, or an anatomical variant that does not match what you expect.
- The procedure is outside your documented training and competency: supervision is not optional.
- The baby's condition changes significantly before or during the procedure: reassess whether to proceed.

In resource-limited settings—whether a district hospital or a smaller regional unit—the answer to 'I cannot do this safely here' is to stabilize the baby and arrange urgent transfer to a facility with the necessary expertise. Attempting a procedure you are not trained for, with equipment you do not have, in isolation, is how babies die from preventable causes.

When to Call Your Senior — No Exceptions

- ★ Two failed attempts at any procedure: stop and call for help.

- ★ Unexpected findings during any procedure: blood, abnormal anatomy, unexpected resistance.
- ★ Baby deteriorating during the procedure: stabilize first, procedure second.
- ★ Outside your training and competency: supervision is not optional, it is mandatory.
- ★ Your instinct says something is wrong: trust your instinct and get eyes on the baby.

Key Clinical Pearls:

This chapter has covered the core procedural skills you need to keep sick neonates alive. A few overarching principles are worth carrying with you every time you pick up a needle, a catheter, or a laryngoscope:

- Know before you go: understand the procedure, the anatomy, the equipment, and the potential complications before the baby needs it, not while the baby is deteriorating.
- Safety check every time: correct patient, correct procedure, correct side, correct equipment. It takes 30 seconds and saves lives.
- Aseptic technique is not situational: 3 AM, understaffed, the most junior person in the room—none of these are reasons to cut corners on sterile technique.
- Pain is real: document your analgesia plan for every procedure. Neonates feel pain and we have tools to manage it.

- Confirm before you use: every central line needs imaging confirmation before first use, especially for hypertonic or vasoactive infusions.
- Two failed attempts, call for help: this is a rule, not a suggestion.
- Document completely: what you did, when, how, what you found, and who supervised.
- Know your limits and your local resources: in Saudi healthcare settings, use your specialized colleagues and PICC teams. If the expertise is not available where you are, arrange transfer rather than improvise dangerously.

Procedures are where safety culture meets clinical skill. Every baby who survives a difficult intubation, a well-placed chest tube, or a perfectly positioned UAC is a testament to the clinician who practiced, who asked for help when needed, and who never stopped treating the procedure as seriously as the disease itself.

Practice safe neonatology. Every time.

Chapter Thirty

QUICK REFERENCE GUIDE: ESSENTIAL ALGORITHMS AND PROTOCOLS

NEONATAL RESUSCITATION ALGORITHM (NRP)

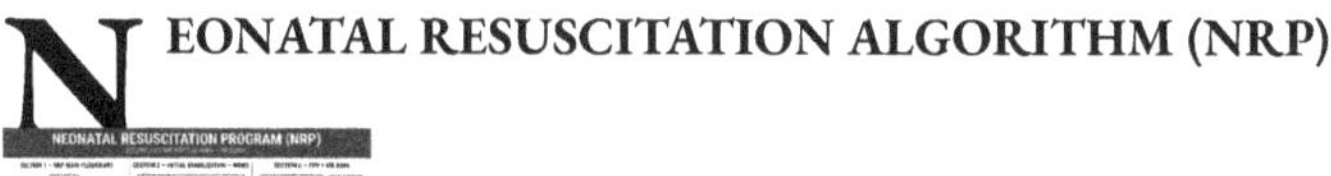

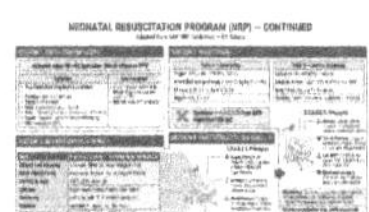

RESPIRATORY DISTRESS ASSESSMENT AND MANAGEMENT

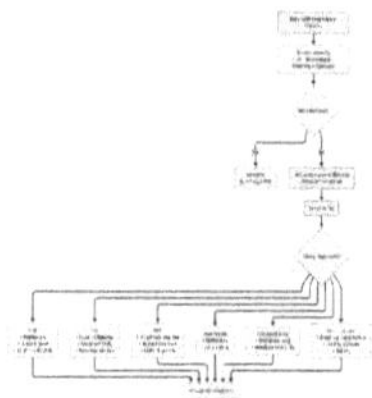

HYPOGLYCEMIA SCREENING AND MANAGEMENT

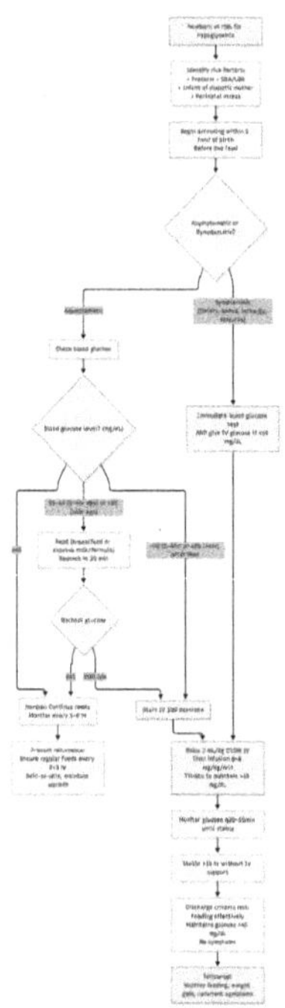

JAUNDICE MANAGEMENT ALGORITHM

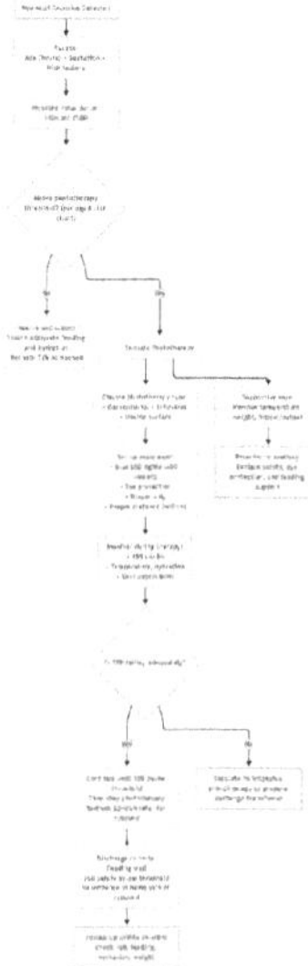

SEPSIS SCREENING AND ANTIBIOTIC PROTOCOL

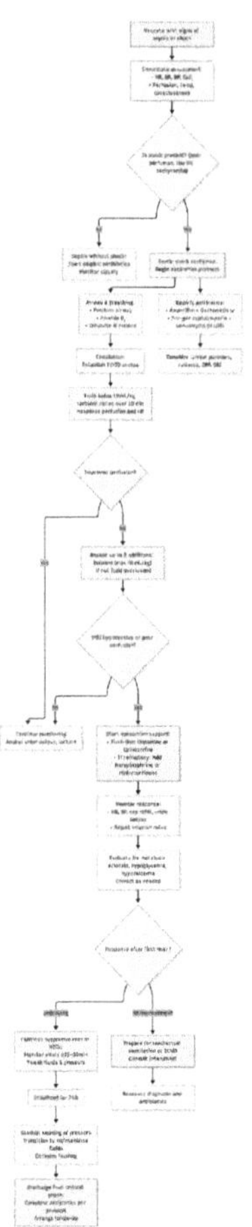

THERAPEUTIC HYPOTHERMIA PROTOCOL (HIE)

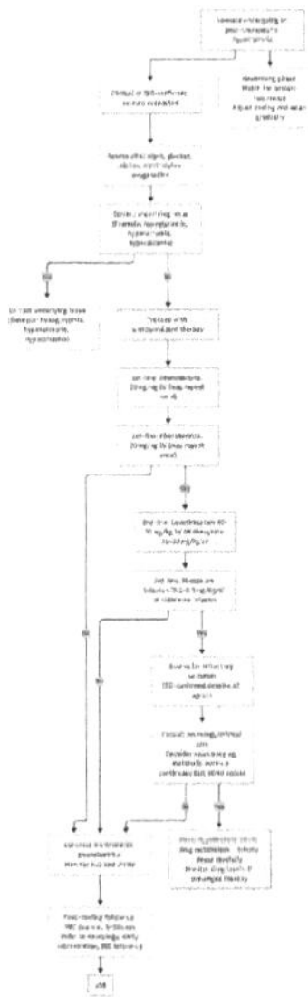

TENSION PNEUMOTHORAX EMERGENCY PROTOCOL

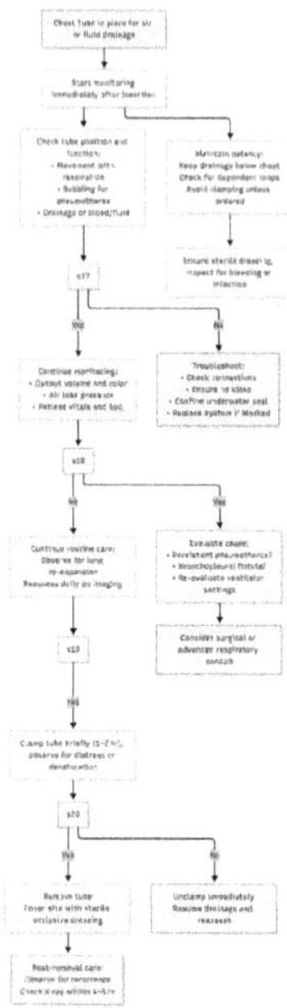

POLYCYTHEMIA MANAGEMENT (Recipient Twin)

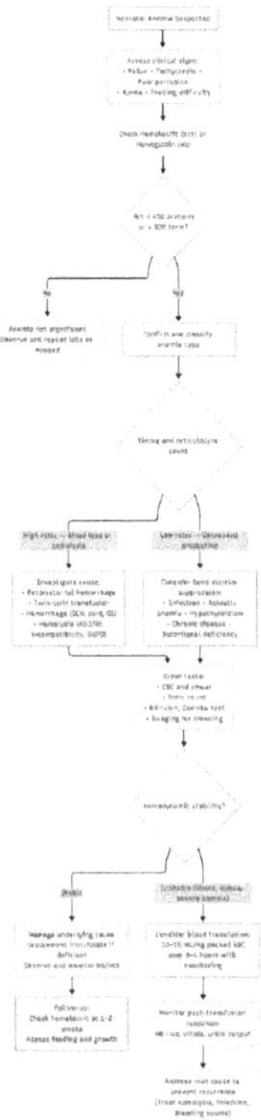

ABDOMINAL WALL DEFECT MANAGEMENT

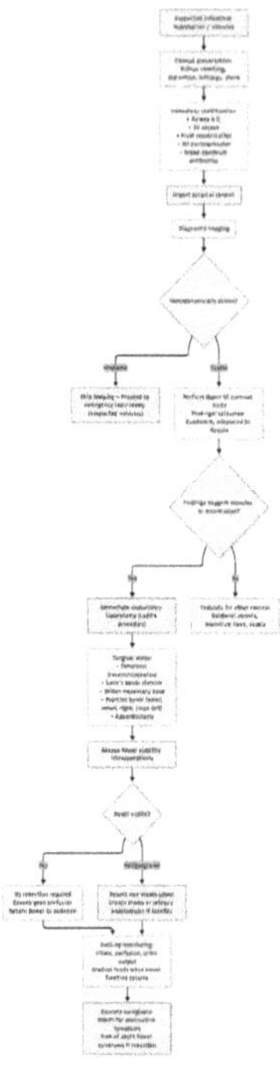

DIAPHRAGMATIC HERNIA PROTOCOL

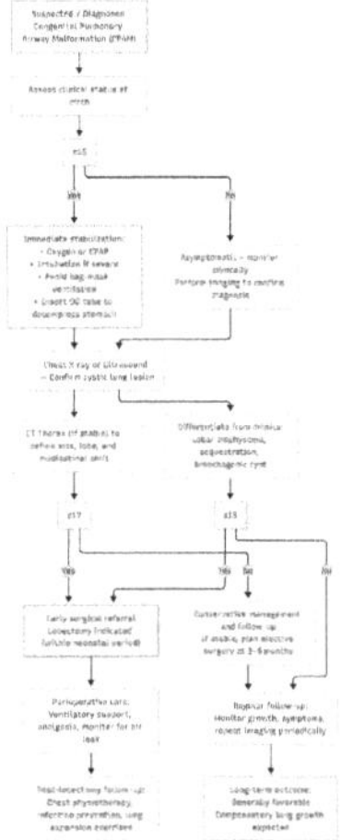

ESOPHAGEAL ATRESIA/TEF PROTOCOL

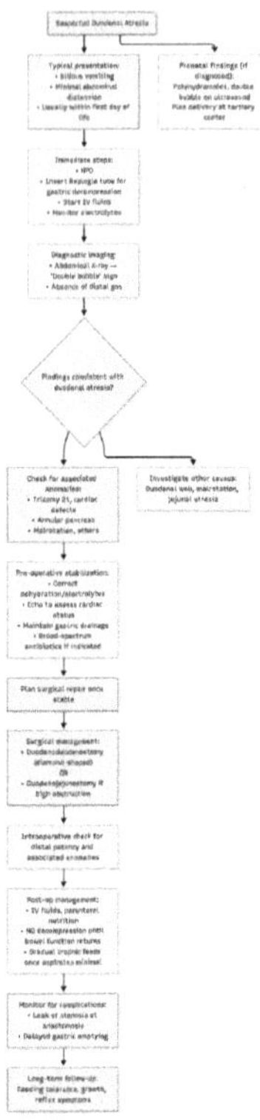

DISCHARGE READINESS CHECKLIST

☐ PHYSIOLOGIC STABILITY:

- ☐ Maintains temperature in open crib
- ☐ Respiratory stable (no apnea/bradycardia)
- ☐ SpO_2 stable on room air or minimal O_2
- ☐ Cardiovascular stable

- ☐ Feeding: full volume by mouth, gaining weight
- ☐ Normal urine/stool output
- ☐ Jaundice resolved or managed with outpatient phototherapy
- ☐ No active infection

☐ NEUROLOGIC STABILITY:

- ☐ Alert and responsive
- ☐ Normal muscle tone
- ☐ No seizures
- ☐ Appropriate feeding behaviors

☐ METABOLIC STABILITY:

- ☐ Normal glucose
- ☐ Normal electrolytes
- ☐ No significant acid-base disturbance

☐ INFECTIOUS DISEASE:

- ☐ Cultures negative (if obtained)

- ☐ Antibiotics completed if indicated
- ☐ Immunizations up to date
- ☐ Screening tests completed or scheduled

☐ PARENTAL READINESS:

- ☐ Parents understand baby's condition
- ☐ Parents can perform necessary care
- ☐ Support system in place
- ☐ Parents know warning signs
- ☐ Follow-up appointments scheduled
- ☐ Prescriptions and resources provided

☐ DISCHARGE PREPARATION:

- ☐ Discharge summary prepared
- ☐ Medications prescribed with clear instructions
- ☐ Equipment arranged and in home
- ☐ Feeding supplies provided
- ☐ Car seat safety reviewed
- ☐ Safe sleep counseling completed

- ☐ Immunization record provided

FOLLOW-UP TIMING BY CONDITION

PRIMARY CARE VISIT: 3-5 days post-discharge

SPECIALTY FOLLOW-UP TIMING:

URGENT (1-2 weeks):

- Cardiac defects
- Significant jaundice
- Seizure disorder
- Severe infection
- Major surgery

IMPORTANT (2-4 weeks):

- Moderate jaundice
- Feeding difficulties
- Mild cardiac findings
- Hearing loss
- Mild developmental concerns

ROUTINE (1-3 months):

- Growth monitoring
- Developmental screening
- Chronic lung disease

- Metabolic follow-up

EARLY INTERVENTION REFERRAL:

High-risk for developmental delay

-Prematurity <32 weeks

-Neurologic impairment

-Genetic/metabolic disorders

-Refer before discharge or at first follow-up

Chapter Thirty-One

BIBLIOGRAPHY AND EVIDENCE-BASED REFERENCES

FOUNDATIONAL GUIDELINES AND CONSENSUS DOCUMENTS

Neonatal Resuscitation and Initial Management

1. Wyckoff MH, Aziz K, Escobedo MB, et al. Part 5: Neonatal Resuscitation: 2015 American Heart Association Guidelines Update for Cardiopulmonary Resuscitation and

Emergency Cardiovascular Care. *Circulation*. 2015;132(18 Suppl 2):S189-S210.

- *Relevance:* Gold standard for NRP algorithm, chest compression techniques, medication dosing
- *Key Updates:* Emphasis on delayed cord clamping, avoiding hyperoxia, gentle ventilation

2. American Academy of Pediatrics & American Heart Association. *Textbook of Neonatal Resuscitation (NRP)*, 8th Edition. 2021.
   - *Relevance:* Comprehensive resource for resuscitation protocols
   - *Clinical Application:* Practical approach to delivery room management
3. Perlman JM, Wyllie J, Kattwinkel J, et al. Part 7: Neonatal Resuscitation: 2015 International Consensus on Cardiopulmonary Resuscitation and Emergency Cardiovascular Care Science with Treatment Recommendations. *Circulation*. 2015;132(16 Suppl 1):S204-S241.
   - *Relevance:* International guidelines for neonatal resuscitation
   - *Key Points:* Evidence-based recommendations for different scenarios

Respiratory Disorders

1. Sweet DG, Carnielli V, Bhuta T, et al. European Consensus Guidelines on the Management of Neonatal Respiratory Distress Syndrome in Preterm Infants. *Neonatology*. 2019;115(4):432-450.

    - *Relevance:* Comprehensive RDS management including surfactant therapy
    - *Key Recommendations:* CPAP vs. intubation, surfactant strategies, ventilation targets

2. Seger N, Soll R. Animal derived surfactant extract versus protein free synthetic surfactant for the prevention and treatment of respiratory distress syndrome. *Cochrane Database Syst Rev*. 2009;(4):CD000144.

    - *Relevance:* Evidence for surfactant therapy efficacy
    - *Outcome Data:* Mortality and morbidity reduction with surfactant

3. Finer NN, Carlo WA, Walsh MC, et al. Early CPAP versus surfactant for extremely preterm infants (SUPPORT trial). *N Engl J Med*. 2010;362(21):1970-1979.

    - *Relevance:* CPAP-first strategy vs. early surfactant
    - *Clinical Implication:* Individualized approach based on baby's response

4. Jobe AH, Bancalari E. Bronchopulmonary dysplasia. *Am J Respir Crit Care Med*. 2019;163(7):1723-1729.

    - *Relevance:* Definition and pathophysiology of BPD

    - *Prevention Strategies:* Gentle ventilation, avoiding oxygen toxicity

5. Verder H, Agertoft L, Pedersen S, et al. Surfactant nebulization is just around the corner. *Arch Dis Child Fetal Neonatal Ed.* 2016;101(2):F175-F177.
    - *Relevance:* Emerging surfactant delivery methods
    - *Future Direction:* Less invasive surfactant administration

Cardiovascular Disorders

1. Kluckow M, Evans N. Low superior vena cava flow and intraventricular haemorrhage in preterm infants. *Arch Dis Child Fetal Neonatal Ed.* 2000;82(3):F188-F194.
    - *Relevance:* Understanding hemodynamic monitoring in preterm infants
    - *Clinical Application:* Echocardiography assessment of cardiac function
2. Schena F, Francescato G, Cappelleri A, et al. Association between hemodynamically significant patent ductus arteriosus and bronchopulmonary dysplasia. *J Pediatr.* 2015;166(6):1488-1492.
    - *Relevance:* PDA management and outcomes
    - *Treatment Options:* Medical vs. surgical closure
3. Benitz WE. Patent ductus arteriosus in preterm infants. *Pe-*

diatrics. 2016;137(1):e20153730.

- *Relevance:* Comprehensive PDA management guidelines
- *Key Points:* When to treat, which medications, monitoring

4. Mahle WT, Newburger JW, Matherne GP, et al. Role of pulse oximetry in examining newborns for congenital heart disease: a scientific statement from the American Heart Association and American Academy of Pediatrics. *Circulation*. 2009;120(5):447-458.
   - *Relevance:* Screening for critical congenital heart disease
   - *Clinical Application:* Pulse oximetry screening protocol

Infections and Sepsis

1. Puopolo KM, Benitz WE, Zaoutis TE. Management of neonates born at ≥35 0/7 weeks' gestation with suspected or proven early-onset bacterial sepsis. *Pediatrics*. 2018;142(6):e20182894.
   - *Relevance:* EOS risk stratification and antibiotic stewardship
   - *Key Algorithm:* Risk-based approach to antibiotic initiation
2. Verani JR, McGee L, Schrag SJ. Prevention of perinatal

group B streptococcal disease: revised guidelines from CDC. *MMWR Recomm Rep.* 2010;59(RR-10):1-36.

- *Relevance:* GBS prevention and intrapartum antibiotic prophylaxis
- *Clinical Application:* Identification of at-risk mothers

3. Polin RA. Management of neonates with suspected or proven early-onset bacterial sepsis. *Pediatrics.* 2012;129(5):1006-1015.
   - *Relevance:* Comprehensive sepsis management protocol
   - *Antibiotic Regimens:* First-line therapy options
4. Wynn JL, Wong HR, Shanley TP, et al. Time for a neonatal-specific consensus definition for sepsis. *Pediatr Crit Care Med.* 2014;15(6):523-528.
   - *Relevance:* Defining sepsis in neonates
   - *Diagnostic Criteria:* Clinical and laboratory markers

Hyperbilirubinemia and Jaundice

1. American Academy of Pediatrics Subcommittee on Hyperbilirubinemia. Management of hyperbilirubinemia in the newborn infant 35 or more weeks of gestation. *Pediatrics.* 2009;124(4):1193-1198.
   - *Relevance:* Phototherapy and exchange transfusion thresholds

- *Key Tool:* Nomogram for bilirubin management

2. Bhutani VK, Johnson LH, Sivieri EM. Predictive ability of a predischarge hour-specific serum bilirubin for subsequent significant hyperbilirubinemia in healthy term and near-term newborns. *Pediatrics*. 1999;103(1):6-14.
   - *Relevance:* Early detection of at-risk infants
   - *Clinical Application:* Predischarge bilirubin screening
3. Maisels MJ, Baltz RD, Bhutani VK, et al. Hyperbilirubinemia in the newborn infant ≥35 weeks' gestation: an update with clarifications. *Pediatrics*. 2009;124(4):1193-1198.
   - *Relevance:* Updated management guidelines
   - *Phototherapy Thresholds:* Age and risk-specific recommendations

Hypoglycemia

1. Adamkin DH. Postnatal glucose homeostasis in late-preterm and term infants. *Pediatrics*. 2011;127(3):575-579.
   - *Relevance:* Pathophysiology of neonatal hypoglycemia
   - *Risk Groups:* Identification of at-risk infants
2. Committee on Fetus and Newborn. Postnatal glucose homeostasis in late-preterm and term infants. *Pediatrics*. 2011;127(3):575-579.

- *Relevance:* Screening and management protocols
- *Treatment Thresholds:* When to treat hypoglycemia

Perinatal Asphyxia and HIE

1. Azzopardi DV, Strohm B, Edwards AD, et al. Moderate hypothermia to treat perinatal asphyxial encephalopathy. *N Engl J Med*. 2009;361(14):1349-1358.
   - *Relevance:* Landmark trial for therapeutic hypothermia efficacy
   - *Outcome Data:* 50% reduction in death or severe disability
2. Gluckman PD, Wyatt JS, Azzopardi D, et al. Selective head cooling with mild systemic hypothermia to improve neurodevelopmental outcome following perinatal asphyxia. *Lancet*. 2005;365(9460):663-670.
   - *Relevance:* CoolCap trial demonstrating hypothermia benefit
   - *Clinical Application:* Cooling protocols and patient selection
3. Shankaran S, Laptook AR, Ehrenkranz RA, et al. Whole-body hypothermia for neonates with hypoxic-ischemic encephalopathy. *N Engl J Med*. 2005;353(15):1574-1584.

- *Relevance:* NICHD trial establishing whole-body cooling efficacy
- *Inclusion Criteria:* Patient selection for hypothermia

4. Sarnat HB, Sarnat MS. Neonatal encephalopathy following fetal distress: a clinical and electroencephalographic study. *Arch Neurol*. 1976;33(10):696-705.
   - *Relevance:* Classic staging of neonatal encephalopathy
   - *Clinical Application:* Grading severity and prognosis

Intraventricular Hemorrhage and Brain Injury

1. Volpe JJ. Neonatal encephalopathy: an inadequate term for hypoxic-ischemic encephalopathy. *Ann Neurol*. 2012;72(2):156-166.
   - *Relevance:* Understanding IVH pathophysiology
   - *Prevention Strategies:* Avoiding fluctuations in cerebral perfusion
2. Papile LA, Burstein J, Burstein R, Koffler H. Incidence and evolution of subependymal and intraventricular hemorrhage: a study of infants with birth weights less than 1,500 gm. *J Pediatr*. 1978;92(4):529-534.
   - *Relevance:* Classic IVH grading system
   - *Clinical Application:* Prognostic assessment

3. Ment LR, Bada HS, Barnes P, et al. Practice parameter: neuroimaging of the neonate. *Neurology*. 2002;58(12):1726-1738.

  - *Relevance:* Neuroimaging indications and timing
  - *Clinical Application:* When to image, interpretation

Necrotizing Enterocolitis

1. Neu J, Walker WA. Necrotizing enterocolitis. *N Engl J Med*. 2011;364(3):255-264.

  - *Relevance:* Comprehensive NEC review
  - *Pathophysiology:* Understanding risk factors and prevention

2. Gephart SM, McGrath JM, Effken JA, Halpern MD. Necrotizing enterocolitis risk: state of the science. *Adv Neonatal Care*. 2012;12(2):77-87.

  - *Relevance:* Risk factors and prevention strategies
  - *Clinical Application:* Feeding protocols for at-risk infants

3. Caplan MS, Jilling T. New concepts in necrotizing enterocolitis. *Curr Opin Pediatr*. 2001;13(2):111-115.

  - *Relevance:* Pathophysiology and risk factors
  - *Prevention:* Probiotics, feeding strategies

4. Bell MJ, Ternberg JL, Feigin RD, et al. Neonatal necrotizing enterocolitis: therapeutic decisions based upon clinical staging. *Ann Surg*. 1978;187(1):1-7.

    - *Relevance:* NEC staging system (Bell classification)
    - *Clinical Application:* Severity assessment and management

Retinopathy of Prematurity

1. International Committee for the Classification of Retinopathy of Prematurity. The International Classification of Retinopathy of Prematurity revisited. *Ophthalmology*. 2005;112(12):1684-1695.

    - *Relevance:* ROP classification and severity
    - *Clinical Application:* Screening and referral criteria

2. Cryotherapy for Retinopathy of Prematurity Cooperative Group. Multicenter trial of cryotherapy for retinopathy of prematurity. *Arch Ophthalmol*. 1988;106(4):471-479.

    - *Relevance:* Treatment efficacy and outcomes
    - *Clinical Application:* When to treat ROP

3. Avery ME, Tooley WH. Establishment of the normal range of blood pH, carbon dioxide tension, and base deficit in normal newborn infants. *Pediatrics*. 1966;37(3):383-391.

    - *Relevance:* Oxygen and ROP risk

- *Prevention:* Target SpO_2 ranges

Genetic and Chromosomal Disorders

1. American Academy of Pediatrics, American College of Obstetricians and Gynecologists. *Guidelines for Perinatal Care*, 8th Edition. 2017.
   - *Relevance:* Screening for genetic disorders
   - *Clinical Application:* Newborn screening protocols
2. Watson MS, Mann MY, Lloyd-Puryear MA, et al. Newborn screening: toward equity in screening across the United States. *Genet Med*. 2006;8(12 Suppl):1S-252S.
   - *Relevance:* Comprehensive newborn screening recommendations
   - *Clinical Application:* Screening algorithms by state
3. Korf BR, Rehm HL. New approaches to molecular diagnosis. *JAMA*. 2013;309(14):1511-1521.
   - *Relevance:* Molecular testing and interpretation
   - *Clinical Application:* Genetic counseling and testing

Congenital Anomalies

1. Cantrell JR, Haller JA, Ravitch MM. A syndrome of congenital defects involving the abdominal wall, sternum,

diaphragm, pericardium, and heart. *Surg Gynecol Obstet.* 1958;107(5):602-614.

- *Relevance:* Classic description of omphalocele and related defects
- *Clinical Application:* Recognition and management

2. Bianchi DW, Crombleholme TM, D'Alton ME. *Fetology: Diagnosis and Management of the Fetal Patient*, 2nd Edition. McGraw-Hill; 2010.
    - *Relevance:* Comprehensive fetal anomaly management
    - *Clinical Application:* Prenatal diagnosis and postnatal planning

Multiple Births

1. Lewi L, Jani J, Blickstein I, et al. The outcome of monochorionic diamniotic twin gestations in the era of invasive fetal diagnosis: a prospective cohort study. *Am J Obstet Gynecol.* 2008;199(5):514.e1-514.e8.
    - *Relevance:* Monochorionic twin complications
    - *Clinical Application:* Recognition of TTTS and management
2. Quintero RA, Morales WJ, Allen MH, et al. Staging of twin-twin transfusion syndrome. *J Perinatol.* 1999;19(8 Pt 1):550-555.

- *Relevance:* TTTS staging and severity assessment
- *Clinical Application:* Prenatal and postnatal management

3. Blickstein I, Keith LG. *Multiple Pregnancy: Epidemiology, Gestation & Perinatal Outcome*, 2nd Edition. Taylor & Francis; 2005.
   - *Relevance:* Comprehensive multiple birth management
   - *Clinical Application:* Prenatal and postnatal care

Neonatal Emergencies and Critical Care

1. Hazinski MF, Nolan JP, Billi JE, et al. Part 1: Executive Summary: 2015 International Consensus on Cardiopulmonary Resuscitation and Emergency Cardiovascular Care Science with Treatment Recommendations. *Circulation*. 2015;132(16 Suppl 1):S2-S39.
   - *Relevance:* Emergency management protocols
   - *Clinical Application:* Systematic approach to emergencies
2. Kaufman J, Almulki L, Castillo L, et al. Improved outcomes using a standardized resuscitation protocol and risk stratification. *Pediatrics*. 2011;128(4):e864-e871.
   - *Relevance:* Protocol-driven emergency management
   - *Outcome Data:* Mortality and morbidity reduction

Discharge Planning and Follow-up

1. American Academy of Pediatrics. Hospital Discharge of the High-Risk Neonate. *Pediatrics*. 2008;122(5):1119-1126.

   - *Relevance:* Discharge criteria and planning
   - *Clinical Application:* Preparation for home care

2. Msall ME, Tremont MR. Measuring functional outcomes after prematurity: developmental impact of very low birth weight and extremely low birth weight status on childhood disability. *Ment Retard Dev Disabil Res Rev*. 2002;8(4):234-242.

   - *Relevance:* Long-term developmental outcomes
   - *Clinical Application:* Follow-up and early intervention

3. Part C of the Individuals with Disabilities Education Act (IDEA). *Early Intervention Program for Infants and Toddlers with Disabilities*. U.S. Department of Education; 2004.

   - *Relevance:* Early intervention services and eligibility
   - *Clinical Application:* Referral and access to services

SYSTEMATIC REVIEWS AND META-ANALYSES

1. Soll RF, Morley CJ. Prophylactic versus selective use of surfactant for preventing morbidity and mortality in preterm

infants. *Cochrane Database Syst Rev*. 2001;(2):CD000510.

- *Relevance:* Evidence for surfactant strategies
- *Outcome Data:* Mortality and morbidity reduction

2. Subramaniam P, Henderson-Smart DJ, Davis PG. Prophylactic nasal continuous positive airway pressure for preventing morbidity and mortality in very preterm infants. *Cochrane Database Syst Rev*. 2016;(6):CD001243.
   - *Relevance:* CPAP efficacy in prevention
   - *Clinical Application:* Early CPAP strategies
3. Ohlsson A, Walia R, Shah SS. Intravenous immunoglobulin for suspected or proven neonatal sepsis: an update with focus on Cochrane reviews. *Neonatology*. 2010;98(4):327-336.
   - *Relevance:* Immunoglobulin therapy in sepsis
   - *Evidence Quality:* Systematic review of efficacy
4. Maguire CM, Walkey GA, Cope Y, et al. Neonatal diagnosis of perinatal asphyxia: a systematic review. *Arch Dis Child Fetal Neonatal Ed*. 2007;92(5):F356-F360.
   - *Relevance:* Diagnostic criteria for asphyxia
   - *Clinical Application:* Identification of at-risk infants

KEY JOURNALS FOR NEONATAL EVIDENCE

Primary Journals

- *The Lancet*
- *New England Journal of Medicine*
- *JAMA*
- *Pediatrics*
- *Archives of Disease in Childhood - Fetal and Neonatal Edition*
- *Journal of Perinatology*
- *Neonatology*
- *Clinics in Perinatology*
- *Seminars in Neonatology*
- *American Journal of Perinatology*

Secondary Journals

- *Pediatric Research*
- *Early Human Development*
- *Biology of the Neonate*
- *Neonatal Network*

- *Newborn and Infant Nursing Reviews*

EVIDENCE-BASED RESOURCES FOR CLINICIANS

Cochrane Neonatal Reviews

Website:

- Systematic reviews of neonatal interventions
- High-quality evidence summaries
- Regular updates on emerging evidence

UpToDate - Pediatrics/Neonatology

Website:

- Evidence-based clinical decision support
- Regularly updated recommendations
- Practical management algorithms

PubMed/MEDLINE

Website:

- Comprehensive medical literature database
- Advanced search capabilities

- Free access to abstracts and many full texts

Google Scholar

Website:

- Academic research search engine
- Citation tracking
- Full-text access to many articles

CLINICAL PRACTICE GUIDELINES BY ORGANIZATION

American Academy of Pediatrics (AAP)

- Newborn screening guidelines
- Hyperbilirubinemia management
- Early-onset sepsis risk stratification
- Congenital heart disease screening
- Discharge planning recommendations

American Heart Association (AHA)

- Neonatal resuscitation guidelines

- Cardiopulmonary resuscitation protocols
- Emergency cardiovascular care

American College of Obstetricians and Gynecologists (ACOG)

- Perinatal care guidelines
- Fetal monitoring recommendations
- Delivery room management

Pediatric Endocrine Society

- Hypoglycemia management protocols
- Metabolic disorder screening

American Academy of Ophthalmology

- Retinopathy of prematurity screening
- Treatment recommendations

American Gastroenterological Association

- Feeding protocols for premature infants

- Necrotizing enterocolitis prevention

ACCESSING EVIDENCE: TIPS FOR CLINICIANS

Stay Current

- Subscribe to journal alerts in your specialty
- Attend conferences and continuing education
- Join professional organizations
- Participate in journal clubs
- Follow evidence-based medicine blogs and podcasts

Evaluate Evidence Quality

- Randomized controlled trials > observational studies
- Systematic reviews > single studies
- Large sample sizes > small studies
- Recent evidence > outdated recommendations
- Multiple confirmatory studies > single positive study

Apply Evidence to Practice

1. Understand the evidence quality
2. Consider patient-specific factors
3. Balance evidence with clinical judgment
4. Involve families in decision-making
5. Implement evidence-based protocols
6. Monitor outcomes and adjust as needed

NOTES ON EVIDENCE HIERARCHY

Level 1 Evidence:

- Randomized controlled trials
- Systematic reviews of RCTs
- Meta-analyses

Level 2 Evidence:

- Cohort studies
- Case-control studies
- Quasi-experimental studies

Level 3 Evidence:

- Observational studies
- Case series
- Case reports

Level 4 Evidence:

- Expert opinion
- Consensus documents
- Editorials

Level 5 Evidence:

- Anecdotal reports
- Personal experience

Note: This book integrates evidence from all levels, prioritizing Level 1 and 2 evidence for recommendations, while acknowledging that clinical judgment and experience (Levels 3-4) remain essential in neonatal care.

Chapter Thirty-Two

SUGGESTED READING LIST

FOUNDATIONAL TEXTS FOR NEONATAL CLINICIANS

Essential Reference Books

1. Avery's Diseases of the Newborn (11th Edition)*Gleason CA, Juul SE (Eds.). Elsevier; 2023.*

- Why Read It: Comprehensive reference covering all major neonatal conditions
- Best For: Deep dives into pathophysiology and management of specific disorders
- Clinical Application: Use as reference when managing com-

plex cases

- Reading Strategy: Don't read cover-to-cover; use as resource for specific topics

2. Gomella's Neonatology: Management, Procedures, On-Call Problems, Diseases, and Drugs (9th Edition)*Gomella TL, Cunningham MD, Eyal FG, et al. McGraw-Hill; 2020.*

- Why Read It: Practical, pocket-sized reference for daily clinical use
- Best For: Quick answers to common problems at the bedside
- Clinical Application: Keep accessible for rapid reference during rounds
- Reading Strategy: Skim entire book to understand organization; refer to specific sections as needed

3. Fanaroff and Martin's Neonatal-Perinatal Medicine (11th Edition)*Fanaroff AA, Martin RJ, Walsh MC (Eds.). Elsevier; 2020.*

- Why Read It: Gold standard comprehensive neonatal textbook
- Best For: Understanding evidence-based management of major conditions
- Clinical Application: Reference for complex cases and evidence-based protocols
- Reading Strategy: Read chapters related to your current cases; build knowledge progressively

4. Cloherty and Stark's Manual of Neonatal Care (9th Edition)*Eichenwald EC, Hansen AR, Martin CR, Stark AR (Eds.) . Wolters Kluwer; 2023.*

- Why Read It: Practical manual with algorithms and protocols
- Best For: Understanding standard approaches to common problems
- Clinical Application: Use protocols as basis for your unit's guidelines
- Reading Strategy: Read relevant chapters before starting new rotation

Specialized Texts by Topic

RESPIRATORY DISORDERS

5. Respiratory Physiology: Understanding Gas Exchange and Ventilation *West JB. Wolters Kluwer; 2012.*

- Why Read It: Deep understanding of respiratory physiology principles
- Best For: Understanding why ventilation strategies work
- Clinical Application: Improve understanding of blood gas interpretation
- Reading Time: 2-3 hours focused reading

6. Assisted Ventilation of the Neonate (6th Edition)*Kacmarek RM, Dimas S, Mack CW. Elsevier; 2016.*

- Why Read It: Comprehensive guide to mechanical ventilation in neonates
- Best For: Understanding ventilation modes, strategies, and weaning
- Clinical Application: Improve ventilator management and troubleshooting
- Reading Time: 4-6 hours for complete understanding

CARDIOVASCULAR DISORDERS

7. Neonatal Hemodynamics: Pathophysiology and Clinical Relevance*Evans N. Arch Dis Child Fetal Neonatal Ed. 2010;95(6):F461-F467.*

- Why Read It: Understanding hemodynamic assessment in neonates
- Best For: Learning echocardiography interpretation and PDA management
- Clinical Application: Improve hemodynamic monitoring at bedside
- Reading Time: 1-2 hours

8. Patent Ductus Arteriosus: A Comprehensive Review*Benitz WE. Pediatrics. 2016;137(1):e20153730.*

- Why Read It: Evidence-based PDA management

- Best For: Understanding when and how to treat PDA
- Clinical Application: Improve decision-making about PDA therapy
- Reading Time: 1 hour

INFECTIONS AND SEPSIS

9. Infectious Diseases of the Fetus and Newborn Infant (8th Edition)*Remington JS, Klein JO, Wilson CB, et al. Elsevier; 2015.*

- Why Read It: Comprehensive coverage of neonatal infections
- Best For: Understanding TORCH infections, GBS, and other pathogens
- Clinical Application: Improve diagnosis and management of infections
- Reading Time: 6-8 hours for key chapters

10. Sepsis in the Newborn: Recognition, Diagnosis, and Management*Puopolo KM, Benitz WE, Zaoutis TE. Pediatrics. 2018;142(6):e20182894.*

- Why Read It: Current evidence-based sepsis management
- Best For: Understanding risk stratification and antibiotic stewardship
- Clinical Application: Implement risk-based sepsis protocols
- Reading Time: 1-2 hours

HYPERBILIRUBINEMIA

11. Bilirubin and Jaundice: A Comprehensive Review*Bhutani VK. Pediatrics. 2011;128(4):e943-e957.*

- Why Read It: Understanding bilirubin metabolism and management
- Best For: Mastering phototherapy thresholds and exchange transfusion
- Clinical Application: Improve jaundice management and reduce severe hyperbilirubinemia
- Reading Time: 1-2 hours

PERINATAL ASPHYXIA AND HIE

12. Therapeutic Hypothermia for Neonatal Encephalopathy*Shankaran S, Laptook AR, Ehrenkranz RA, et al. N Engl J Med. 2005;353(15):1574-1584.*

- Why Read It: Landmark trial establishing hypothermia efficacy
- Best For: Understanding patient selection and protocols for cooling
- Clinical Application: Implement therapeutic hypothermia protocols
- Reading Time: 1 hour

13. Neonatal Encephalopathy and Neurologic Outcomes*Volpe JJ. N Engl J Med. 2009;360(6):576-588.*

- Why Read It: Understanding long-term neurologic outcomes after asphyxia
- Best For: Counseling families about prognosis
- Clinical Application: Improve prognostic assessment and family communication
- Reading Time: 1-2 hours

NECROTIZING ENTEROCOLITIS

14. Necrotizing Enterocolitis: Pathophysiology, Prevention, and Management*Neu J, Walker WA. N Engl J Med. 2011;364(3):255-264.*

- Why Read It: Comprehensive NEC review with prevention strategies
- Best For: Understanding NEC pathophysiology and prevention
- Clinical Application: Implement feeding protocols to reduce NEC risk
- Reading Time: 1-2 hours

RETINOPATHY OF PREMATURITY

15. Retinopathy of Prematurity: Screening, Prevention, and Treatment*International Committee for the Classification of Retinopathy of Prematurity. Ophthalmology. 2005;112(12):1684-1695.*

- Why Read It: Understanding ROP classification and treatment
- Best For: Learning screening criteria and referral thresholds
- Clinical Application: Ensure appropriate ROP screening and follow-up
- Reading Time: 1 hour

GENETIC DISORDERS

16. Genetics in Clinical Practice: A Practical Approach*Korf BR, Rehm HL. JAMA. 2013;309(14):1511-1521.*

- Why Read It: Understanding genetic testing and interpretation
- Best For: Improving genetic counseling and testing knowledge
- Clinical Application: Better communication with families about genetic disorders
- Reading Time: 1-2 hours

CONGENITAL ANOMALIES

17. Fetology: Diagnosis and Management of the Fetal Patient (3rd Edition)*Bianchi DW, Crombleholme TM, D'Alton ME. McGraw-Hill; 2010.*

- Why Read It: Comprehensive fetal anomaly management
- Best For: Understanding prenatal diagnosis and postnatal planning
- Clinical Application: Improve coordination with obstetrics and planning for delivery
- Reading Time: 4-6 hours for relevant chapters

MULTIPLE BIRTHS

18. Twin-Twin Transfusion Syndrome: Current Understanding and Management*Lewi L, Jani J, Blickstein I, et al. Am J Obstet Gynecol. 2008;199(5):514.e1-514.e8.*

- Why Read It: Understanding TTTS pathophysiology and complications
- Best For: Recognizing and managing TTTS complications at delivery
- Clinical Application: Improve outcomes in monochorionic twin pregnancies
- Reading Time: 1-2 hours

NEONATAL RESUSCITATION

19. Textbook of Neonatal Resuscitation (NRP), 8th Edition*American Academy of Pediatrics & American Heart Association. 2021.*

- Why Read It: Gold standard for delivery room management
- Best For: Mastering resuscitation algorithms and techniques
- Clinical Application: Prepare for NRP certification and re-certification
- Reading Time: 6-8 hours; ongoing review

20. Delivery Room Resuscitation: Beyond the Guidelines*Wyckoff MH. Clin Perinatol. 2010;37(1):175-189.*

- Why Read It: Practical approach to resuscitation beyond algorithms
- Best For: Understanding when to deviate from standard protocols
- Clinical Application: Improve clinical decision-making in complex resuscitations
- Reading Time: 1-2 hours

JOURNAL ARTICLES: LANDMARK STUDIES TO READ

Must-Read Landmark Trials

1. SUPPORT Trial*Finer NN, Carlo WA, Walsh MC, et al. Early CPAP versus surfactant for extremely preterm infants. N Engl J Med. 2010;362(21):1970-1979.*

- Key Finding: CPAP-first strategy reduces surfactant use without increasing mortality
- Clinical Impact: Supports less invasive respiratory support
- Reading Time: 30 minutes

2. Cooling for Asphyxia Trial (CoolCap)*Gluckman PD, Wyatt JS, Azzopardi D, et al. Selective head cooling with mild systemic hypothermia to improve neurodevelopmental outcome following perinatal asphyxia. Lancet. 2005;365(9460):663-670.*

- Key Finding: Head cooling reduces death or severe disability by 50%
- Clinical Impact: Establishes therapeutic hypothermia as standard care
- Reading Time: 30 minutes

3. NICHD Neonatal Research Network Hypothermia Study*Shankaran S, Laptook AR, Ehrenkranz RA, et al. Whole-body hypothermia for neonates with hypoxic-ischemic encephalopathy. N Engl J Med. 2005;353(15):1574-1584.*

- Key Finding: Whole-body cooling reduces death or severe disability
- Clinical Impact: Confirms efficacy of therapeutic hypothermia
- Reading Time: 30 minutes

4. Cryotherapy for Retinopathy of Prematurity (CRYO-ROP)*Cryotherapy for Retinopathy of Prematurity Cooperative Group. Multicenter trial of cryotherapy for retinopathy of prematurity. Arch Ophthalmol. 1988;106(4):471-479.*

- Key Finding: Cryotherapy reduces unfavorable outcomes in ROP
- Clinical Impact: Establishes ROP treatment efficacy
- Reading Time: 30 minutes

5. Prevention of Respiratory Distress Syndrome Trial*Soll RF, Morley CJ. Prophylactic versus selective use of surfactant for preventing morbidity and mortality in preterm infants. Cochrane Database Syst Rev. 2001;(2):CD000510.*

- Key Finding: Prophylactic surfactant reduces mortality and pneumothorax
- Clinical Impact: Supports early surfactant use in RDS
- Reading Time: 30 minutes

ONLINE RESOURCES AND TOOLS

Essential Websites

1. UpToDate ()
- Content: Evidence-based clinical decision support
- Best For: Quick answers to clinical questions

- Frequency: Access regularly for current recommendations
- Cost: Subscription (often available through institution)

2. PubMed Central ()
   - Content: Free full-text access to medical literature
   - Best For: Accessing research articles
   - Frequency: Use for literature searches
   - Cost: Free

3. Cochrane Neonatal Reviews ()
   - Content: Systematic reviews of neonatal interventions
   - Best For: Finding best available evidence
   - Frequency: Check for relevant topics
   - Cost: Free

4. AAP Pediatrics Official Journal ()
   - Content: Official journal of American Academy of Pediatrics
   - Best For: Latest evidence-based recommendations
   - Frequency: Subscribe to email alerts
   - Cost: Free access to many articles

5. New England Journal of Medicine ()
   - Content: High-impact medical research
   - Best For: Landmark studies and clinical reviews

- Frequency: Check weekly for neonatal content
- Cost: Subscription or institutional access

READING BY CAREER STAGE

For Medical Students and Junior Residents

Essential Reading (Start Here):

- Gomella's Neonatology (skim entire book)
- NRP Textbook (read thoroughly)
- Cloherty and Stark's Manual (read relevant chapters)
- AAP guidelines on common conditions

Recommended Reading (Build Knowledge):

- Avery's Diseases of the Newborn (read specific chapters)
- Journal articles on conditions you encounter
- Landmark trials mentioned above

Advanced Reading (Deepen Expertise):

- Fanaroff and Martin's Neonatology (read thoroughly)
- Specialty texts (respiratory, cardiovascular, etc.)
- Recent literature on your area of interest

Time Commitment: 30-60 minutes daily of focused reading

For Senior Residents and Fellows

Essential Reading:

- Fanaroff and Martin's Neonatology (read thoroughly)
- Specialty texts in your area of focus
- Recent literature (current year publications)
- Landmark trials and systematic reviews

Recommended Reading:

- UpToDate for current recommendations
- Journal clubs and case conferences
- Mentorship from experienced clinicians

Advanced Reading:

- Research methodology and statistics
- Health services and outcomes research
- Leadership and management literature

Time Commitment: 60-90 minutes daily of focused reading

For Practicing Clinicians

Essential Reading (Maintenance):

- Journal alerts in specialty areas
- UpToDate updates on relevant topics

- Continuing education courses
- Unit-specific protocols and guidelines

Recommended Reading (Professional Development):

- Landmark trials and systematic reviews
- New guidelines from professional organizations
- Literature on your specific patient population
- Leadership and quality improvement literature

Advanced Reading (Expertise Development):

- Specialty texts in your area of focus
- Research literature on your area of interest
- Teaching and mentorship resources

Time Commitment: 20-30 minutes daily of focused reading

JOURNAL CLUBS AND LEARNING GROUPS

How to Start a Journal Club

1. Select Articles:

- Choose 1-2 recent, high-quality articles
- Select articles relevant to your patient population
- Mix landmark trials with current research

2. Distribute in Advance:
   - Send articles 1 week before meeting
   - Include brief summary of key points
   - Suggest discussion questions
3. Facilitate Discussion:
   - Review study design and methods
   - Discuss key findings and implications
   - Consider applicability to your practice
   - Identify evidence gaps
4. Document and Share:
   - Record key points and decisions
   - Share with team members who couldn't attend
   - Implement changes based on evidence

Topics for Journal Club

- Respiratory support strategies
- Sepsis management and antibiotic stewardship
- Feeding protocols and NEC prevention
- Jaundice management
- Neurologic outcomes and follow-up

- Quality improvement initiatives
- New diagnostic or therapeutic technologies

PROFESSIONAL ORGANIZATIONS AND RESOURCES

American Academy of Pediatrics (AAP)

- Website: www.aap.org
- Resources: Guidelines, policy statements, educational materials
- Membership Benefits: Journal access, continuing education, networking

American Heart Association (AHA)

- Website: www.heart.org
- Resources: Resuscitation guidelines, training programs
- NRP Certification: Required for neonatal clinicians

Pediatric Academic Societies (PAS)

- Website: www.pas-meeting.org

- Resources: Annual conference, research abstracts
- Professional Development: Networking and education

Society for Maternal-Fetal Medicine (SMFM)

- Website: www.smfm.org
- Resources: Perinatal guidelines, continuing education
- Collaboration: Coordination between obstetrics and neonatology

American College of Obstetricians and Gynecologists (ACOG)

- Website: www.acog.org
- Resources: Perinatal care guidelines, delivery room management
- Collaboration: Joint guidelines with pediatrics

READING STRATEGIES FOR BUSY CLINICIANS

Efficient Reading Techniques

1. Skim First, Read Second:
    - Read abstract and conclusion first
    - Skim methods and results
    - Read in detail only if relevant to your practice
2. Active Reading:
    - Highlight key points
    - Take notes in margins
    - Write summary after reading
    - Discuss with colleagues
3. Spaced Reading:
    - Read one article per week
    - Review notes after 1 month
    - Implement changes gradually
    - Revisit topics quarterly
4. Focused Reading:
    - Read only articles relevant to your current cases
    - Search literature for specific questions
    - Follow authors doing research in your area
    - Subscribe to journal alerts
5. Group Learning:
    - Participate in journal clubs

- Attend conferences and lectures
- Join study groups
- Teach others (reinforces learning)

STAYING CURRENT: CONTINUOUS LEARNING RESOURCES

Podcasts and Audio Resources

1. Neonatology Today Podcast
    - Content: Clinical cases and expert interviews
    - Frequency: Weekly
    - Length: 15-30 minutes
    - Best For: Learning during commute or exercise
2. Journal Club Podcasts
    - Content: Discussion of recent literature
    - Frequency: Weekly to monthly
    - Length: 30-45 minutes
    - Best For: Staying current with evidence
3. Medical Education Podcasts
    - Content: Teaching on various topics

- Frequency: Varies
- Length: 20-60 minutes
- Best For: Deep dives into specific topics

Webinars and Online Courses

1. American Academy of Pediatrics Online Learning
    - Content: Accredited continuing education
    - Cost: Varies by course
    - Time: Self-paced
2. University-Based Neonatology Courses
    - Content: Comprehensive neonatology education
    - Cost: Varies
    - Time: Weeks to months
3. Specialty Society Webinars
    - Content: Expert-led education on specific topics
    - Cost: Free to members, fee for non-members
    - Time: 1-2 hours

CREATING YOUR PERSONAL LEARNING PLAN

Assessment

1. Identify Knowledge Gaps:
    - Reflect on challenging cases
    - Ask colleagues for feedback
    - Take practice exams
    - Review your error patterns
2. Set Learning Goals:
    - Specific: "Improve management of polycythemia in twins"
    - Measurable: "Read 3 articles on TTTS by month's end"
    - Achievable: "Realistic given my schedule"
    - Relevant: "Applies to my patient population"
    - Time-bound: "Complete by specific date"

Implementation

1. Schedule Reading Time:
    - Block 30 minutes daily for reading
    - Choose consistent time (morning, lunch, evening)
    - Minimize distractions
    - Track your reading

2. Select Resources:
    - Choose high-quality sources
    - Mix textbooks, journals, and online resources
    - Align with your learning goals
    - Build knowledge progressively
3. Apply Learning:
    - Implement new knowledge in practice
    - Discuss with colleagues
    - Present at journal club
    - Teach others

Evaluation

1. Assess Progress:
    - Improved clinical decision-making
    - Better patient outcomes
    - Increased confidence
    - Positive feedback from colleagues
2. Adjust Plan:
    - Modify based on progress
    - Add new topics as needed

- Maintain momentum
- Celebrate accomplishments

FINAL THOUGHTS ON READING AND LEARNING

The field of neonatology is constantly evolving. New evidence emerges regularly, and guidelines are updated frequently. Commitment to continuous learning—through reading, discussion, and reflection—is essential for providing the best care to your patients.

Remember:

- Quality over quantity: Reading deeply and thoughtfully is more valuable than skimming broadly
- Apply learning: Knowledge only matters when implemented in practice
- Teach others: Teaching reinforces your own learning
- Stay humble: Medicine is complex; there's always more to learn
- Balance evidence and experience: Use evidence as guide, but trust clinical judgment

Your commitment to learning will directly benefit your patients and your team.

Chapter Thirty-Three

QUICK REFERENCE: KEY MEDICATIONS AND DOSAGES

RESUSCITATION MEDICATIONS

EPINEPHRINE (Adrenaline)

- IV/IO Dose: 0.01-0.03 mg/kg (0.1-0.3 mL/kg of 1:10,000 solution)
- Endotracheal Dose: 0.1 mg/kg (0.1 mL/kg of 1:1,000 solution)

- Frequency: Every 3-5 minutes during resuscitation
- Route: IV preferred (umbilical vein), IO if no IV access
- Indication: Asystole, bradycardia <60 despite ventilation
- Key Point: Higher dose (0.1 mg/kg) if IO route used
- Concentration: Use 1:10,000 for IV; 1:1,000 for ET

SODIUM BICARBONATE

- Dose: 1 mEq/kg IV
- Concentration: 4.2% solution (0.5 mEq/mL)
- Frequency: Once during resuscitation if indicated
- Route: IV only (umbilical vein preferred)
- Indication: Severe metabolic acidosis (pH <7.0)
- Key Point: Give slowly; can cause hypernatremia and hyperosmolarity
- Caution: Incompatible with many drugs; flush line between medications

DEXTROSE (Glucose)

- Dose: 250-500 mg/kg IV
- Concentration: 10% dextrose = 100 mg/mL

- Volume: 2.5-5 mL/kg of 10% dextrose
- Route: IV only (central line preferred for >12.5% dextrose)
- Indication: Hypoglycemia during resuscitation
- Key Point: Recheck glucose 15 minutes after administration
- Caution: Hyperglycemia increases cerebral injury risk; avoid excessive dosing

CALCIUM GLUCONATE (Hyperkalemia/Hypocalcemia)

- Dose: 100-200 mg/kg IV
- Concentration: 10% solution = 100 mg/mL
- Volume: 1-2 mL/kg
- Route: IV only (central line preferred)
- Indication: Hyperkalemia (peaked T waves on ECG), hypocalcemia
- Key Point: Stabilizes cardiac membrane in hyperkalemia; doesn't lower K^+
- Caution: Can cause tissue necrosis if extravasated; give slowly

CARDIOVASCULAR MEDICATIONS

DOPAMINE (Inotrope/Vasopressor)

- Dose: 5-20 mcg/kg/min IV infusion
- Concentration: Mix 6 mg/mL in normal saline
- Route: Central or peripheral IV
- Indication: Hypotension, poor perfusion, low cardiac output

Dosing Effects:

- 2-5 mcg/kg/min: Renal vasodilation
- 5-10 mcg/kg/min: Inotropic effect
- 10 mcg/kg/min: Vasopressor effect
- Key Point: Titrate to effect; monitor BP, HR, urine output
- Caution: Extravasation causes tissue necrosis; use central line if possible

DOBUTAMINE (Inotrope)

- Dose: 5-20 mcg/kg/min IV infusion
- Concentration: Mix 12.5 mg/mL in normal saline
- Route: Central or peripheral IV
- Indication: Cardiogenic shock, poor cardiac contractility

- Key Point: Increases contractility without increasing afterload
- Caution: May cause hypotension; often combined with dopamine

EPINEPHRINE (Low-Dose Infusion)

- Dose: 0.1-1 mcg/kg/min IV infusion
- Concentration: Mix 1 mg/mL in normal saline
- Route: Central line preferred
- Indication: Severe shock, refractory hypotension
- Key Point: Use after dopamine/dobutamine failure
- Caution: Causes vasoconstriction; monitor perfusion closely

MILRINONE (Inodilator)

- Dose: 0.25-0.75 mcg/kg/min IV infusion
- Concentration: Mix 0.2 mg/mL in normal saline
- Route: Central or peripheral IV
- Indication: Heart failure, pulmonary hypertension
- Key Point: Increases contractility and causes vasodilation

- Caution: Can cause systemic hypotension; monitor BP

HYDRALAZINE (Vasodilator)

- Dose: 0.15-0.3 mg/kg IV/IM every 4-6 hours
- Route: IV or IM
- Indication: Hypertension, afterload reduction
- Key Point: Onset 10-30 minutes
- Caution: Can cause reflex tachycardia and hypotension

SODIUM NITROPRUSSIDE (Potent Vasodilator)

- Dose: 0.5-10 mcg/kg/min IV infusion
- Route: Central line only (light-sensitive)
- Indication: Severe hypertension, acute heart failure
- Key Point: Rapid onset and offset
- Caution: Risk of cyanide toxicity with prolonged use; limit to 4 hours

INDOMETHACIN (PDA Closure)

- Dose: 0.1 mg/kg IV every 12-24 hours × 3 doses

- Route: IV only
- Indication: Patent ductus arteriosus (hemodynamically significant)
- Key Point: Contraindicated if active infection, bleeding, NEC, renal failure
- Caution: Monitor renal function, platelet count, urine output

IBUPROFEN (PDA Closure)

- Loading Dose: 10 mg/kg IV
- Maintenance: 5 mg/kg IV at 24 and 48 hours
- Route: IV only
- Indication: Patent ductus arteriosus
- Key Point: Similar efficacy to indomethacin with fewer renal effects
- Caution: Avoid if thrombocytopenia or NEC risk

PROSTAGLANDIN E1 (Ductal Patency)

- Dose: 0.05-0.1 mcg/kg/min IV infusion
- Route: Central line preferred
- Indication: Ductal-dependent lesions (TGA, severe coarctation)

- Key Point: Keep ductus arteriosus open until definitive surgery
- Caution: Apnea common; have intubation ready

RESPIRATORY MEDICATIONS

SURFACTANT (Exosurf, Survanta, Curosurf)

- Dose: 100-200 mg/kg (varies by product)
- Volume: 4-6 mL/kg
- Route: Endotracheal tube only
- Indication: Respiratory distress syndrome, meconium aspiration
- Key Point: Give within first 15 minutes of life if possible
- Dosing Schedule: May repeat at 6-12 hours if needed
- Administration: Stop ventilation, instill via ET tube, resume ventilation

ALBUTEROL (Beta-2 Agonist)

- Nebulized Dose: 0.1-0.15 mg/kg per dose (max 2.5 mg)
- Frequency: Every 4-6 hours as needed

- Route: Nebulized inhalation
- Indication: Bronchospasm, chronic lung disease
- Key Point: Onset 5-15 minutes
- Caution: Can cause tachycardia, tremor, hyperglycemia

IPRATROPIUM (Anticholinergic)

- Dose: 0.25 mg per dose
- Frequency: Every 6-8 hours
- Route: Nebulized inhalation (often combined with albuterol)
- Indication: Chronic lung disease, bronchospasm
- Key Point: Often used with albuterol for synergistic effect
- Caution: Minimal systemic absorption in neonates

BUDESONIDE (Inhaled Corticosteroid)

- Dose: 0.25-0.5 mg twice daily
- Route: Nebulized inhalation
- Indication: Chronic lung disease, prevention of BPD
- Key Point: Local effect; minimal systemic absorption

- Caution: Long-term use requires monitoring for growth

DEXAMETHASONE (Systemic Corticosteroid)

- Dose: 0.5 mg/kg/day divided into 2-4 doses
- Frequency: Taper over 7-10 days
- Route: IV or oral
- Indication: Severe BPD, airway edema
- Key Point: Use cautiously; risk of hyperglycemia, infection, GI bleeding
- Caution: Long-term use associated with neurodevelopmental effects

METHYLXANTHINES (Apnea Prevention)

- Caffeine Base: 20 mg/kg loading dose, then 5-10 mg/kg/day maintenance
- Route: IV or oral
- Indication: Apnea of prematurity
- Key Point: Narrow therapeutic window; monitor levels
- Caution: Can cause tachycardia, jitteriness, feeding intolerance

ANTIBIOTICS (First-Line)

AMPICILLIN (Early-Onset Sepsis)

- Dose: 50 mg/kg IV/IM every 12 hours (≤7 days old)
- Dose: 50 mg/kg IV/IM every 8 hours (>7 days old)
- Route: IV or IM
- Indication: GBS, gram-positive coverage in EOS
- Key Point: Combine with gentamicin for broad coverage
- Caution: Rash possible; discontinue if occurs

GENTAMICIN (Early-Onset Sepsis)

- Dose: 7.5 mg/kg IV/IM once daily (preferred) or 2.5 mg/kg every 8 hours
- Route: IV or IM
- Indication: Gram-negative coverage in EOS
- Key Point: Monitor renal function and drug levels
- Caution: Ototoxic and nephrotoxic; adjust for renal function

VANCOMYCIN (Resistant Organisms)

- Dose: 15-20 mg/kg IV every 8-12 hours
- Route: IV only
- Indication: MRSA, resistant gram-positive organisms
- Key Point: Trough level 10-15 mcg/mL; peak 25-40 mcg/mL
- Caution: Monitor renal function; red man syndrome possible

CEFOTAXIME (Meningitis/Sepsis)

- Dose: 50 mg/kg IV/IM every 8-12 hours
- Route: IV or IM
- Indication: Gram-negative coverage, meningitis
- Key Point: Good CNS penetration
- Caution: Cross-reactivity with penicillin allergy

ACYCLOVIR (HSV/VZV)

- Dose: 20 mg/kg IV every 8 hours
- Route: IV only
- Indication: Herpes simplex virus, varicella-zoster

- Key Point: Start empirically if HSV suspected
- Caution: Nephrotoxic; maintain hydration

FLUCONAZOLE (Candida)

- Dose: 6-12 mg/kg IV/oral once daily
- Route: IV or oral
- Indication: Candida sepsis, prophylaxis in high-risk infants
- Key Point: Good CNS penetration
- Caution: Monitor liver function

ANTICONVULSANTS

PHENOBARBITAL (First-Line)

- Loading Dose: 20 mg/kg IV/IM
- Maintenance: 5 mg/kg/day divided into 1-2 doses
- Route: IV, IM, or oral
- Indication: Neonatal seizures, HIE prophylaxis
- Key Point: Slow onset (20-30 minutes)
- Caution: Respiratory depression; monitor closely

LEVETIRACETAM (Alternative)

- Loading Dose: 20-50 mg/kg IV
- Maintenance: 10-20 mg/kg twice daily
- Route: IV or oral
- Indication: Neonatal seizures, alternative to phenobarbital
- Key Point: Faster onset than phenobarbital
- Caution: Behavioral changes possible; monitor mood

LORAZEPAM (Acute Seizures)

- Dose: 0.05-0.1 mg/kg IV
- Frequency: Can repeat every 15 minutes if needed
- Route: IV only
- Indication: Status epilepticus, acute seizure cluster
- Key Point: Rapid onset (1-3 minutes)
- Caution: Respiratory depression; have intubation ready

MIDAZOLAM (Sedation/Seizures)

- Loading Dose: 0.15 mg/kg IV

- Infusion: 0.5-2 mcg/kg/min
- Route: IV
- Indication: Sedation, seizure management
- Key Point: Rapid onset; reversible with flumazenil
- Caution: Respiratory depression; monitor closely

GASTROINTESTINAL MEDICATIONS

OMEPRAZOLE (Gastric Acid Suppression)

- Dose: 1-2 mg/kg once daily
- Route: Oral (capsule opened, mixed with breast milk)
- Indication: GERD, gastric ulcer prevention
- Key Point: Give 30 minutes before feeds
- Caution: Long-term use may reduce calcium absorption

RANITIDINE (H2 Blocker)

- Dose: 2 mg/kg IV/oral every 6-8 hours
- Route: IV or oral
- Indication: GERD, gastric ulcer prevention

- Key Point: Less potent than omeprazole
- Caution: Monitor for thrombocytopenia

METOCLOPRAMIDE (Prokinetic)

- Dose: 0.1-0.2 mg/kg IV/oral every 6-8 hours
- Route: IV or oral
- Indication: Gastroesophageal reflux, feeding intolerance
- Key Point: Enhances gastric motility
- Caution: Risk of tardive dyskinesia with long-term use

DOMPERIDONE (Prokinetic)

- Dose: 0.3-0.4 mg/kg oral three times daily
- Route: Oral only
- Indication: Gastroesophageal reflux, feeding intolerance
- Key Point: Peripheral dopamine antagonist
- Caution: Limited availability in some countries

PROBIOTICS (Gut Health)

- Dose: Varies by product (typically 10^8-10^9 CFU daily)

- Route: Oral
- Indication: NEC prevention (controversial), microbiome support
- Key Point: Evidence mixed; use varies by institution
- Caution: Avoid in immunocompromised infants

METABOLIC/ELECTROLYTE MEDICATIONS

CALCIUM GLUCONATE (Hypocalcemia)

- Dose: 100-200 mg/kg IV
- Concentration: 10% solution (100 mg/mL)
- Volume: 1-2 mL/kg
- Route: IV (central line preferred)
- Indication: Hypocalcemia, tetany, seizures from low calcium
- Key Point: Give slowly; monitor heart rate
- Caution: Tissue necrosis if extravasated

POTASSIUM CHLORIDE (Hypokalemia)

- Dose: 0.5-1 mEq/kg/day IV or oral

- Concentration: Dilute in maintenance fluids
- Route: IV (diluted) or oral
- Indication: Hypokalemia, diuretic-induced losses
- Key Point: Never give as IV bolus; risk of cardiac arrhythmia
- Caution: Monitor K^+ levels; recheck after 4-6 hours

SODIUM CHLORIDE (Hyponatremia Correction)

- Dose: Calculate based on deficit
- Formula: Na^+ deficit = 0.6 × BW(kg) × (desired Na – actual Na)
- Route: IV
- Indication: Severe symptomatic hyponatremia
- Key Point: Correct slowly (8-10 mEq/L per 24 hours) to avoid seizures
- Caution: Overcorrection causes hypernatremia and brain injury

MAGNESIUM SULFATE (Hypomagnesemia)

- Dose: 25-50 mg/kg IV/IM
- Concentration: 50% solution

- Route: IV or IM
- Indication: Hypomagnesemia, seizures, cardiac arrhythmias
- Key Point: Often used with calcium for hypocalcemia
- Caution: Respiratory depression possible; monitor closely

INSULIN (Hyperglycemia)

- Dose: 0.05-0.1 unit/kg/hour IV infusion
- Route: IV infusion only
- Indication: Hyperglycemia (glucose >180-200 mg/dL)
- Key Point: Use in combination with dextrose adjustment
- Caution: Risk of hypoglycemia; monitor glucose frequently

DIURETICS

FUROSEMIDE (Loop Diuretic)

- Dose: 1-2 mg/kg IV/oral every 6-24 hours
- Route: IV or oral
- Indication: Pulmonary edema, heart failure, fluid overload
- Key Point: Rapid onset; potent effect

- Caution: Monitor electrolytes (K^+, Na^+, Cl^-), renal function

HYDROCHLOROTHIAZIDE (Thiazide Diuretic)

- Dose: 1-2 mg/kg/day oral divided into 2 doses
- Route: Oral only
- Indication: Chronic diuretic therapy, BPD with fluid retention
- Key Point: Longer duration than furosemide
- Caution: Monitor electrolytes; hypokalemia common

SPIRONOLACTONE (Potassium-Sparing Diuretic)

- Dose: 1-3 mg/kg/day oral divided into 1-2 doses
- Route: Oral only
- Indication: Combined with loop diuretics to prevent hypokalemia
- Key Point: Slow onset (3-5 days)
- Caution: Monitor K^+ levels; risk of hyperkalemia

VITAMINS AND SUPPLEMENTS

VITAMIN A

- Dose: 5,000 IU IM three times weekly
- Route: IM only
- Indication: BPD prevention in extremely preterm infants
- Key Point: Start early; continue for 28 days
- Caution: High doses toxic; monitor liver function

VITAMIN D

- Dose: 400-1,000 IU daily oral
- Route: Oral
- Indication: Bone health, calcium absorption
- Key Point: Important for growth and development
- Caution: Excessive supplementation causes hypercalcemia

VITAMIN E

- Dose: 15-25 IU/kg/day oral
- Route: Oral
- Indication: Antioxidant, ROP prevention (controversial)
- Key Point: Often included in multivitamins

- Caution: Evidence for efficacy limited

IRON SUPPLEMENTATION

- Dose: 2-4 mg/kg/day elemental iron oral
- Route: Oral
- Indication: Anemia prevention, especially in premature infants
- Key Point: Start at 2-4 weeks of age
- Caution: Can cause GI upset, dark stools; monitor hemoglobin

FOLIC ACID

- Dose: 0.05 mg/kg/day oral (max 1 mg/day)
- Route: Oral
- Indication: Hemolytic anemia, anticonvulsant use
- Key Point: Often combined with vitamin B_{12}
- Caution: Deficiency causes megaloblastic anemia

IMPORTANT REMINDERS

✓ Always verify: Drug name, dose, route, patient weight

✓ Calculate carefully: Use weight-based dosing; double-check math

✓ Check compatibility: Some drugs incompatible; flush lines between medications

✓ Monitor closely: Watch for adverse effects and therapeutic response

✓ Document: Record medication, dose, time, route, response

✓ Communicate: Ensure team knows what medications baby is receiving

✓ Update regularly: Medications change as baby grows and improves

✓ Ask questions: If unsure, consult pharmacist or senior clinician

This is a quick reference guide. Always consult your institution's protocols, drug formulary, and pharmacist for specific questions.

Chapter Thirty-Four

CRITICAL CLINICAL POINTS TO REMEMBER

GENERAL PRINCIPLES

1. Anticipation Prevents Panic

Know which deliveries are high-risk BEFORE the baby arrives. Review maternal history, imaging, and delivery circumstances. A prepared team responds faster and makes better decisions than a surprised one.

2. The Golden Hour Matters Most

The first 60 minutes of life determine outcomes more than any other single period. Optimize this window—delayed interventions compound problems exponentially.

3. Normal Newborns Don't Need Intervention

Resist the urge to "do something." Healthy term infants need warmth, drying, stimulation, and observation. Unnecessary interventions introduce iatrogenic complications.

4. Assume the Worst Until Proven Otherwise

A baby who "looks okay" may be deteriorating. Serial assessments trump single reassuring observations. Trust your gut—if something feels wrong, it probably is.

5. Document Everything in Real-Time

Memory fails under stress. Write down times, interventions, responses, and decision points immediately. This protects the baby, your team, and your documentation.

RESUSCITATION & EMERGENCY

6. Meconium-Stained Amniotic Fluid ≠ Automatic Suctioning

Routine endotracheal suctioning for meconium-stained fluid does NOT improve outcomes and delays positive pressure ventilation (PPV). Only suction if meconium is thick and the baby is NOT vigorous AND needs PPV. Most meconium-stained babies do fine with routine care.

7. Start PPV by 1 Minute of Life

Delayed PPV is the #1 preventable cause of poor neonatal outcomes. Don't wait for the perfect setup—begin with what you have. A room-air breath is better than no breath.

8. Chest Compressions = Last Resort, Not First Response

Compressions are only indicated if HR <60 bpm AFTER 15 seconds of adequate PPV. Most babies respond to PPV alone. Premature compressions waste time and cause injury.

9. The 3-Step Mantra: Dry, Stimulate, Reassess

Before jumping to PPV, ensure the baby is dried, positioned correctly, and stimulated. Many babies respond to these simple steps alone. Reassess HR and respiratory effort after each intervention.

10. Apgar Score ≠ Resuscitation Guide

Apgar scores are descriptive, not prescriptive. They do NOT tell you when to start or stop resuscitation. Use clinical signs (HR, respiratory effort, tone) to guide interventions, not Apgar numbers.

11. Know When to Stop

If no HR is detected after 10 minutes of adequate resuscitation in a term infant, stopping is reasonable. Continuing futile resuscitation causes family trauma and resource waste. Document the decision and timeline clearly.

RESPIRATORY CARE

12. Respiratory Distress Doesn't Always Mean Lung Disease

Tachypnea, grunting, and retractions can signal sepsis, metabolic acidosis, pneumothorax, or cardiac disease. Don't reflexively intubate—diagnose first. A chest X-ray and blood gas guide management.

13. Early CPAP Prevents Intubation

Starting CPAP early in respiratory distress syndrome (RDS) reduces intubation rates by 50%. Even preterm infants benefit. CPAP is your friend—use it liberally before reaching for the tube.

14. Surfactant Timing is Critical

Give surfactant early (within 2 hours of birth) in preterm infants with RDS. Delayed surfactant increases barotrauma and chronic lung disease risk. Don't wait for "confirmation" of RDS—clinical suspicion is enough.

15. Pneumothorax Can Kill Silently

A baby can deteriorate suddenly from tension pneumothorax with minimal warning signs. High suspicion in any baby with sudden decompensation, especially on mechanical ventilation. Needle aspiration (2nd intercostal space, midclavicular line) can be life-saving.

16. Extubation Readiness ≠ Passing a Trial

Babies can pass spontaneous breathing trials but still fail extubation. Consider overall clinical status, metabolic stability, and feeding tolerance. Premature extubation leads to reintubation, which worsens outcomes.

17. Ventilator Settings Cause Harm

High tidal volumes (>6 mL/kg) and high pressures cause volutrauma and barotrauma. Use gentle ventilation: target Vt 4-6 mL/kg, permissive hypercapnia ($PaCO_2$ 45-55 mmHg), and low FiO_2. Lung protection prevents chronic lung disease.

CARDIOVASCULAR

18. Hypotension Doesn't Always Need Treatment

Many preterm infants have "low" blood pressure but excellent perfusion. Don't treat numbers—treat the baby. Signs of poor perfusion (delayed cap refill, poor urine output, metabolic acidosis) guide therapy, not BP alone.

19. Patent Ductus Arteriosus (PDA) is Often Benign

A PDA murmur is common and often closes spontaneously. Treat only if hemodynamically significant (pulmonary edema, steal physiology, worsening respiratory status). Unnecessary treatment causes renal dysfunction and NEC.

20. Inotropes Before Fluids in Septic Shock

In septic shock, aggressive fluid resuscitation can worsen outcomes. Give 10-15 mL/kg crystalloid, then reassess. If still hypotensive, start inotropes (dopamine or epinephrine) rather than pushing more fluid. Excessive fluids cause pulmonary edema and worsen mortality.

21. Bradycardia = Hypoxia Until Proven Otherwise

A slow heart rate in a baby is a sign of severe hypoxia, not a primary cardiac problem. Immediately improve oxygenation and ventilation. Don't start pacing—fix the lungs first.

22. Pulse Oximetry Targets Matter

For preterm infants <28 weeks, target SpO_2 90-95%. Higher targets increase ROP risk; lower targets increase mortality and NEC. Use postnatal age-based targets (lower in first week, higher by week 2-3).

INFECTIONS & SEPSIS

23. Maternal Fever ≠ Neonatal Infection

Maternal chorioamnionitis increases neonatal infection risk but doesn't guarantee it. Asymptomatic, well-appearing babies with maternal fever may not need antibiotics. Use clinical judgment and risk stratification, not automatic treatment.

24. Early Sepsis Mimics RDS

Bacterial sepsis presents with tachypnea, grunting, and retractions—identical to RDS. Sepsis often coexists with RDS. Always get blood cultures and consider antibiotics in at-risk infants, even if you give surfactant.

25. Antibiotics Should Be Stopped by 48 Hours if Cultures Negative

Continuing antibiotics in culture-negative, asymptomatic babies increases antibiotic resistance and disrupts microbiome. If the baby is well and cultures are negative at 48 hours, stop antibiotics. Unnecessary antibiotics cause harm.

26. Group B Streptococcus (GBS) Prevention Matters

Mothers with GBS colonization or risk factors should receive intrapartum antibiotics. Neonates born to inadequately treated mothers need close observation and empiric antibiotics if symptomatic. Prevention is far easier than treatment.

27. Fungal Sepsis is Sneaky

Candida sepsis often presents late (>5 days) with subtle signs: feeding intolerance, hyperglycemia, thrombocytopenia. High suspicion in preterm infants on prolonged antibiotics or with central lines. Start antifungal therapy early if suspected—mortality is high if delayed.

METABOLIC & FEEDING

28. Hypoglycemia Causes Permanent Neurologic Damage

Prolonged or severe hypoglycemia (<40 mg/dL) causes seizures and brain injury. Screen at-risk infants (preterm, growth-restricted, maternal diabetes) within 1 hour of birth. Treat aggressively: IV dextrose if unable to feed, target >50 mg/dL initially.

29. Hyperglycemia is a Marker of Illness

Babies with hyperglycemia (>150 mg/dL) often have sepsis, NEC, or severe stress. Investigate the cause rather than reflexively giving insulin. Insulin use in neonates is controversial and may worsen outcomes.

30. Early Feeding Prevents NEC

Delayed feeding increases NEC risk. Start trophic feeds (10-20 mL/kg/day) as soon as the baby is stable, even on mechanical ventilation. Human milk is superior to formula—use it whenever possible.

31. Rapid Feeding Advancement Causes NEC

Aggressive feeding advancement (>35 mL/kg/day) increases NEC risk in preterm infants. Advance slowly (10-20 mL/kg/day) and watch for feeding intolerance. Patience prevents catastrophe.

32. Necrotizing Enterocolitis (NEC) is Unpredictable

NEC can strike suddenly in any preterm infant. Classic signs (abdominal distention, blood in stool, apnea) may come late. Maintain high suspicion—stop feeds, get imaging, start antibiotics at the first sign of concern. Early diagnosis improves outcomes.

33. Electrolyte Imbalances Cause Seizures

Hyponatremia, hypernatremia, hypocalcemia, and hypomagnesemia all cause seizures. Don't assume seizures are primary neurologic—check electrolytes and glucose first. Correcting metabolic abnormalities stops seizures faster than antiepileptic drugs.

NEUROLOGIC

34. Hypothermia Protects the Brain After Asphyxia

Therapeutic hypothermia (33.5°C for 72 hours) reduces death and disability in moderate-to-severe hypoxic-ischemic encephalopathy (HIE). Initiate within 6 hours of birth in eligible infants. This is one of the few proven neuroprotective interventions.

35. Seizures in Neonates Are Often Subtle

Neonatal seizures may not look like typical convulsions—watch for eye deviation, lip smacking, pedaling movements, or apnea. EEG is gold standard for diagnosis. Many "seizures" are actually jitteriness; EEG differentiates them.

36. Intraventricular Hemorrhage (IVH) Prevention Starts Immediately

Head ultrasound screening at 3-5 days identifies IVH. Prevention includes: avoid hypercarbia, maintain stable BP, avoid rapid fluid shifts, minimize suctioning. Severe IVH (grade 3-4) causes long-term disability—prevention is paramount.

37. Bilirubin Neurotoxicity is Real

Kernicterus still occurs. Know phototherapy and exchange transfusion thresholds for each age and risk group. Don't underestimate indirect hyperbilirubinemia—it causes permanent brain damage. Treat aggressively in at-risk infants.

38. Avoid Unnecessary Head Imaging

Head ultrasound is the imaging of choice for preterm infants (no radiation, portable). MRI is superior for term infants with suspected HIE but requires transport and sedation. CT has no role in routine neonatal brain imaging.

DISCHARGE & FOLLOW-UP

39. Screening Tests are Non-Negotiable

Newborn screening (metabolic panel, hearing, pulse oximetry for CCHD) identifies treatable conditions. Missed screening causes preventable disability and death. Ensure all screening is completed BEFORE discharge.

40. Retinopathy of Prematurity (ROP) Screening Saves Vision

Preterm infants <30 weeks or <1500g need ROP screening starting at 4 weeks of age. Treatable ROP (stage 3+ with plus disease) can be reversed with anti-VEGF therapy or laser. Missed ROP causes blindness.

41. Follow-Up Appointments Are Critical

Neurodevelopmental follow-up at 18-24 months identifies cerebral palsy and developmental delay. Early intervention services improve outcomes dramatically. Don't discharge without scheduling follow-up—many families don't return without a reminder.

42. Immunizations Protect Preterm Infants

Vaccinate by chronologic age, not corrected age, starting at birth. Preterm infants are at higher risk for vaccine-preventable diseases.

RSV prophylaxis (palivizumab) is indicated for high-risk preterm infants during RSV season.

43. Communication Prevents Readmissions

Provide clear discharge instructions, medication lists, and follow-up plans. Poor communication leads to missed appointments, medication errors, and preventable readmissions. Spend extra time with families—it's time well invested.

FINAL WISDOM

44. Humility Saves Lives

You will make mistakes. Ask for help early. Consult specialists when unsure. Second opinions prevent errors. The best clinicians know what they don't know.

45. Listen to the Nurses

Nurses spend the most time with babies. They notice subtle changes before anyone else. If a nurse is concerned, investigate. Nurse intuition is often right.

46. The Baby Always Wins

Your job is to keep the baby alive, healthy, and growing. Every decision should be filtered through this lens. When in doubt, choose the option that's best for the baby, not the easiest for the team.

47. Family-Centered Care Improves Outcomes

Parents are the baby's best advocates. Include them in decisions, explain your reasoning, and respect their values. Babies with engaged families have better long-term outcomes.

48. Never Stop Learning

Neonatology evolves constantly. Yesterday's standard is today's contraindication. Read journals, attend conferences, question old practices. The best clinicians are lifelong learners.

Chapter Thirty-Five

INDEX

INDEX

A

B

C

D

E

F

G

H

U

V

Chapter Thirty-Six

AUTHOR CONTACT INFORMATION

AUTHOR CONTACT INFORMATION

Dr. Ahmed Badawy | EBP | EPIC Diploma

- Email: a.m.b.hassane@gmail.com
- Institution: King Fahd Central Hospital, Jazan, Saudi Arabia
- Professional Affiliations:
  - Member, Royal College of Paediatrics and Child Health (United Kingdom)
  - Certified, European Board of Paediatrics
  - Certified, European Board of Paediatrics and Neonatal

Intensive Care Diploma

Correspondence Address:Dr. Ahmed Badawy ,Department of Neonatology, King Fahd Central Hospital Jazan, Saudi Arabia

For permissions, feedback, or collaboration inquiries:Please use the email address above. The author welcomes questions, case discussions, and suggestions for future editions.

Chapter Thirty-Seven

PUBLICATION INFORMATION

PUBLICATION INFORMATION

Title: *Practice Safe Neonatology: A Clinical Survival Guide*

Author: Dr. Ahmed Badawy (, EBP, EPIC Dip.)

Edition: First Edition, 2026

Publisher: Talented LLC

- Registered Office: Wyoming, USA
- EIN: 32-0853753

ISBN: 979-8-9963420-0-6 (Paperback)

Library of Congress Control Number (LCCN): 2026913882

Publication Date: 2026

Distribution: Worldwide

Format: Print (softcover) and Digital (eBook)

Subject Classification:

- Neonatology (MED070000)
- Pediatrics (MED069000)
- Critical Care Medicine (MED015000)
- Clinical Practice Guidelines (MED029000)
- Medical Education (MED024000)

Target Audience:

- Neonatal practitioners and neonatologists
- Pediatric residents and fellows
- Medical students (pediatrics rotation)
- Neonatal nurses and advanced practice providers
- Healthcare providers managing critically ill newborns in tertiary settings

Copyright: © 2026 Dr. Ahmed Badawy. All rights reserved.

Disclaimer: This book is intended as an educational clinical reference. It is not a substitute for professional clinical judgment, institutional protocols, or direct patient assessment. See full disclaimer on page [ii].

Cover Design: Professional layout by Talented LLC

Printing and Binding: Printed in the United States of America

Available from:

- Talented LLC (direct)
- Major medical book distributors

www.ingramcontent.com/pod-product-compliance
Lightning Source LLC
LaVergne TN
LVHW052338100826
845147LV00021B/1113

* 9 7 9 8 9 9 6 3 4 2 0 0 6 *